OCULAR INFECTIONS
Prophylaxis and Management

OCULAR INFECTIONS
Prophylaxis and Management

Editors

Namrata Sharma
MD DNB MNAMS
Professor
Cornea, Cataract and Refractive Surgery Services
Dr Rajendra Prasad Centre for Ophthalmic Sciences
All India Institute of Medical Sciences
New Delhi, India

Neelima Aron
MD DNB FICO
Senior Resident
Cornea, Cataract and Refractive Surgery Services
Dr Rajendra Prasad Centre for Ophthalmic Sciences
All India Institute of Medical Sciences
New Delhi, India

Atul Kumar
MD FAMS
Chief, Professor and Head
Vitreoretina, Uvea and Retinopathy of Prematurity (ROP) Services
Dr Rajendra Prasad Centre for Ophthalmic Sciences
All India Institute of Medical Sciences
New Delhi, India

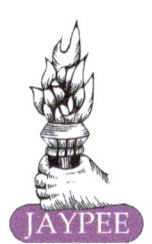

JAYPEE   *The Health Sciences Publisher*
New Delhi | London | Panama

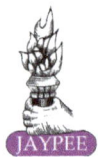 **Jaypee Brothers Medical Publishers (P) Ltd.**

Headquarters
Jaypee Brothers Medical Publishers (P) Ltd.
4838/24, Ansari Road, Daryaganj
New Delhi 110 002, India
Phone: +91-11-43574357
Fax: +91-11-43574314
E-mail: jaypee@jaypeebrothers.com

Overseas Offices

J.P. Medical Ltd.
83, Victoria Street, London
SW1H 0HW (UK)
Phone: +44-20 3170 8910
Fax: +44 (0)20 3008 6180
E-mail: info@jpmedpub.com

Jaypee-Highlights Medical Publishers Inc.
City of Knowledge, Bld 235, 2nd Floor
Clayton, Panama City, Panama
Phone: +1 507-301-0496
Fax: +1 507-301-0499
E-mail: cservice@jphmedical.com

Jaypee Brothers Medical Publishers (P) Ltd.
17/1-B, Babar Road, Block-B
Shaymali, Mohammadpur
Dhaka-1207, Bangladesh
Mobile: +08801912003485
E-mail: jaypeedhaka@gmail.com

Jaypee Brothers Medical Publishers (P) Ltd.
Bhotahity, Kathmandu, Nepal
Phone: +977-9741283608
E-mail: kathmandu@jaypeebrothers.com

Website: www.jaypeebrothers.com
Website: www.jaypeedigital.com

© 2017, Jaypee Brothers Medical Publishers

The views and opinions expressed in this book are solely those of the original contributor(s)/author(s) and do not necessarily represent those of editor(s) of the book.

All rights reserved. No part of this publication may be reproduced, stored or transmitted in any form or by any means, electronic, mechanical, photocopying, recording or otherwise, without the prior permission in writing of the publishers.

All brand names and product names used in this book are trade names, service marks, trademarks or registered trademarks of their respective owners. The publisher is not associated with any product or vendor mentioned in this book.

Medical knowledge and practice change constantly. This book is designed to provide accurate, authoritative information about the subject matter in question. However, readers are advised to check the most current information available on procedures included and check information from the manufacturer of each product to be administered, to verify the recommended dose, formula, method and duration of administration, adverse effects and contraindications. It is the responsibility of the practitioner to take all appropriate safety precautions. Neither the publisher nor the author(s)/editor(s) assume any liability for any injury and/or damage to persons or property arising from or related to use of material in this book.

This book is sold on the understanding that the publisher is not engaged in providing professional medical services. If such advice or services are required, the services of a competent medical professional should be sought.

Every effort has been made where necessary to contact holders of copyright to obtain permission to reproduce copyright material. If any have been inadvertently overlooked, the publisher will be pleased to make the necessary arrangements at the first opportunity.

Inquiries for bulk sales may be solicited at: jaypee@jaypeebrothers.com

Ocular Infections: Prophylaxis and Management

First Edition: **2017**

ISBN: 978-93-86322-88-3

Dedicated to

My parents, Dr Ramesh C Sharma and Mrs Maitreyi Pushpa, husband Dr Subhash Chandra and daughter Vasavdatta

—Namrata Sharma

My parents, Mr Rakesh Aron and Mrs Anshu Aron and husband Dr Kanav Kaushal

—Neelima Aron

My late parents, Mr Sanat Kumar and Mrs Swarna Kumar, wife Mrs Parul Kumar and children Aman and Aarshi

—Atul Kumar

Contributors

Amar Pujari MD
Senior Resident
Oculoplasty and Pediatric
Ophthalmology Services
Dr Rajendra Prasad Centre for
Ophthalmic Sciences
All India Institute of Medical
Sciences (AIIMS)
New Delhi, India

Amreen Aslam MD
Senior Resident
Cornea, Cataract and
Refractive Surgery Services
Dr Rajendra Prasad Centre for
Ophthalmic Sciences
All India Institute of Medical Sciences
New Delhi, India

Ankit Singh Tomar MBBS
Junior Resident
Dr Rajendra Prasad Centre for
Ophthalmic Sciences
All India Institute of Medical Sciences
New Delhi, India

Anubha Rathi MD
Senior Resident
Cornea, Cataract and
Refractive Surgery Services
Dr Rajendra Prasad Centre for
Ophthalmic Sciences
All India Institute of Medical Sciences
New Delhi, India

Archita Singh MD FICO
Senior Resident
Cornea, Cataract and
Refractive Surgery Services
Dr Rajendra Prasad Centre for
Ophthalmic Sciences
All India Institute of Medical Sciences
New Delhi, India

Atul Kumar MD FAMS
Chief, Professor and Head
Vitreoretina, Uvea and Retinopathy of
Prematurity (ROP) Services
Dr Rajendra Prasad Centre for
Ophthalmic Sciences
All India Institute of Medical Sciences
New Delhi, India

Deepali Singhal MD
Senior Resident
Cornea, Cataract and
Refractive Surgery Services
Dr Rajendra Prasad Centre for
Ophthalmic Sciences
All India Institute of Medical Sciences
New Delhi, India

Divya Agarwal MBBS
Junior Resident
Dr Rajendra Prasad Centre for
Ophthalmic Sciences
All India Institute of Medical Sciences
New Delhi, India

Divya Singh MD DNB
Senior Resident
Cornea, Cataract and
Refractive Surgery Services
Dr Rajendra Prasad Centre for
Ophthalmic Sciences
All India Institute of Medical Sciences
New Delhi, India

Gita Satpathy MD
Professor
Department of Ocular Microbiology
Dr Rajendra Prasad Centre for
Ophthalmic Sciences
All India Institute of Medical Sciences
New Delhi, India

Jayanand Urkude MD
Senior Resident
Cornea, Cataract and
Refractive Surgery Services
Dr Rajendra Prasad Centre for
Ophthalmic Sciences
All India Institute of Medical Sciences
New Delhi, India

Karthikeya R MD
Senior Resident
Vitreoretina, Uvea and Retinopathy of
Prematurity (ROP) Services
Dr Rajendra Prasad Centre for
Ophthalmic Sciences
All India Institute of Medical Sciences
New Delhi, India

Manthan Chaniyara MD DNB FICO
Senior Resident
Cornea, Cataract and
Refractive Surgery Services
Dr Rajendra Prasad Centre for
Ophthalmic Sciences
All India Institute of Medical Sciences
New Delhi, India

Mrittika Sen MBBS
Junior Resident
Dr Rajendra Prasad Centre for
Ophthalmic Sciences
All India Institute of Medical Sciences
New Delhi, India

Mukesh Patil MD FICO
Senior Resident
Cornea, Cataract and
Refractive Surgery Services
Dr Rajendra Prasad Centre for
Ophthalmic Sciences
All India Institute of Medical Sciences
New Delhi, India

Namrata Sharma MD DNB MNAMS
Professor
Cornea, Cataract and
Refractive Surgery Services
Dr Rajendra Prasad Centre for
Ophthalmic Sciences
All India Institute of Medical Sciences
New Delhi, India

Neelam Pushker MD
Professor
Oculoplasty and Pediatric
Ophthalmology Services
Dr Rajendra Prasad Centre for
Ophthalmic Sciences
All India Institute of Medical Sciences
New Delhi, India

Neelima Aron MD DNB FICO
Senior Resident
Cornea, Cataract and
Refractive Surgery Services
Dr Rajendra Prasad Centre for
Ophthalmic Sciences
All India Institute of Medical Sciences
New Delhi, India

Neha Midha MD DNB FICO
Senior Resident
Glaucoma Services
Dr Rajendra Prasad Centre for
Ophthalmic Sciences
All India Institute of Medical Sciences
New Delhi, India

Nishat Hussain Ahmed MD
Assistant Professor
Department of Microbiology
Dr Rajendra Prasad Centre for
Ophthalmic Sciences
All India Institute of Medical Sciences
New Delhi, India

Prafulla K Maharana MD
Assistant Professor
Cornea, Cataract and
Refractive Surgery Services
Dr Rajendra Prasad Centre for
Ophthalmic Sciences
All India Institute of Medical Sciences
New Delhi, India

Pranita Sahay MD
Senior Resident
Cornea, Cataract and
Refractive Surgery Services
Dr Rajendra Prasad Centre for
Ophthalmic Sciences
All India Institute of Medical Sciences
New Delhi, India

Prasad Gupta MBBS
Junior Resident
Dr Rajendra Prasad Centre for
Ophthalmic Sciences
All India Institute of Medical Sciences
New Delhi, India

Prateek Kakkar MD DNB FICO FAICO
Senior Resident
Vitreoretina, Uvea and Retinopathy of
Prematurity (ROP) Services
Dr Rajendra Prasad Centre for
Ophthalmic Sciences
All India Institute of Medical Sciences
New Delhi, India

Rachna Meel MS
Assistant Professor
Squint, Neuro-ophthalmology, Pediatric
Ophthlamoplasty and Squint Services
Dr Rajendra Prasad Centre for
Ophthalmic Sciences
All India Institute of Medical Sciences
New Delhi, India

Raghav Ravani MD FICO
Senior Resident
Vitreoretina, Uvea and Retinopathy of
Prematurity (ROP) Services
Dr Rajendra Prasad Centre for
Ophthalmic Sciences
All India Institute of Medical Sciences
New Delhi, India

Rajesh Sinha MD DNB FIACLE FRCS
Professor
Cornea, Cataract and
Refractive Surgery Services
Dr Rajendra Prasad Centre for
Ophthalmic Sciences
All India Institute of Medical Sciences
New Delhi, India

Reena Singh MD DNB FICO FAICO
Senior Resident
Cornea, Cataract and
Refractive Surgery Services
Dr Rajendra Prasad Centre for
Ophthalmic Sciences
All India Institute of Medical Sciences
New Delhi, India

Renu Venugopal MSc
PhD Scholar
Dr Rajendra Prasad Centre for
Ophthalmic Sciences
All India Institute of Medical Sciences
New Delhi, India

Ritika Mukhija MBBS
Junior Resident
Dr Rajendra Prasad Centre for
Ophthalmic Sciences
All India Institute of Medical Sciences
New Delhi, India

Rohan Chawla MD FRCS (Glasg)
Assistant Professor
Vitreoretina, Uvea and Retinopathy of
Prematurity (ROP) Services
Dr Rajendra Prasad Centre for
Ophthalmic Sciences
All India Institute of Medical Sciences
New Delhi, India

Rohit Saxena MD PhD
Professor
Squint and Neuro-ophthalmology Services
Dr Rajendra Prasad Centre for
Ophthalmic Sciences
All India Institute of Medical Sciences
New Delhi, India

Ruchita Falera MD DNB FICO
Senior Resident
Cornea, Cataract and
Refractive Surgery Services
Dr Rajendra Prasad Centre for
Ophthalmic Sciences
All India Institute of Medical Sciences
New Delhi, India

Sagnik Sen MBBS
Junior Resident
Dr Rajendra Prasad Centre for
Ophthalmic Sciences
All India Institute of Medical Sciences
New Delhi, India

Saranya Devi K MD DNB FICO
Senior Resident
Squint and Neuro-ophthalmology Services
Dr Rajendra Prasad Centre for
Ophthalmic Sciences
All India Institute of Medical Sciences
New Delhi, India

Srikant Kumar Padhy MBBS
Junior Resident
Dr Rajendra Prasad Centre for
Ophthalmic Sciences
All India Institute of Medical Sciences
New Delhi, India

Talvir Sidhu MD DNB
Senior Resident
Glaucoma Services
Dr Rajendra Prasad Centre for
Ophthalmic Sciences
All India Institute of Medical Sciences
New Delhi, India

Tanuj Dada MD
Professor
Glaucoma Services
Dr Rajendra Prasad Centre for
Ophthalmic Sciences
All India Institute of Medical Sciences
New Delhi, India

Vaishali MBBS
Junior Resident
Dr Rajendra Prasad Centre for
Ophthalmic Sciences
All India Institute of Medical Sciences
New Delhi, India

Preface

Post-surgical ocular infections are serious vision-threatening complications of any intra- or extraocular surgery which are avoidable. The infections vary in terms of time of onset, severity and course. They may range from a small infiltrate to the most serious of these complications such as post-operative endophthalmitis or panophthalmitis leading to loss of the eye. We, as ophthalmic surgeons, have the major responsibility of taking all measures to reduce this risk to a minimum. The onus is on us to bring down the incidence of post-operative infections and achieve successful visual outcomes. Various books on management of infections in ophthalmic practices are available; however, none provides in detail the basic precautions to be followed and steps to be taken pre-operatively, intra-operatively and post-operatively to prevent the occurrence of ophthalmic infections. With the rising number of dedicated centres for ophthalmic practice both in the government and private sector and increase in the number of ocular surgeries being performed, the incidence of infection and endophthalmitis is on a rise which is a dreaded complication and a nightmare for ophthalmologists. This calls for a certain set of criterion to be followed at every step to prevent such avertable complications. This book attempts to lay down guidelines for the prophylaxis of ocular infections which must be followed and are useful not only for the ophthalmic surgeons but also for the nursing staff, ophthalmic assistants and postgraduate students. The first half of the book enlists the prophylactic measures to be taken to prevent post-operative infections. The second part of the book deals with the management of cases of infection after various ophthalmic surgeries when they occur, despite taking all precautions. The book has been written in a user-friendly style with a precise format assisted by suitable illustrations and tables, wherever appropriate for easy understanding. We hope that the book will serve its purpose of providing useful guidelines to the ophthalmic community to prevent post-surgical ocular infections and reduce ocular morbidity.

Namrata Sharma
Neelima Aron
Atul Kumar

Contents

1. **Introduction** — 1
   Nishat Hussain Ahmed, Gita Satpathy
   - History *1*
   - Cleaning, Disinfection and Sterilization *2*
   - Cleaning *4*
   - Sterilization and Disinfection *5*

2. **Operation Theatre: Design and Layout** — 15
   Ritika Mukhija, Neelima Aron, Namrata Sharma, Atul Kumar
   - History *15*
   - Setting up an Operation Theatre *15*
   - Layout *16*
   - Lighting *19*
   - Temperature and Humidity *19*
   - Scrub Room *19*
   - Recovery Room *19*
   - Minor Operation Theatre *20*

3. **Air Flow System in Ophthalmic Operation Theatre** — 22
   Prateek Kakkar, Neelima Aron, Atul Kumar
   - Ventilation/Air Conditioning *22*
   - Laminar Air Flow *23*
   - Air Change Per Hour *23*
   - Air Velocity *23*
   - Positive Pressure *24*
   - Air Filtration *24*
   - Maintenance of Air Flow System *24*

4. **Water Requirement in Ophthalmic Operation Theatre** — 26
   Mrittika Sen, Neelima Aron, Namrata Sharma, Atul Kumar
   - Handwashing *26*
   - Instruments *26*

5. **Operation Theatre List and Record Maintenance** — 29
   Pranita Sahay, Srikant Kumar Padhy, Neelima Aron
   - The Operation Theatre List *29*
   - Recommendations *29*
   - Special Considerations while Preparing an Operation Theatre List *30*
   - Distribution of the Operation Theatre List *31*
   - Record Maintenance in Operation Theatre *31*

6. **Pre-operative Patient Preparation** 33
   Mukesh Patil, Neelima Aron, Namrata Sharma, Atul Kumar
   - Pre-operative Measures *33*
   - Operation Theatre Attire *34*
   - Marking and Cleaning of the Surgical Area *34*
   - Shifting the Patient to Operation Theatre *35*
   - Surgical Preparation *35*
   - *High Risk:* HIV, HBsAg, HCV *36*

7. **Pre-operative Preparation of Operation Theatre Personnel** 38
   Archita Singh, Sagnik Sen, Ankit Singh Tomar, Neelima Aron
   - Operation Theatre Occupancy *38*
   - Operation Theatre Attire *38*
   - Components of the Attire *39*
   - *Special Cases:* HIV, Hepatitis B and C *41*
   - Surgical Scrubbing *42*
   - Gowning and Gloving *43*

8. **OT Protocol: Codes of Conduct** 47
   Sagnik Sen, Neelima Aron, Vaishali, Namrata Sharma
   - General Considerations *47*
   - Scrubbed Surgeon and Assistant *47*
   - Nursing Staff *48*
   - Operation Theatre Assistant *49*
   - Observer in the Operation Theatre *50*
   - Visitors in the Operation Theatre *50*
   - Intra-operative and Post-operative Practices *50*
   - Practices in the use of Intra-operative Adjuncts *51*

9. **Operation Theatre Sterilization** 52
   Ruchita Falera, Sagnik Sen, Neelima Aron
   - Operation Theatre Cleaning *52*
   - Operation Theatre Disinfection and Sterilization *53*
   - Cleaning Schedule *55*
   - Septic Operation Theatre *55*
   - Special Cases: HIV, Hepatitis B, Hepatitis C *56*

10. **Ophthalmic Instrument Sterilization** 57
    Nishat Hussain Ahmed, Manthan Chaniyara, Sagnik Sen, Neelima Aron, Gita Satpathy
    - Instrument Processing *57*
    - Sterilization *59*
    - Instrument Sterilization in Ophthalmic OT *64*

11. **Waste Disposal in Ophthalmic Operation Theatre** 68
    Reena Singh, Rajesh Sinha
    - Categorization of Waste in Operation Theatre *69*
    - Segregation and Accumulation of Categorized Waste *69*
    - Packaging of Segregated Wastes *70*
    - Transportation of Packed Wastes from OT to Final Site of Treatment or Disposal *71*
    - Treatment of Waste *71*
    - Training of Staff Handling Waste Disposal in Operation Theatre *72*

12. Quality Control and Surveillance 73
Nishat Hussain Ahmed, Gita Satpathy, Neelima Aron
- Quality Control *73*
- Microbiological Sampling *78*
- Hospital Sterilization and Disinfection Policy *82*

13. Post-Cataract Surgery Endophthalmitis 87
Anubha Rathi, Rohan Chawla, Atul Kumar
- Microbial Spectrum of Post-operative Endophthalmitis *87*
- *MRSA and MRSE:* Increasing Resistance to Topical Antibiotics *87*
- Risk Factors and Incidence of Post-cataract Surgery Endophthalmitis *88*
- Prophylaxis of Post-cataract Surgery Endophthalmitis *88*
- Diagnosis and Management *90*

14. Post-Intravitreal Injection Infections 94
Raghav Ravani, Rohan Chawla, Atul Kumar
- Incidence and Risk Factors *94*
- Clinical Presentation *94*
- Diagnosis and Management *95*
- Prophylaxis *96*

15. Endophthalmitis after Pars Plana Vitrectomy 101
Karthikeya R, Rohan Chawla, Atul Kumar
- Clinical Features *101*
- Risk Factors *101*
- Prophylaxis *102*
- Management *103*
- Outcomes *103*

16. Post-LASIK Infections 105
Divya Singh, Neelima Aron, Prafulla K Maharana, Namrata Sharma
- Microbial Spectrum *105*
- Risk Factors *105*
- Clinical Diagnosis *106*
- Prophylaxis *107*
- *Treatment:* Medical and Surgical Therapy *108*

17. Infections after Intrastromal Corneal Ring Segments 110
Deepali Singhal, Neelima Aron, Prasad Gupta, Rajesh Sinha
- Risk Factors *110*
- Etiological Organisms *110*
- Pathogenesis *111*
- Differential Diagnosis *111*
- Clinical Features *111*
- Microbiological Work-up *112*
- Treatment *112*
- Complications and Sequelae *112*
- Prophylaxis *112*

18. Post-Collagen Cross-Linking Infections — 114
Jayanand Urkude, Neelima Aron, Anubha Rathi, Prafulla K Maharana, Namrata Sharma
- Incidence *114*
- Risk Factors *114*
- Microbial Profile of Post-collagen Cross-linking Infection *115*
- Prophylaxis *115*
- Diagnosis and Management *116*

19. Post-Keratoplasty Infections — 119
Neelima Aron, Prafulla K Maharana, Namrata Sharma
- Risk Factors for Graft Infection and Prevention *119*
- Clinical Features *121*
- Investigations *123*
- Microbiological Spectrum *124*
- Management *124*
- Prevention *125*
- Outcomes *125*

20. Bleb-Related Infections — 128
Neha Midha, Talvir Sidhu, Tanuj Dada
- Incidence *128*
- Classification *128*
- Risk Factors *129*
- Microbial Spectrum *129*
- Prophylaxis *131*
- Diagnosis and Management *132*
- Visual Outcome and Prognosis *132*
- Patient Education and Counseling *133*

21. Post-Strabismus Surgery Infections — 136
Saranya Devi K, Rohit Saxena
- Incidence and Prevalence *136*
- Microbial Flora and Risk Factors *136*
- Endophthalmitis *137*
- Orbital and Preseptal Cellulitis *137*
- Scleritis *137*
- Surgically-induced Necrotizing Scleritis *138*
- Prophylaxis and Management *138*

22. Post-Pterygium Surgery Infections — 143
Neelima Aron, Divya Agarwal, Prafulla K Maharana, Namrata Sharma
- Incidence and Microbial Spectrum *143*
- Risk Factors *143*
- Pathogenesis *143*
- Clinical Presentation *144*
- Investigations *145*
- Management *145*
- Prophylaxis *147*

23. Infections after Ocular Surface Reconstruction Surgery 149
Amreen Aslam, Renu Venugopal, Neelima Aron, Prafulla K Maharana, Namrata Sharma
- Incidence *149*
- Risk Factors *150*
- Clinical Features *150*
- Investigations *151*
- Prophylaxis *152*
- Treatment *153*
- Coexisting Endophthalmitis *153*

24. Infections after Oculoplasty Surgery 155
Amar Pujari, Rachna Meel, Neelam Pushker
- Pre-operative Assessment *155*
- Intra-operative Precautions *155*
- Post-operative Care and Antibiotic Prophylaxis *156*
- Microbiology Profile *156*
- Antibiotics for Prophylaxis *156*
- Diagnosis and Management *157*

Index *159*

CHAPTER 1

Introduction

Nishat Hussain Ahmed, Gita Satpathy

The theme behind operation theatre sterilization and disinfection is: 'The first requirement of a hospital is that it should do the sick no harm'. This is a paraphrase of the favorite aphorism of Florence Nightingale—*'primum non nocere'* (first of all do no harm).[1] Principally, the suggestion in the dictum is of harm caused to the patient as a result of hospital acquired infections.

Sight is the most valued of all assets possessed by the mortals. Modern ophthalmic interventions have come a long way in managing a variety of ophthalmic conditions, which were previously considered fatal in terms of visual loss. However, like all powers, the capability to be able to venture into intricate procedures comes with the responsibility to care for the unfavorable consequences which might arise from matters and objects other than the skill of surgery. Prevention of pre-, intra- and post-procedural infection is one such responsibility; which if overlooked can twist the whole outcome of an otherwise impeccable procedure. Sterilization and disinfection of operating rooms and instruments, and carrying out the procedures as per the infection control guidelines thus have a key role in determining the ultimate success of a procedure.

HISTORY

Long back, around 500 BC, the hygienic standards for care of the sick existed in civilized world, particularly in India, Egypt, Palestine and Greece. These standards were mainly based on religious concepts of practicing purity for its believed intimacy with godliness. The earliest available advice on hospital construction and hygiene is contained in the *Charaka-Samhita*, a Sanskrit Textbook of Medicine.[2]

The civilizations of fifth century BC, including ancient Greeks and Jews had high standard inflexible laws for prevention of infections in their hospitals. Similar were the standards of hospitals and intervention places of ancient Romans.[3,4]

By the commencement of Medieval period (5th to the 15th century AD), most of the early standards of hygiene and infection prevention were forgotten.[5] The pre-renaissance era saw few surgeons understanding the importance of cleanliness and asepsis in procedures, however for the most part, these concepts were looked down upon.[6,7]

The scientific study of hospital infections began in first half of eighteenth century. A number of physicians and surgeons came forward with insistence on hospital infection control and procedural antisepsis. Notable are the achievements of John Pringle (1740–1780), who pioneered 'antiseptics' and gave the concept of 'hospital fever'; Francis Home, Thomas Young, Alexander Hamilton and Alexander Gordon, who worked on understanding the nature of and preventing puerperal fever from 1750 to 1800; and John Bell (1790–1820), who gave valuable observations on surgical sepsis.[8]

As the acquaintance was building up in understanding and prevention of infections, it was understood by many that use of carbolic acid in surgical wounds can prevent infection. This knowledge achieved its first practical expression in the work of Joseph Lister (1865–1868). He demonstrated the role of bacteria in surgical sepsis, and that sepsis could be avoided by excluding bacteria from a surgical wound. This work pioneered the way to the principles of antiseptic, and later, aseptic surgeries.[9,10] At around the same time in 1860s, Louis Pasteur was able to confirm that heat kills microbes, and sterilization came of age. The later years, with advancements in every aspect of medical, surgical and diagnostic fields; saw development of more interest in taking care of hospital acquired and surgical infections. Concepts of infection control in hospitals and thorough sterilization and disinfection of patient care devices and areas were agreed upon to be all important for successful outcome of patient interventions. This led to customization and development of different sterilization and disinfection practices especially in patient intervention areas like critical care units and operation theatres. Major milestones reached in the subject matter are shown in **Table 1.1**.

CLEANING, DISINFECTION AND STERILIZATION

Cleaning, disinfection and sterilization are the key components for favorable outcomes, in terms of infective complications; of procedures taking place in operating rooms. As the interventions and thus the devices and instruments used for them are becoming more and more complex, ever increasing is the demand to treat the devices and instruments in manners which render them safe for use in such interventions. As sterilizing all the equipment and surroundings of patient intervention is unnecessary and expensive, a methodical knowledge of the various methods of sterilization, disinfection and cleaning is important to guide the correct treatment of a place or article depending on its intended use.

A Rational Approach

In 1968, Earle H Spaulding devised a rational approach to disinfection and sterilization of patient-care items

S.No.	Year	Milestone
1.	1683	Antonie van Leeuwenhoek (**Fig. 1.1**) developed the microscope and proved the existence of microorganisms
2.	1847	Ignaz Semmelweis, an Hungarian obstetrician, advocated handwashing and fingernail scrubbing for infection prevention
3.	1862	Louis Pasteur (**Fig. 1.2**) gave the 'germ' theory of infections, later he developed the pasteurization process
4.	1867	Joseph Lister (**Fig. 1.3**) pioneered the way to antiseptic surgeries by initially using carbolic acid on surgical wounds and hands of surgeons
5.	1876	The first steam autoclave was made and process of tyndallization was discovered
6.	1881	Boiling as a method of sterilization for surgical drapes, gowns, dressings, instruments, etc. was used
7.	1885 to 1900	Germans made many notable contributions to the principles governing steam sterilization and chemical disinfection
8.	1900	Dry heat sterilization practice was started
9.	Early 1900's	Use of 'ozone' for potable water treatment in Europe
10.	1929	Recognition of ethylene oxide as an antibacterial agent
11.	Early 1940's	Ethylene oxide (EtO) employed as a sterilizing agent in hospitals; thereafter sterilization by irradiation developed
12.	Late 1940's	Discovery of microwave energy
13.	1963	Glutaraldehyde was introduced as a sterilizing agent for heat-sensitive instruments
14.	1968	Earle H Spaulding proposed how an object should be disinfected or sterilized depended on the object's intended use (Spaulding's classification system)
15.	1989	Ozone sterilizers introduced for healthcare applications
16.	1993	Plasma sterilizing systems were introduced

Table 1.1 Major milestones in history of sterilization and disinfection for prevention of surgical infections

Introduction

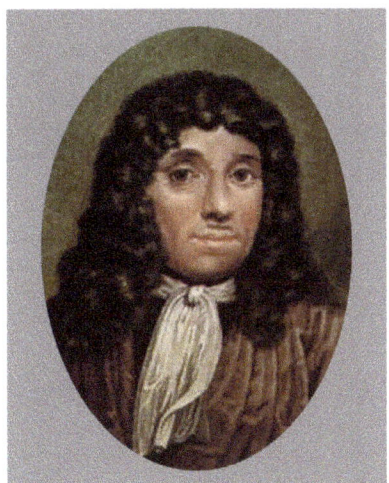

Figure 1.1 Antonie van Leeuwenhoek

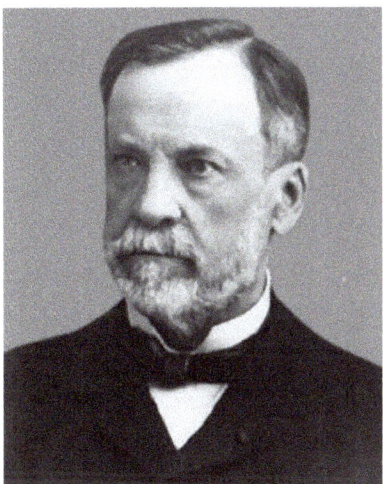

Figure 1.2 Louis Pasteur

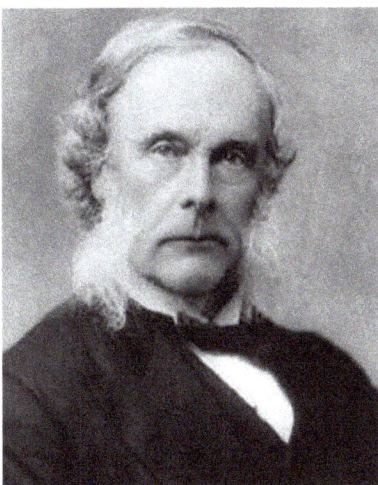

Figure 1.3 Joseph Lister

and equipment. Spaulding categorized the instruments and items of patient care as critical, semicritical, and noncritical according to the degree of risk for infection involved in use of the items. The treatment of the items was recommended to be based on the above categorization. Although more than forty decades old, the classification still retains its logic even in the modern treatment amenities of patient care articles.[11] **Table 1.2** shows the Spaulding's classification of patient care devices and the recommended treatments.

Critical items confer a high-risk for infection, if they are contaminated with any microorganism. These items enter sterile tissue or the vascular system, and hence must be sterile before use. This category includes surgical instruments, cardiac and urinary catheters, implants, and ultrasound probes used in sterile body cavities. Most of the critical items should be procured as sterile or be sterilized with steam, if possible. Heat-sensitive objects can be treated with EtO, hydrogen peroxide gas plasma; or if above are not suitable, by liquid chemical sterilants.[12]

Semicritical items contact mucous membranes or nonintact skin. They include respiratory therapy and anesthesia equipment, endoscopes, laryngoscope blades, manometry probes, cystoscopes, diaphragm fitting rings, etc. They should be free from all microorganisms before use. However, as intact mucous membranes, such as those of the lungs and the gastrointestinal tract are generally resistant to infection by common bacterial spores-small numbers of bacterial spores are permissible. Thus, semicritical items at the least require high-level disinfection using chemical disinfectants.[13,14]

Noncritical items come in contact with intact skin but not mucous membranes. Intact skin acts as an effective barrier to most microorganisms; therefore, the sterility of items coming in contact with intact skin is not critical. Noncritical items can be divided into noncritical patient care items, such as bedpans, blood pressure cuffs, crutches etc.; and noncritical environmental surfaces such as table tops, computers etc. Almost no risk has been documented for transmission of infectious agents to patients through noncritical items, as long as they do not contact non-intact skin and/or mucous membranes.[15,16]

Definitions[12,17,18]

Cleaning is the physical removal of all visible soil, dust, and other foreign material (e.g. organic and inorganic

Table 1.2 Spaulding's classification of patient care devices					
Device classification	Definition based on intended use	Examples	Risk of infections	Recommended treatment
Critical	A device that enters normally sterile tissue or the vascular system or through which blood flows	Implants, scalpels, needles, phacoemulsification machine handpiece, forceps, scissors, hooks, cannulas	High	Sterilization
Semi-critical	A device that comes into contact with intact mucous membranes and does not ordinarily penetrate sterile tissue	Laryngoscopes, endoscopes, endotracheal tubes, manometry probes	High or intermediate	Sterilization desirable, high level disinfection acceptable
Non-critical	A device that does not ordinarily touch the patient or touches only intact skin	Stethoscopes, blood pressure cuffs, tabletops	Low	Intermediate or low level disinfection

material) from objects and surfaces and normally is accomplished manually or mechanically using water with detergents or enzymatic products. Thorough cleaning is essential before high-level disinfection and sterilization because inorganic and organic materials that remain on the surfaces of instruments interfere with the effectiveness of these processes.

Decontamination removes pathogenic microorganisms from objects so that they are safe to handle, use, or discard. Technically, it involves cleaning with detergent and/ or treatment with germicides.

Disinfection is a process that eliminates many or all pathogenic microorganisms, except bacterial spores, on inanimate objects. In healthcare settings, objects usually are disinfected by liquid chemicals or wet pasteurization. Unlike sterilization, disinfection is not sporicidal. A few disinfectants will kill spores with prolonged exposure times (e.g. 2% glutaraldehyde in 3–12 hours); these are called chemical sterilants. At similar concentrations but with shorter exposure periods (e.g. 20 minutes for 2% glutaraldehyde), these same disinfectants will kill all microorganisms except large numbers of bacterial spores; they are called high-level disinfectants.

Thus, high level disinfection (HLD) is a process that kills all microorganisms except large number of bacterial spores. Thus HLD destroys enveloped and nonenveloped viruses, gram-positive and gram negative bacteria, fungi, *Mycobacteria*, trophozoites and cysts.

Intermediate level disinfection (ILD) is a process which destroys mycobacteria, vegetative bacteria, trophozoites, most viruses, and most fungi but not bacterial or fungal spores.

Low-level disinfection (LLD) destroys most vegetative bacteria, some fungi, and some viruses in a practical period of time (<10 minutes).

Sterilization is a process that destroys or eliminates all forms of microbial life, including most resistant spores. It is a closely monitored, validated process carried out in healthcare facilities by physical or chemical methods. Steam under pressure, dry heat, ethylene oxide (EtO) gas, hydrogen peroxide gas plasma, and liquid chemicals are the principal sterilizing agents used in healthcare facilities. When chemicals are used to destroy all forms of microbiologic life, they can be called chemical sterilants. Sterilization destroys enveloped and non-enveloped viruses, gram-positive and gram-negative bacteria including bacterial spores, fungi and their spores, *Mycobacteria*, trophozoites, cysts and coccidia.

CLEANING[12,19-21]

Cleaning of Patient Care Items

Cleaning is the first and most important step before disinfection and sterilization can occur. Presoaking may be necessary to prevent soils and proteins from drying on surgical instruments/other patient care articles. Presoaking softens the organic matter and should be done immediately after using the item. Manual cleaning follows presoaking; thorough cleaning is required to remove all organic matter and other residue, which might interfere with the later steps of disinfection or sterilization as per the category of item. While cleaning, appropriate personal protective equipment such as gloves, masks, gowns, and protective eye wear must be used; and wherever suitable, cleaning of appliances and machines should be done so as to prevent potential exposure to microorganisms through aerosolization and splashing. The cleaning process must be carried out in a controlled environment using standard precautions. Proper ventilation, humidity control and temperature should be maintained in the cleaning area. The work flow should be unidirectional. Instructions should be visibly and clearly labelled in the cleaning area, appliances and machines, and on cleaning agents; and compliance should be strictly maintained to ensure the proper procedure for given articles. After cleaning, the items must be inspected for cleanliness and absence of defects. Items to be sterilized should also be tested for functional integrity when applicable.

At the place of using the patient care items, clean and dirty items must be kept separate at all times. Clean supplies should be maintained in a different room or area away from soiled instruments. All used supplies and equipment are considered contaminated even when contamination might not be visible to the eye. Contaminated items, should be collected into a container. The container must be covered, and the contents must be transported to decontamination area in a manner that minimizes potential contamination of staff, patients, or the environment.

STERILIZATION AND DISINFECTION

Sterilization and disinfection are the processes used in healthcare settings for making an article/area safe for use in patient care. These processes differ from each other in the level of freedom from microorganisms they provide; however, the agents used to accomplish the processes and the mechanisms with which the agents destroy the microorganisms are overlapping. For example, 2% glutaraldehyde is a chemical sterilant if the exposure time is 3–6 hours; however, with shorter exposure period of 20 minutes, it is a high level disinfectant. Understandably, factors which influence the effectiveness of sterilization and disinfection processes are also the same **(Table 1.3)**.[12] The methods of sterilization (and disinfection) can be physical or chemical methods. While some of the methods, e.g. steam under pressure are used primarily as means of sterilization, and some other, e.g. alcoholic

Table 1.3 Factors affecting the efficacy of sterilization and disinfection[12]	
Factor	Effect
Cleaning	Failure to adequately clean instrument results in higher bioburden, protein load, and salt concentration. These will decrease sterilization efficacy
Type of pathogen	Bacterial and fungal spores, mycobacteria and non-enveloped viruses are more resistant to sterilizing agents than vegetative bacteria and fungi and enveloped viruses
Biofilm	Biofilms reduce the efficacy of sterilization by impairing exposure of the sterilant to the microbial cell
Lumen length	Increasing lumen length impairs sterilant penetration. May require forced flow through lumen to achieve sterilization
Lumen diameter	Decreasing lumen diameter impairs sterilant penetration. May require forced flow through lumen to achieve sterilization
Restricted flow	Sterilant must come into contact with microorganisms. Device designs that prevent or inhibit this contact (e.g. sharp bends, blind lumens) will decrease sterilization efficacy
Device design and construction	Materials used in construction may affect compatibility with different sterilization processes and affect sterilization efficacy. Design issues (e.g. screws, hinges) will also affect sterilization efficacy
Temperature	Activity of most disinfectants increases as the temperature increases, but some exceptions exist. Too much increase in temperature causes the disinfectant to degrade and weakens its germicidal activity and thus might produce a potential health hazard
pH	An increase in pH improves the antimicrobial activity of some disinfectants (e.g. glutaraldehyde, quaternary ammonium compounds) but decreases the antimicrobial activity of others (e.g. phenols, hypochlorites, and iodine)
Humidity	Relative humidity is an important factor influencing the activity of gaseous disinfectants/sterilants, such as EtO, chlorine dioxide, and formaldehyde
Hardness of water	Water hardness reduces the effectiveness of certain disinfectants because high concentration of divalent cations (e.g. magnesium, calcium) in the hard water interact with the disinfectant to form insoluble precipitates

hand rubs for the most part are used as disinfectants; many methods with different standardizations (e.g. of exposure time, concentration, etc.) can be used as either. An understanding of different sterilizing agents is vital in applying them for different categories of patient care items and areas.

Sterilization Practices[12]

The quality of sterilization procedure as a service in patient care depends not only on the effectiveness of the sterilization process but also on other things including proper precleaning, disassembling and packaging of the device, loading the sterilizer, monitoring, appropriateness of the cycle for the load contents, and quality assurance of the procedures. The sterilization practices should be devised in manners so that they can be strictly adhered to by the personnel involved, there should be absolute protection of the patients from infections, there should be minimum risks to staff and the value of the items should be preserved. Ensuring consistency of sterilization practices requires a comprehensive program that ensures operator competence and proper methods of cleaning and wrapping instruments, loading the sterilizer, operating the sterilizer, and monitoring of the entire process. The details of pre-sterilization components, various methods of sterilization and their monitoring and quality assurance will be dealt with elsewhere.

The Methods of Disinfection

The Ideal Disinfectant

An ideal disinfectant does not exist. However, it is important to know the most desirable characteristics of a perfect disinfectant, against which any disinfectant needs to be weighed to know whether the specific criteria are being met or not by that particular disinfectant. This helps in understanding the potential uses; in calculating the dilutions which are least detrimental to the patient and cleaning personnel; and in deciding the points of specific precautions for that disinfectant. **Table 1.4** shows the characteristics of an ideal disinfectant.[12,22]

Many disinfectants are used alone or in combinations in the health-care setting. These include alcohols, chlorine and chlorine compounds, formaldehyde, glutaraldehyde, ortho-phthalaldehyde, hydrogen peroxide, iodophors, peracetic acid, phenolics, and quaternary ammonium compounds.

Disinfectants are not interchangeable, and incorrect concentrations and inappropriate disinfectants can result in improper disinfection and increased costs. Cleaning personnel should take due precautions to minimize exposure to disinfectants as many of them are associated with harmful effects to the exposed persons.[23,24] An understanding of the performance characteristics of various disinfectants is vital to select

Table 1.4 Properties of an ideal disinfectant[12,51]	
Spectrum	It should have a wide antimicrobial spectrum, and be effective against all microorganisms
Action	It should be fast acting to produce a rapid kill
Penetration	It should have high penetrating power
Effect of environmental factors	It should be active in the presence of organic matter (e.g. blood, sputum, feces) and compatible with soaps, detergents, and other chemicals encountered in use
Toxicity	It should be nontoxic, safe for the user and patient
Interference with healing	It should not interfere with healing
Surface compatibility	It should not corrode instruments and metallic surfaces and should not cause the deterioration of cloth, rubber, plastics, and other materials
Usage	Easy to use with clear label directions
Residual effect	It should leave an antimicrobial film on the treated surface.
Odor	It should have no odor or a pleasant odor to facilitate its routine use
Economical	It should not be expensive and should be easily available
Solubility	It should be soluble in water
Stability	It should be stable in concentrated stocks and in working dilutions
Cleaning action	It should have good cleaning properties
Environment friendly	It should not spoil the environment on disposal

an appropriate disinfectant for any item and use it in the most efficient way **(Table 1.5)**.

Alcohols[12,17,24-26]

Alcohols refer to two water-soluble disinfectants, ethyl alcohol and isopropyl alcohol. These alcohols are rapidly bactericidal against vegetative forms of bacteria; they also are tuberculocidal, fungicidal, and virucidal but do not destroy bacterial spores. Their optimum bactericidal concentration is 60–90% solutions in water, and the cidal activity drops sharply when diluted below 50%.

Mode of action: The most reasonable explanation for the cidal (killing) action of alcohol is denaturation of proteins. This is supported by the observation that absolute ethyl alcohol, a dehydrating agent, is less

Table 1.5 Summary of commonly used disinfectants			
Disinfectant	Advantages	Disadvantages	Uses
Alcohols	• Minimal toxicity • Fast acting • Fast drying • Nonstaining and nonallergic	• Low penetration in organic matter • Deleterious effects on some materials such as metals, lensed instruments, rubbers, plastics • Inflammable • Causes drying of skin	• Mainly used as ILD or LLD • Small surface disinfection, e.g. trolleys, etc. • Surface disinfection of noncritical items, e.g. stethoscopes, ambu bags, medicine vial stoppers, ultrasound probes, etc. • Used in hand rubs
Chlorine and chlorine compounds	• Inexpensive • Fast acting • Relatively nontoxic • Noninflammable • Unaffected by water hardness • Nonstaining	• Poor material compatibility • Corrosive • Inactivated by organic matter • Diluted form unstable • Bleaches fabrics • Irritant	• Used for HLD/ILD/LLD, based on concentration of free chlorine and contact time • Decontamination of spills • Surface decontamination • Disinfection of water • Disinfection of soiled laundry
Formaldehyde	• Active in presence of organic matter • Good biocide	• Very pungent • Exposure related to dermatitis, asthma and other systemic effects • Potential carcinogen	• Vaccine preparation • Embalming/ tissue and specimen preservation • Previously used for fumigation of critical care areas • Decontamination of biological safety cabinets
Glutaraldehyde	• Active in presence of organic matter • Good material compatibility • Excellent biocide • Moderate residual activity	• Coagulates blood and fixes proteins to surfaces • Irritant to eyes, skin and airways • Chronic exposure related to cases of dermatitis, colitis, keratopathy • Relatively costly	• Used as a chemical sterilant/HLD • Sterilization/HLD of endoscopes, dialysers, respiratory equipment, transducers, etc. • Should not be used for noncritical articles
Hydrogen peroxide	• Low toxicity • Active in presence of organic matter • Environment friendly • Good material compatibility • Odorless, noncorrosive • Fast acting • Strong biocide	• Cannot be used with some endoscopes • Irritation and colitis can occur with chronic exposure • Corneal damage	• Used as a chemical sterilant/HLD • Used for disinfecting semicritical and critical patient care items, e.g. endoscopes, ventilators, soft contact lenses, tonometer biprisms, etc. • Vaporized form is used for gas plasma sterilization

Contd...

Contd...

Disinfectant	Advantages	Disadvantages	Uses
Iodophors	• Rapid action • Relatively less toxic	• Inactivated by organic matter • Corrosive • Irritants for eyes • Gram-negative bacteria can grow in them	• Used as ILD/LLD • Used as skin antiseptics • Noncritical surface decontamination • Disinfection of thermometers, hydrotherapy tanks, etc.
Ortho-phthalaldehyde	• Excellent biocide • Fast acting • Active in presence of organic matter • Good material compatibility	• Stains proteins and skin gray • Irritant for the eyes • Expensive • Slow sporicidal activity	• Used as a chemical sterilant/HLD • Useful for equipment at places where glutaraldehyde resistance has emerged
Peracetic acid	• Low toxicity • Active in presence of organic matter • May enhance removal of organic matter • Environment friendly • Leaves no residues • Fast acting • Strong biocide	• Unstable in diluted form • Corrosive for metals, harmful for rubber • Irritant for skin and eyes • Costly	• Used as a chemical sterilant/HLD • Used for disinfection of endoscopes and dental equipment • In combination with hydrogen peroxide used for disinfection of hemodialyzer
Phenolics	• Active in presence of organic matter • Inexpensive • Noncorrosive • Stable	• Leave residual film on surfaces • Irritant to eyes and skin • Corrosive • Skin pigmentation • Gram-negative bacteria can grow in them	• Used as ILD/LLD • To be used only on noncritical surfaces and items
Quaternary ammonium compounds	• Nonstaining • Odorless • Noncorrosive • Relatively nontoxic	• Inactivated by hard water and organic matter • Irritant to skin and eyes • Poor bactericidal • Narrow spectrum • Leave sticky residues • Gram-negative bacteria can grow in them	• Used as LLD • Good cleansing agents • To be used only on noncritical surfaces and items

bactericidal than mixtures of alcohol and water because proteins are denatured more quickly in the presence of water. The bacteriostatic (keeping the metabolism at such a low level that the organism does not multiply, nor is it able to cause disease) action is believed to be caused by inhibition of the production of metabolites essential for rapid cell division.

Uses: Alcohols are not recommended for sterilizing medical and surgical materials principally because they lack sporicidal action and they cannot penetrate protein-rich materials. They have been used effectively to disinfect oral and rectal thermometers, hospital pagers, scissors, and stethoscopes. Alcohol towelettes are used for years to disinfect small surfaces such as rubber stoppers of multiple-dose medication vials or vaccine bottles.

Alcohols have some detrimental effects on equipment, they damage the shellac mountings of lensed instruments, tend to swell and harden rubber and certain plastic tubing after prolonged and repeated use, bleach rubber and plastic tiles and damage tonometer tips (by deterioration of the glue) if used routinely. They also evaporate rapidly, thus extended exposure time is difficult to achieve unless the items are immersed.

Chlorine and Chlorine Compounds[12,17,27-32]

Hypochlorites are the most widely used of the chlorine disinfectants. They are available as liquid (e.g. sodium hypochlorite) and solid (e.g. calcium hypochlorite) preparations. They have a broad spectrum of antimicrobial activity, do not leave toxic residues, are unaffected by water hardness, are inexpensive and fast acting, remove dried or fixed organisms and biofilms from surfaces, and have a low incidence of serious toxicity. Unfavorable effects include ocular irritation and oropharyngeal, esophageal, and gastric burns. Other disadvantages are corrosiveness to metals in high concentrations (>500 ppm), inactivation by organic matter, bleaching of fabrics, and release of toxic chlorine gas when mixed with ammonia or acid (e.g. household cleaning agents).

The microbicidal activity of chlorine is attributed largely to undissociated hypochlorous acid (HOCl). The disinfecting efficacy of chlorine decreases with an increase in pH. Alternative compounds that release chlorine and are used in the healthcare setting include demand-release chlorine dioxide, sodium dichloroisocyanurate, and chloramine-T. The advantage of these compounds over the hypochlorites is that they retain chlorine longer and so exert a more prolonged bactericidal effect. Sodium dichloroisocyanurate tablets are stable, the total available chlorine is released in phases, and the solutions of sodium dichloroisocyanurate are acidic, thus making it a better disinfectant.

A new disinfectant, "superoxidized water," with the concept of electrolyzing saline to create a disinfectant has been developed. The main products of this water are hypochlorous acid (e.g. at a concentration of about 144 mg/L) and chlorine. This method is inexpensive and end product—water is not detrimental to the environment. Although superoxidized water is intended to be generated fresh at the point of use, when tested under clean conditions the disinfectant was effective from 5 minutes to 48 hours after preparation. In 2002, the FDA cleared superoxidized water as a high-level disinfectant.

Mode of action: The exact mechanism by which free chlorine destroys microorganisms is not completely understood. Role of oxidation of sulfhydryl enzymes and amino acids; ring chlorination of amino acids; loss of intracellular contents; decreased uptake of nutrients; inhibition of protein synthesis; decreased oxygen uptake; oxidation of respiratory components; decreased adenosine triphosphate production; breaks in DNA; and depressed DNA synthesis has been proposed. The actual mechanism of action might involve a combination of these factors.

Uses: Hypochlorites are widely used in healthcare facilities in different dilutions for a variety of disinfection purposes. Disinfection of countertops and floors; decontamination of blood spills; as an irrigating agent in endodontic treatment; as a disinfectant for manikins, laundry, dental appliances, hydrotherapy tanks; in treatment of medical waste before disposal; and decontaminating water distribution system in hemodialysis centers and hemodialysis machines.

Formaldehyde[12,17,28,33-35]

Formaldehyde is used as a disinfectant and sterilant in both its liquid and gaseous states. Formaldehyde is used principally as a water-based solution called formalin, which is 37% formaldehyde by weight. The aqueous solution is a bactericide, tuberculocide, fungicide, virucide and sporicide. Formaldehyde should be handled in the workplace as a potential carcinogen and its exposure should be limited to an 8-hour time-weighted average exposure concentration of 0.75 ppm. Ingestion of formaldehyde can be fatal; and long-term exposure to low levels in the air or on the skin can cause asthma-like respiratory problems and skin irritation, such as dermatitis and itching. For these reasons, employees should have limited direct contact with formaldehyde; and these considerations limit its role in sterilization and disinfection processes.

Mode of action: Formaldehyde inactivates micro-organisms by alkylating the amino and sulfhydral groups of proteins and ring nitrogen atoms of purine bases.

Uses: Although formaldehyde-alcohol is a chemical sterilant and formaldehyde is a high-level disinfectant, the healthcare uses of formaldehyde are limited by its irritating fumes and its pungent odour even at very low levels (<1 ppm). For these reasons and its role as a suspected human carcinogen, its use is limited in healthcare settings; when it is used, direct exposure to employees is generally avoided. Formaldehyde is used in the healthcare setting to prepare viral vaccines (e.g. poliovirus and influenza); as an embalming agent; and to preserve anatomic specimens. Previously, it was used for fumigation of operation theatres and critical care areas; however, that has almost been replaced by other methods. Paraformaldehyde, a solid polymer of formaldehyde, which can be vaporized by heat, is used for the gaseous decontamination of laminar flow biologic safety cabinets.

Glutaraldehyde[12,17,36-39]

Glutaraldehyde is a saturated dialdehyde that has gained popularity as a high-level disinfectant and chemical sterilant. Aqueous solutions of glutaraldehyde are acidic and generally in this state are not sporicidal. Only when the solution is "activated" by use of alkylating agents and made alkaline to pH 7.5–8.5 does the solution become sporicidal. Once activated, these solutions have a shelf-life of 14 days. New glutaraldehyde formulations (e.g. glutaraldehyde-phenol-sodium phenate, potentiated acid glutaraldehyde, stabilized alkaline glutaraldehyde) have a shelf-life of up to 30 days.

Mode of action: The biocidal activity of glutaraldehyde results from its alkylation of sulfhydryl, hydroxyl, carboxyl, and amino groups of microorganisms, which alters RNA, DNA, and protein synthesis.

Uses: Glutaraldehyde is most commonly used as a high-level disinfectant for medical equipment such as endoscopes, spirometry tubing, dialyzers, transducers, anesthesia, hemodialysis proportioning and dialysate delivery systems, respiratory therapy equipment and reuse of laparoscopic disposable plastic trocars. It is noncorrosive to metal and does not damage lensed instruments, plastics or rubber. It should not be used for cleaning noncritical surfaces because it is too toxic and expensive.

Colitis from residual glutaraldehyde in endoscopes; keratopathy and corneal decompensation from improperly rinsed ophthalmic instruments; dermatitis, mucositis and pulmonary symptoms with chronic exposure have been reported.

Hydrogen Peroxide[12,17,40-42]

Hydrogen peroxide has been ascribed good bactericidal, virucidal, sporicidal, and fungicidal activities. Many products containing hydrogen peroxide are used as liquid chemical sterilants and high-level disinfectants. Concentrations of hydrogen peroxide from 6% to 25% show promise as chemical sterilants. The product marketed as a sterilant is a premixed, ready-to-use chemical that contains 7.5% hydrogen peroxide and 0.85% phosphoric acid to maintain a low pH. A new, rapid-acting 13.4% hydrogen peroxide formulation (that is not yet FDA-cleared) has demonstrated sporicidal, fungicidal, mycobactericidal and virucidal efficacy. Manufacturer data demonstrate that this solution sterilizes in 30 minutes and provides high-level disinfection in 5 minutes.

Mode of action: Hydrogen peroxide works by producing destructive hydroxyl free radicals that can attack membrane lipids, DNA, and other essential cell components. Catalase which is produced by aerobes and facultative anaerobes that possess cytochrome systems, can protect cells from metabolically produced hydrogen peroxide by degrading hydrogen peroxide to water and oxygen. This defense needs to be overcome by the concentrations used for disinfection.

Uses: Commercially available 3% hydrogen peroxide is a stable and effective disinfectant when used on inanimate surfaces. It is commonly used in concentrations of 3–6% for disinfecting soft contact lenses, tonometer biprisms, ventilators, fabrics, and endoscopes. Some cases of enteritis and colitis due to residual hydrogen peroxide in endoscopes have been reported.

Iodophors[12,17,43-45]

Iodine solutions or tinctures have long been used as antiseptics on skin or tissue. An iodophor is a combination of iodine and a solubilizing agent or carrier; the resulting complex provides a sustained-release reservoir of iodine and releases small amounts of free iodine in aqueous solution. The best-known and most commonly used iodophor is povidone-iodine, a compound of polyvinylpyrrolidone with iodine. Iodophors retain the germicidal efficacy of iodine but unlike iodine generally are nonstaining and relatively nontoxic and nonirritant. Iodophors have been used both as antiseptics and disinfectants. FDA has not cleared any liquid chemical sterilant or high-level disinfectants with iodophors as the main active ingredient. Free iodine (I_2) contributes to the bactericidal activity of iodophors and dilutions of iodophors demonstrate more rapid bactericidal action than does a full-strength povidone-iodine solution. Therefore, iodophors must be diluted according to the manufacturers' directions to achieve antimicrobial activity.

Mode of action: Iodine can penetrate the microbial cell wall quickly, and the lethal effects are believed to result from disruption of protein and nucleic acid structure and synthesis.

Uses: Besides their use as an antiseptic, iodophors have been used for disinfecting blood culture bottles and medical equipment, such as hydrotherapy tanks, thermometers, and endoscopes. Antiseptic iodophors are not suitable as hard-surface disinfectants because of concentration differences. Iodophors formulated as antiseptics contain less free iodine than those formulated as disinfectants. Iodine or iodine-based antiseptics should not be used on silicone catheters because they can adversely affect the silicone tubing.

Ortho-phthalaldehyde[12,17,46-48]

Ortho-phthalaldehyde (OPA) is a high-level disinfectant that received FDA clearance in October 1999. It contains 0.55% 1,2-benzenedicarboxaldehyde. OPA solution is a clear, pale-blue liquid with a pH of 7.5.

Mode of action: Proposed mechanism is interaction with amino acids and affecting proteins of the microorganisms. The sporicidal activity of OPA is attributed to the blockage of the spore germination process.

Uses: OPA has several potential advantages over glutaraldehyde. It has excellent stability over a wide pH range (pH 3-9), is not a known irritant to the eyes and nasal passages, has a barely perceptible odor, does not require exposure monitoring, and requires no activation. It has excellent material compatibility. A disadvantage of OPA is that it stains proteins gray (including unprotected skin) and thus must be handled with caution. OPA residues remaining on inadequately water-rinsed transesophageal echo probes can stain the patient's mouth. Personal protective equipment should be worn while working and equipment must be thoroughly rinsed postdisinfection to prevent discoloration of skin or mucous membrane.

Recently, cases have been reported of anaphylaxis-like reactions in patients who underwent repeated cystoscopy with the scopes which had been reprocessed using OPA.

Peracetic Acid[12,17,49-52]

Peracetic, or peroxyacetic, acid is characterized by rapid action against all microorganisms. Advantages of peracetic acid are that the decomposition products, i.e. acetic acid, water, oxygen and hydrogen peroxide are not harmful; it enhances removal of organic material; and leaves no residue. It remains effective in the presence of organic matter and is sporicidal even at low temperatures. Peracetic acid can corrode copper, bronze, brass, plain steel, and galvanized iron but these effects can be reduced by additives and pH modifications. It is considered unstable, especially when diluted; for example, a 1% solution loses half its strength through hydrolysis in 6 days, whereas 40% peracetic acid loses 1-2% of its active ingredients per month.

Mode of action: Similar to other oxidizing agents, the proposed mechanism is denaturation of proteins, disruption of the cell wall permeability, and oxidation of sulfhydryl and sulfur bonds in proteins, enzymes, and other metabolites.

Uses: Peracetic acid is used to chemically sterilize medical (e.g. endoscopes, arthroscopes), surgical, and dental instruments. The sterilant, 35% peracetic acid, is diluted to 0.2% with filtered water at 50°C. Simulated-use and clinical trials have demonstrated excellent microbicidal activity.

Peracetic Acid and Hydrogen Peroxide[12,17,52,53]

Two chemical sterilants are available that contain peracetic acid plus hydrogen peroxide in different percentages. It has been demonstrated that this combination inactivated all microorganisms including glutaraldehyde resistant *Mycobacteria*, except bacterial spores within 20 minutes.

Phenolics[12,17,54]

Joseph Lister in his revolutionary work on antiseptic surgery, used phenol as a germicide to prevent surgical infections. In the past few decades, work has been done on the phenol derivatives or phenolics and their antimicrobial properties. Phenol derivatives originate when a functional group (e.g. alkyl, phenyl, benzyl, halogen) replaces one of the hydrogen atoms on the aromatic ring of phenol. Two phenol derivatives commonly found as constituents of hospital disinfectants are ortho-phenylphenol and ortho-benzyl-para-chlorophenol. The antimicrobial properties of these compounds and many other phenol derivatives are much improved over those of the parent chemical. Phenolics are absorbed by porous materials, and the residual disinfectant can irritate tissue. In 1970, depigmentation of the skin was reported to be caused by phenolic germicidal detergents containing para-tertiary butylphenol and para-tertiary amylphenol.

Mode of action: In high concentrations, phenol acts as a protoplasmic poison, penetrating and disrupting the cell wall and precipitating the cell proteins. Low concentrations of phenol and higher molecular-weight phenol derivatives lead to bacterial death by inactivation of essential enzyme systems and leakage of essential metabolites from the cell wall.

Uses: Many phenolic germicides are used as disinfectants for use on environmental surfaces (e.g. bedside tables, laboratory surfaces and bedrails) and noncritical medical devices. Phenolics are not FDA-cleared as high-level disinfectants for use with semicritical items but could be used to preclean or decontaminate critical and semicritical devices before terminal sterilization or high-level disinfection.

Quaternary Ammonium Compounds[12,17,55,56]

Quaternary ammonium compounds are widely used as disinfectants. Increased water hardness decreases their microbicidal activity due to formation of insoluble precipitates; and materials such as cotton and gauze pads can absorb the active ingredients thus decreasing their efficacy. As with several other disinfectants, (e.g. phenolics, iodophors) gram-negative bacteria can survive or grow in them. A few case reports have documented occupational asthma as a result of exposure to benzalkonium chloride.

Mode of action: The bactericidal action of the quaternaries has been attributed to the inactivation of energy-producing enzymes, disruption of the cell membranes and denaturation of essential cell proteins.

Uses: The quaternaries commonly are used in ordinary environmental sanitation of noncritical surfaces, such as floors, walls and furniture. EPA-registered quaternary ammonium compounds are appropriate to use for disinfecting medical equipment that contacts intact skin (e.g. blood pressure cuffs).

Heavy Metals[12,57-59]

The anti-infective activity of some heavy metals has been known for long. Silver has been used for prophylaxis of conjunctivitis of the newborn, bonding to indwelling catheters and topical therapy for burn wounds. The use of heavy metals as antiseptics or disinfectants is again being explored. Preliminary data suggests that metals are effective against a wide variety of microbes.

Ultraviolet Radiation[12,22]

The wavelength of ultraviolet (UV) radiation ranges from 328 nm to 210 nm (3280 A to 2100 A). The maximum bactericidal effect occurs at 240–280 nm. Mercury vapor lamps emit more than 90% of their radiation at 253.7 nm, which is near the maximum microbicidal activity. Inactivation of microorganisms results from nucleic acid through induction of thymine dimers. UV radiation has been employed in the disinfection of drinking water, air, contact lenses and titanium implants. Bacteria and viruses are more readily killed by UV light than are bacterial spores. The application of UV radiation in the healthcare environment (i.e. operating rooms, biologic safety cabinets and isolation rooms) is limited to destruction of airborne organisms or inactivation of microorganisms on surfaces.

REFERENCES

1. Nightingale F. Notes on hospitals, 3rd edn. London: Longmans 1863. (A complete revision of the 1st edn of 1859).
2. Anon. *Charaka-Samhita* (c. 4th Century BC); English translation from Sanskrit by Kavipatna AC. Calcutta: Privately Printed. 1888;1:168-9.
3. Caton R. Two lectures on the temples and ritual of Asklepios at Epiduuros and Athens. Delivered at the Royal Institution of Great Britain; 1899. pp. 4-30.
4. Snowman J. A short history of Talmudic medicine. London: Bale and Danielssohn; 1935. pp. 46.
5. Samuel G. Kosher tests. J Royal Sot of Medicine. 1990;83:477.
6. Major RH. A history of medicine, Vol 1. Oxford: Blackwell. 1954;294321.
7. Bell J. The principles of surgery. Edinburgh: Cadell and Davies; 1801. pp. 107-17.
8. Selwy S. Hospital infection: The first 2500 years. J Hosp Infect. 1991;18(Suppl A):5-64.
9. Lister J. On the antiseptic principle in the practice of surgery. Lancet. 1867;2:353-6.
10. Lister J. An address on the effect of the antiseptic treatment upon the general salubrity of surgical hospitals. Br Med J. 1875;2:769-71.
11. Spaulding EH. Chemical disinfection of medical and surgical materials. In: Lawrence C, Block SS, eds. Disinfection, sterilization, and preservation. Philadelphia: Lea & Febiger; 1968. pp. 517-31.

12. Ruthala WA, Weber DJ, and the Healthcare Infection Control Practices Advisory Committee (HICPAC), Centre for Disease Control and Prevention, Atlanta, USA. Guideline for Disinfection and Sterilization in Healthcare Facilities, 2008.
13. Bhattachatyya M, Kepnes LJ. The effectiveness of immersion disinfection for flexible fiberoptic laryngoscopes. Otolaryngol Head Neck. 2004;130:681-5.
14. Hamasuna R, Nose K, Sueyoshi T, Nagano M, Hasui Y, Osada Y. High-level disinfection of cystoscopic equipment with ortho-phthalaldehyde solution. J Hosp Infect. 2004;57:346-8.
15. Weber DJ, Rutala WA. Environmental issues and nosocomial infections. In: Wenzel RP (Ed). Prevention and control of nosocomial infections. Baltimore: Williams and Wilkins; 1997. pp. 491-514.
16. Sehulster L, Chinn RYW. Healthcare Infection Control Practices Advisory Committee. Guidelines for environmental infection control in health-care facilities. MMWR. 2003;52:1-44.
17. Mathur P. Cleaning, disinfection and Sterilization. Hospital acquired infections-Prevention and Control, 1st edition. Published Wolters Kluver Health, India; 2010. pp. 143-220.
18. Rutala WA, Weber DJ. Disinfection and sterilization in health care facilities: what clinicians need to know. Clin Infect Dis. 2004;39:702-9.
19. AORN Standards, Recommended Practices, and Guidelines: Recommended Practices for Cleaning and Caring for Surgical Instruments and Powered Equipment, 2005.
20. Mathur P. Operating Rooms. Hospital Acquired Infections-Prevention and Control, 1st edition. Published Wolters Kluver health, India; 2010. pp. 249-74.
21. Mangram AJ, Horan TC, Pearson ML, Silver LC, Jarvis WR. Guideline for Prevention of Surgical Site Infection. Centers for Disease Control and Prevention (CDC) Hospital Infection Control Practices Advisory Committee. Am J Infect Control. 1999;27(2):97-132.
22. Sterilization and disinfection. In: Kapil A, ed. Ananathnarayan and Paniker's textbook of microbiology, 9th edition. India: Universities Press Pvt Ltd; 2014. pp. 28-38.
23. Hansen KS. Occupational dermatoses in hospital cleaning women. Contact Dermatitis. 1983;9:343-51.
24. Melli MC, Giorgini S, Sertoli A. Sensitization from contact with ethyl alcohol. Contact Dermatitis. 1986;14:315.
25. Ali Y, Dolan MJ, Fendler EJ, Larson EL. Alcohols. In: Block SS (Ed). Disinfection, sterilization, and preservation. Philadelphia: Lippincott Williams & Wilkins; 2001. pp. 229-54.
26. Spaulding EH. Alcohol as a surgical disinfectant. AORN J. 1964;2:67-71.
27. Hoffman PN, Death JE, Coates D. The stability of sodium hypochlorite solutions. In: Collins CH, Allwood MC, Bloomfield SF, Fox A (Eds). Disinfectants: their use and evaluation of effectiveness. London: Academic Press; 1981. pp. 77-83.
28. Gamble MR. Hazard: formaldehyde and hypochlorites. Lab. Anim. 1977;11:61.
29. Coates D. Comparison of sodium hypochlorite and sodium dichloroisocyanurate disinfectants: neutralization by serum. J Hosp Infect. 1988;11:60-7.
30. Coates D, Wilson M. Use of sodium dichloroisocyanurate granules for spills of body fluids. J Hosp Infect. 1989;13:241-51.
31. Tanaka H, Hirakata Y, Kaku M, et al. Antimicrobial activity of superoxidized water. J Hosp Infect. 1996;34:43-9.
32. Sampson MN MA. Not all super-oxidized waters are the same. J Hosp Infect. 2002;52:227-8.
33. Occupational Health and Safety Administration. OSHA Fact Sheet: Formaldehyde: Occupational Safety and Health Administration, US Department of Labor, 2002.
34. Centers for Disease Control. Occupational exposures to formaldehyde in dialysis units. MMWR. 1986;35:399-01.
35. Centers for Disease Control. Formaldehyde exposures in a gross anatomy laboratory—Colorado. MMWR. 1983;52:698-700.
36. Scott EM, Gorman SP. Glutaraldehyde. In: Block SS (Ed). Disinfection, sterilization, and preservation. Philadelphia: Lippincott Williams & Wilkins; 2001. pp. 361-81.
37. Dauendorffer JN, Laurain C, Weber M, Dailloux M. Evaluation of the bactericidal efficiency of a 2% alkaline glutaraldehyde solution on *Mycobacterium xenopi*. J Hosp Infect. 2000;46:73-6.
38. Overton D, Burgess JO, Beck B, Matis B. Glutaraldehyde test kits: evaluation for accuracy and range. Gen Dent. 1989;37:126-8.
39. Cooke RPD, Goddard SV, Chatterley R, Whymant-Morris A, Cheale J. Monitoring glutaraldehyde dilution in automated washer/disinfectors. J Hosp Infect. 2001;48:242-6.
40. Block SS. Peroxygen compounds. In: Block SS (Ed). Disinfection, sterilization, and preservation. Philadelphia: Lippincott Williams & Wilkins; 2001. pp. 185-204.
41. Sattar SA, Springthorpe VS, Rochon M. A product based on accelerated and stabilized hydrogen peroxide: Evidence for broad-spectrum germicidal activity. Canadian J Infect Control; 1998. pp. 123-30.
42. Omidbakhsh N, Sattar SA. Broad-spectrum microbicidal activity, toxicologic assessment, and materials compatibility of a new generation of accelerated hydrogen peroxide-based environmental surface disinfectant. Am J Infect Control. 2006;34:251-7.

43. Gottardi W. Iodine and iodine compounds. In: Block SS (Ed). Disinfection, sterilization, and preservation. Philadelphia: Lippincott Williams & Wilkins; 2001. pp. 159-84.
44. Berkelman RL, Holland BW, Anderson RL. Increased bactericidal activity of dilute preparations of povidone-iodine solutions. J Clin Microbiol. 1982;15:635-9.
45. Craven DE, Moody B, Connolly MG, Kollisch NR, Stottmeier KD, McCabe WR. Pseudobacteremia caused by povidone-iodine solution contaminated with *Pseudomonas cepacia*. N Engl J Med. 1981;305:621-3.
46. Simons C, Walsh SE, Maillard JY, Russell AD. A note: ortho-phthalaldehyde: proposed mechanism of action of a new antimicrobial agent. Lett Appl Microbiol. 2000;31:299-302.
47. Cabrera-Martinez RM, Setlow B, Setlow P. Studies on the mechanisms of the sporicidal action of orthophthalaldehyde. J Appl Microbiol. 2002;92:675-80.
48. Walsh SE, Maillard JY, Russell AD. Ortho-phthalaldehyde: a possible alternative to glutaraldehyde for high level disinfection. J Appl Microbiol. 1999;86:1039-46.
49. Malchesky PS. Medical applications of peracetic acid. In: Block SS (Ed). Disinfection, sterilization, and preservation. Philadelphia: Lippincott Williams & Wilkins, 2001. pp. 979-96.
50. Mannion PT. The use of peracetic acid for the reprocessing of flexible endoscopes and rigid cystoscopes and laparoscopes. J Hosp Infect. 1995;29:313-5.
51. Duc DL, Ribiollet A, Dode X, Ducel G, Marchetti B, Calop J. Evaluation of the microbicidal efficacy of Steris System I for digestive endoscopes using GERMANDE and ASTM validation protocols. J Hosp Infect. 2001;48:135-41.
52. Alasri A, Roques C, Michel G, Cabassud C, Aptel P. Bactericidal properties of peracetic acid and hydrogen peroxide, alone and in combination, and chlorine and formaldehyde against bacterial water strains. Can J Microbiol. 1992;38:635-42.
53. Stanley P. Destruction of a glutaraldehyde-resistant mycobacterium by a per-oxygen disinfectant.(Abstract). Am J Infect. Control. 1998;26:185.
54. Goddard PA, McCue KA. Phenolic compounds. In: Block SS (Ed). Disinfection, sterilization, and preservation. Philadelphia: Lippincott Williams & Wilkins; 2001. pp. 255-81.
55. Merianos JJ. Surface-active agents. In: Block SS (Ed). Disinfection, sterilization, and preservation. Philadelphia: Lippincott Williams & Wilkins; 2001. pp. 283-320.
56. Purohit A, Kopferschmitt-Kubler MC, Moreau C, Popin E, Blaumeiser M, Pauli G. Quaternary ammonium compounds and occupational asthma. International Archives of Occupational and Environmental Health. 2000;73:423-7.
57. Weber DJ, Rutala WA. Use of metals as microbicides in preventing infections in healthcare. In: Block SS (Ed). Disinfection, sterilization, and preservation. Philadelphia: Lippincott Williams & Wilkins; 2001. pp. 415-30.
58. Brady MJ, Lisay CM, Yurkovetskiy AV, Sawan SP. Persistent silver disinfectant for the environmental control of pathogenic bacteria. Am J Infect. Control. 2003;31:208-14.
59. Bright KR, Gerba CP, Rusin PA. Rapid reduction of *Staphylococcus aureus* populations on stainless steel surfaces by zeolite ceramic coatings containing silver and zinc ions. J Hosp Infect. 2002;52:307-9.

CHAPTER 2

Operation Theatre: Design and Layout

Ritika Mukhija, Neelima Aron, Namrata Sharma, Atul Kumar

INTRODUCTION

Operating theatre or operating room, sometimes also referred to as surgical suite is a specially designed area, isolated from other sections of the hospital where various surgical procedures are carried out by highly trained personnel under aseptic conditions. The name 'theatre' stems from the traditional design which consisted of semicircular amphitheatres to allow students and other spectators to observe the surgical procedures.

HISTORY

In the initial days, it was very common for the financially well-endowed patients to have surgical procedures done by private practitioners at their residences, and hospitals were often associated with infection and poverty, which was unfortunately often the case. Operating rooms in the early 18th century were basically large rooms crowded with patients and cluttered with medical supplies and waste. Post-operative infections and difficult recovery periods for patients were the result of wards serving as both surgical spaces and recovery quarters. In the second half of the 18th century, operating rooms were separated from other areas in the hospital and surgery became a specialization with surgeons having their own space, equipment and nurses. It was in the 19th century that the concept of operation theatres originated, which were designed to have a raised table at the centre for performing surgeries, surrounded by several rows of seats allowing students and other spectators to observe the case in progress. One of the oldest surviving operating theatres is the old operating theatre in London, which was built in 1822, and is now a museum of surgical history, amongst a few other surviving theatres.

Patient care and safety has always been the main focus in the development of operating rooms over time. Maintaining a separate sterile area for performing surgeries, using sterile gowns and instruments, and sustaining a clean environment with ambient temperature and humidity have played a major role in decreasing the morbidity and mortality associated with surgical procedures. Therefore, architectural layout and design of an operation theatre are essential in determining the productivity, quality of care, and cost effectiveness of any surgical specialty hospital.

SETTING UP AN OPERATION THEATRE

The surgical suite on an average consumes 9–10% of the hospital budget. The setting up of an operation theatre complex requires meticulous planning and execution by a specialized team consisting of health care personnel, engineers (civil, mechanical, electrical and technical) and hospital administration staff. Theatre managers, infection control team, surgeons and anesthetists should be involved in the planning of the theatre design from the onset.[1]

The **main objectives** of planning should be:
- To promote high standards of asepsis
- Ensure maximum standard of safety
- Optimise utilization of OT and staff time
- Ensure patient and staff comfort in terms of thermal, acoustic and lighting requirements

- Minimize maintenance
- Ensure functional separation of spaces
- Provide soothing environment
- Regulate flow of traffic.

Design and Principles

The vital principles in planning the layout and design of any operation theatre should be the ability to exclude contamination from outside, maintain a clear segregation of clean and contaminated areas within the OT and to maintain proper flow of traffic. The location of the theatre complex should allow easy access to the surgical wards, intensive care unit (ICU), blood bank, and laboratory services. There must always be a provision for future expansion/alterations that may be required in accordance with the changing trends and technology.[2,3]

There should be no unrelated hospital traffic flow in and around the theatre area, and if possible, traffic within the operating suite must be regulated via a security lock system which only allows access to staff, patients and equipment from different entrances and exits. There should be a zone-wise distribution of the area, so as to avoid crisscross movements of men and machine. The design should be such as to ensure avoidance of any outdoor source of noise.[4] There should be a provision for emergency exit.

LAYOUT

The OT complex can be broadly divided into 4 zones depending upon the varying degrees of cleanliness (**Table 2.1 and Flow chart 2.1**).[5] In **Figure 2.1**, the red line marks the boundary between rest of the hospital and the protective zone. As a rule, the bacteriological count should decrease as one goes from the outer to inner zones (operating area). The differential decreasing positive pressure ventilation gradient from the inner zone to the outer zone plays an important role in this.

There should be a one-way traffic of waste products from inside the OT to outside.

Operating Room

As per the National Accreditation Board for Hospitals and Healthcare Providers (NABH) guidelines, standard OT size of 20' × 20' × 10' is recommended. Height below the false ceiling is considered. A minimum space of 180 square feet is desired for one operation table.

Table 2.1 Operation theatre layout

Level-I Protective zone	• Restricted entry • Changing rooms/patient waiting area/toilets (**Figs 2.2 and 2.3**) • Shoes/footwear to be removed and clothes changed • Transfer bay for patient, material and equipment • Rooms for administrative staff • Stores and records
Level-II Clean zone	• Entry only after changing for both patients and staff • Caps/masks/separate slippers to be worn • Administration of peribulbar blocks/pre-medication
Level-III Aseptic zone	• Sterile area • Entry restricted to minimal staff • Fumigated areas • Scrub room/gloving and gowning
Level-IV Disposal zone	• Corridor from where used instruments and OT debris is taken out • Sterilization room • Instrument maintenance (under supervision of the Staff Nurse/OT Technician)

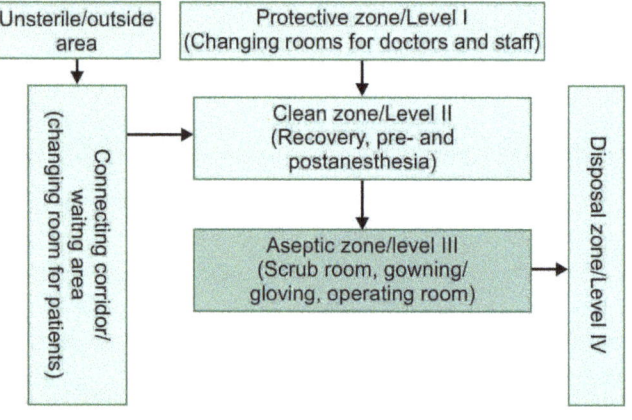

Flow chart 2.1 Zones of an operation theatre

There should be not more than 2 operation tables per OT (**Fig. 2.4**). Standard occupancy of 5–8 persons and equipment load of 5–7 kW at any given point of time inside the OT is considered acceptable. Corridors should not be less than 2.85 m (approx. 10 feet) width for easy movement of men, stretchers and machines and separate corridors for other uses should be set-up (**Fig. 2.5**).

Doors

Sliding type doors of adequate width (1.2–1.5 m) or swing doors (self-closing) are recommended especially

Operation Theatre: Design and Layout

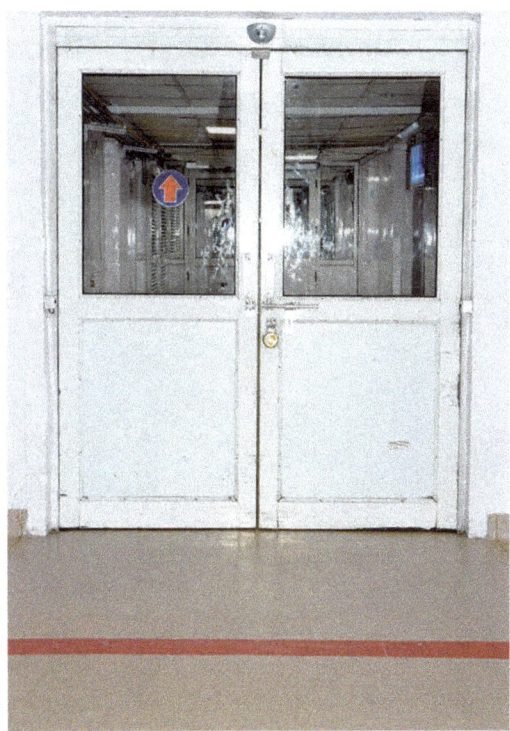

Figure 2.1 A red demarcation line between the protective zone and hospital area

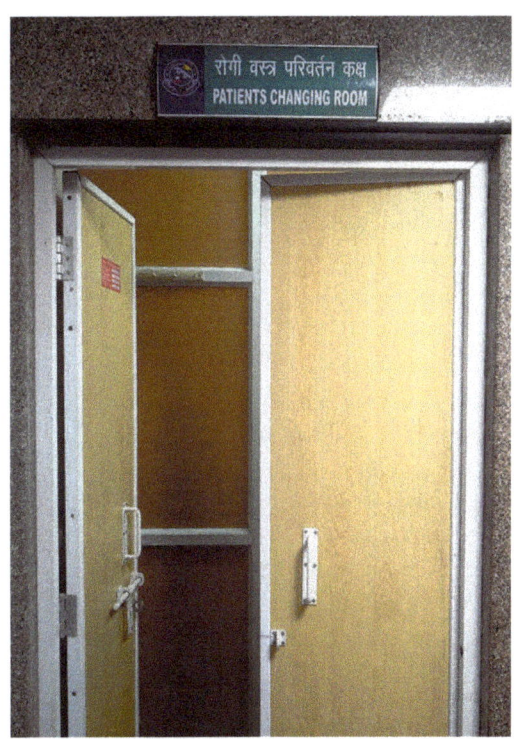

Figure 2.2 Patient's changing room

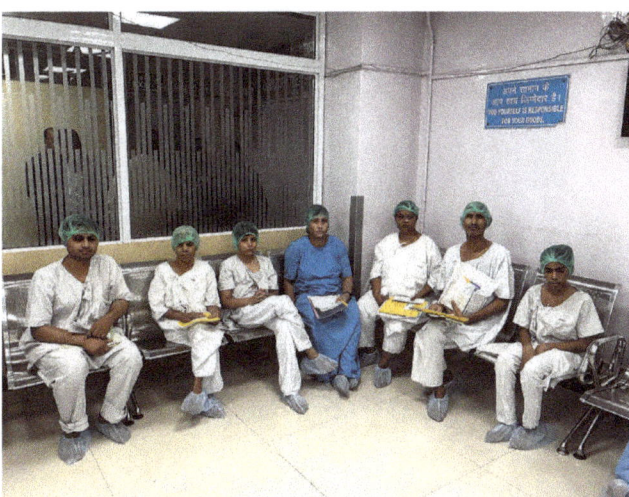

Figure 2.3 Patients and attendants sitting in the waiting area

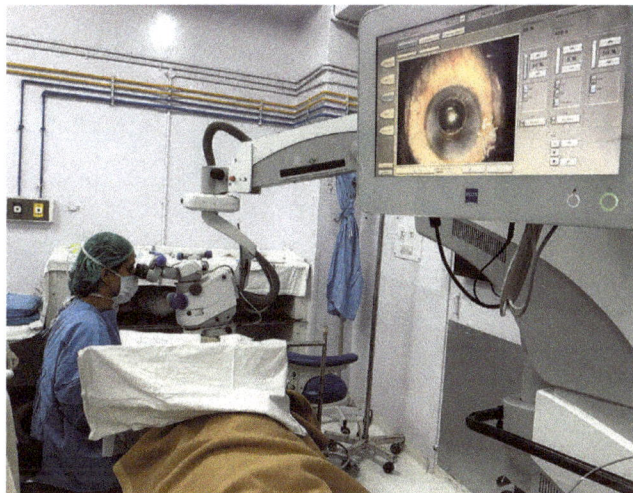

Figure 2.4 Standard operating room with one operating table

in areas where patient movement is anticipated like in operation theatres, pre-operative and post-operative rooms. The sliding doors are preferred to the double action leaf type since they save space, prevent air turbulences and are more user-friendly. Doors must remain closed at all times, particularly during the surgery because the microbial count in the air rises every time doors swing open from either direction. There must be a clear glass viewing window in the door to prevent frequent opening and closing of the door. The door from the semi-restricted corridor into the operating room should be at least 6 ft. wide and located in such a way as to permit the bed/trolley to move as directly as possible from the corridor to the side of

Ocular Infections: Prophylaxis and Management

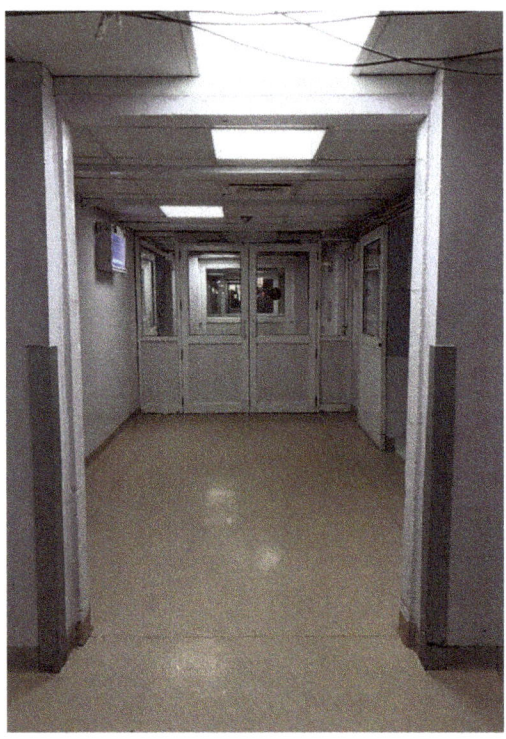

Figure 2.5 Operation theatre corridors (more than 6 feet wide)

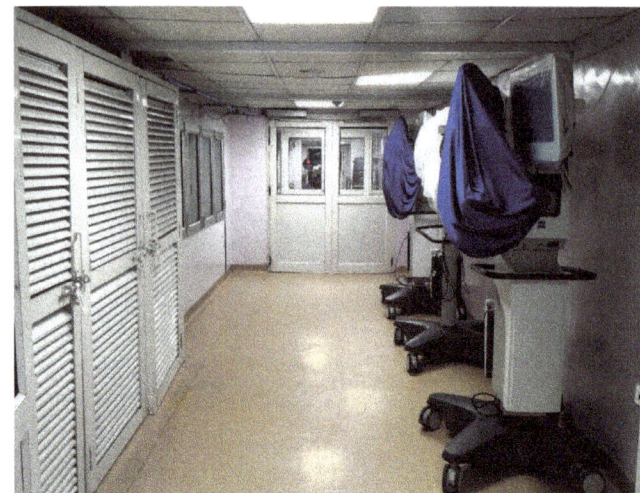

Figure 2.6 Wide doors for trolleys and operating microscopes to pass by

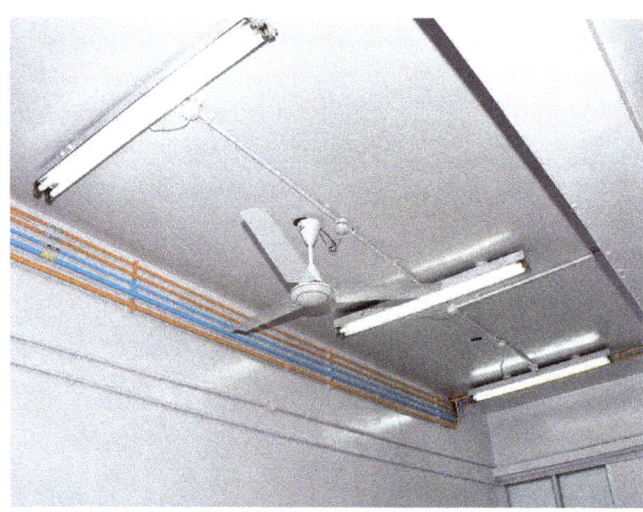

Figure 2.7 Ceiling with various pipelines for oxygen and other gases

the operating room table (Fig. 2.6). For this reason, these doors are typically located toward the foot of the operating table away from the anesthesia equipment for ophthalmic machinery. For doors between the clean zone and the operating rooms, a double acting door, 4 ft. wide, with a small view window is required.

Walls and Ceiling (Fig. 2.7)

It is recommended that all surface materials should be hard, nonporous, fire resistant, waterproof, stain proof, seamless and easy to clean. Washable epoxy resin paint for the walls is ideal, because it lasts a long time and can withstand a daily washing programme. Cheaper paint has a tendency to break off and may fall in an open surgical wound. One of the low budget alternatives for the walls is the vitrified tiles. Collusion corners and joints should be covered with steel or aluminum plates or epoxy resin. The color of paint should allow reflection of light and yet be soothing to the eyes. Light color (light blue or green) washable paint will be ideal. A semi-matt wall surface reflects less light than a highly gloss finish and is less tiring to the eyes of the OT team. The final prepared surface may be treated with antibacterial paint.

Ceiling should be painted with washable paint and corners of the rooms should be rounded off to prevent collection of dirt and dust. The walls and ceiling often are used to mount essential devices and equipment to reduce crowding of the floor area therefore the walls must be solid and robust enough to carry the weight of equipment. The walls must be fitted with outlets for oxygen, other medical gases and vacuum, and where possible, an anesthetic gas scavenging system should be fitted at floor level. There is also a need to fit multiple electric outlets on the walls, preferably at a height of less than 1.5 m from the floor.

Floor

Floor should be smooth, without cracks and breaks, nonslip, made of suitably hard material and should not endanger the safety of personnel **(Fig. 2.8)**. The floor covering should be specified, such as continuous thick and tough vinyl, and the manufacturer's guidelines for cleaning and maintaining the floor must be available in the cleaning policy. Kota stone flooring is hard, tough, nonwater absorbent, nonslippery, cheap and easy to maintain and hence is recommended. Conductive copper mesh and self-leveling epoxy flooring may be done. The floor covering should be curved up the wall to 2.5 cm, thus ensuring that edges are coved and easier to clean than right angled floors.

LIGHTING

Lighting should be evenly distributed throughout the room, also ensuring sufficient light for the anesthetist. Most OT lights are white fluorescent because they cast minimal shadow. Color corrected fluorescent lamps (recessed or surface ceiling mounted) to produce even illumination of at least 500 Lux at working height, with minimal glare are preferred. To minimize eye fatigue, the ratio of intensity of general room lighting to that at the surgical site should not exceed 1:5, preferably 1:3. This contrast should be maintained in corridors and scrub areas, as well as in the room itself, so that the surgeon becomes accustomed to the light before entering the sterile field.

TEMPERATURE AND HUMIDITY

The temperature should be maintained at $21 \pm 3°C$ inside the OT all the time with a corresponding relative humidity (RH) between 40 and 60%, though the ideal RH is considered to be 55%. Appropriate devices to monitor and display these conditions inside the OT may be installed.

SCRUB ROOM

This should be built within the restricted area and as close to the operating room as possible **(Fig. 2.9)**. Elbow, knee or foot operated taps/water source are recommended, electronically controlled or those activated by infrared sensors are ideal **(Fig. 2.10)**. It is extremely important to have nonslippery flooring in this area.

RECOVERY ROOM

In an ophthalmic operation theatre, recovery room is the area where patients undergoing surgeries in general anesthesia are observed for a short duration in the post-operative period before shifting them to the wards, and where patients undergoing surgeries in local anesthesia receive peribulbar or retrobulbar anesthesia **(Fig. 2.11)**. It has various equipment such as vitals monitor (blood pressure, pulse, oxygen saturation), weighing machine and drugs required pre-operatively and post-operatively **(Fig. 2.12)**. Dilatation required for various

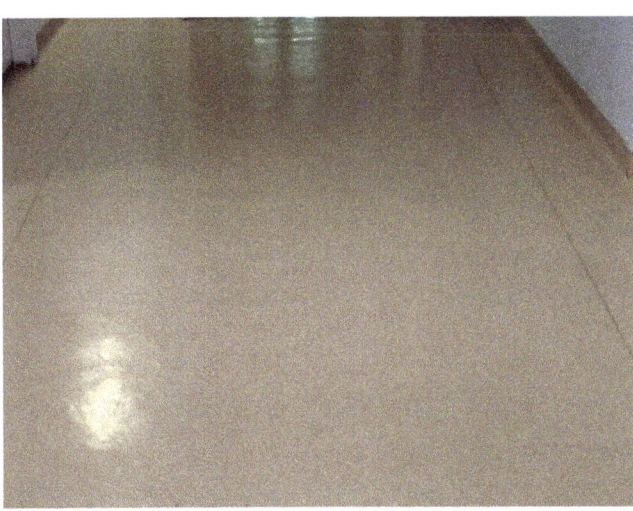

Figure 2.8 Nonslip smooth flooring without cracks and breaks

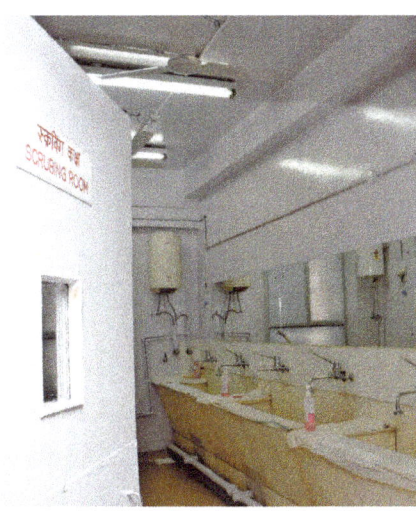

Figure 2.9 Separate scrubbing area

Ocular Infections: Prophylaxis and Management

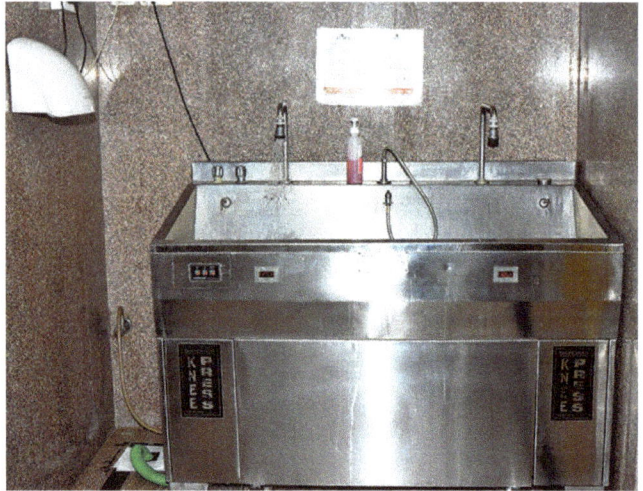

Figure 2.10 Foot operated taps in scrubbing area

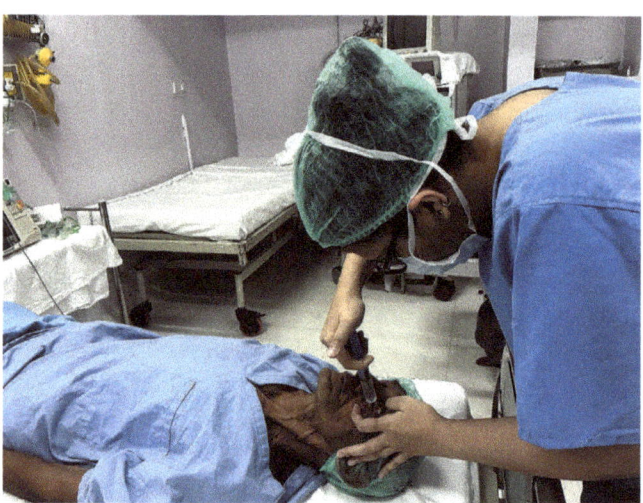

Figure 2.11 Administration of peribulbar anesthesia in recovery room

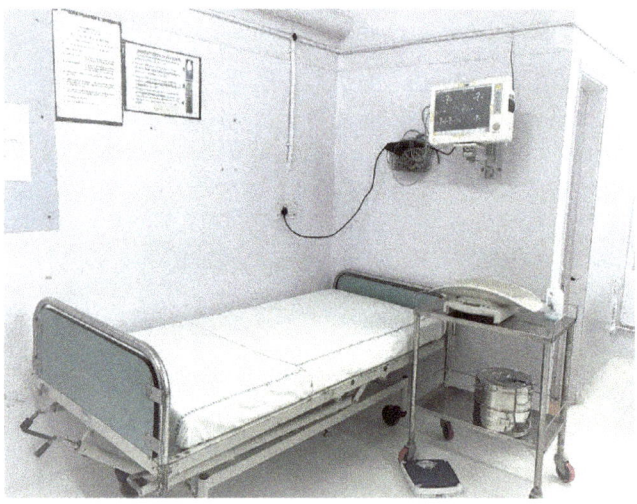

Figure 2.12 Recovery room with necessary equipment (weighing machine, vitals monitor)

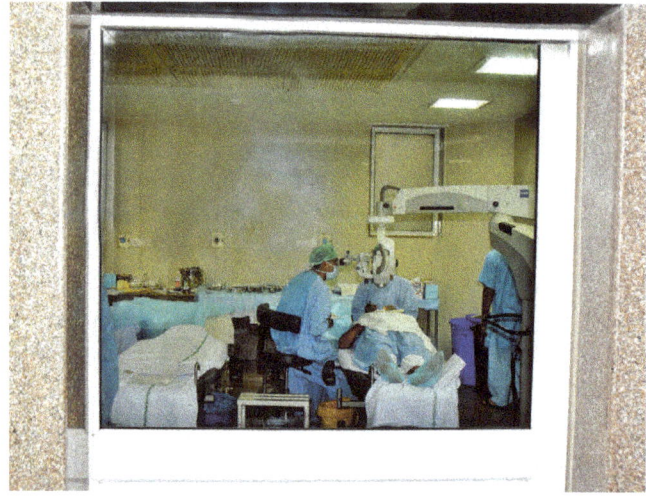

Figure 2.13 Minor operation theatre with lid surgery being performed

procedures like cataract surgery and vitreoretinal procedures is also done in the recovery room. Various types of cryotherapy (cyclocryotherapy, anterior retinal cryotherapy, etc.) and other surface procedures like diode laser cyclophotocoagulation, electrolysis of trichiatic eyelashes may also be undertaken in the recovery room itself, provided there is patient privacy and consent.

MINOR OPERATION THEATRE

There are various minor ophthalmic procedures which do not necessarily require a dedicated operating theatre. A suitably equipped and sufficiently large room with air conditioning may suffice for such procedures. To name a few, excision biopsy or cauterization of eyelid lesions, e.g. chalazion, intravitreal injections, lacrimal sac washouts, subconjunctival and subtenon injections may be carried out under aseptic conditions in a minor operation theatre **(Fig. 2.13)**. The following specifications should be adhered to:[6,7]

- Ceilings and walls should be made of nonporous material and should be cleaned and disinfected at regular intervals.
- There should be no windows on the walls. If at all windows are present, they should be non-openable.

- Doors should be self-closing with a vision panel.
- Flooring should be durable and strong enough to withhold various types of machinery and should be cleaned and disinfected as per norms.
- Single use instruments should be used wherever feasible. Dedicated and secure facilities should be provided for the storage and collection of re-usable instruments if preferred, though unlike for conventional operating theatres, a separate area for the laying up of instruments is not required.
- Proper scrub facilities should be there as in the general OT; taps or faucets should be hands-free and disposable towels should be used.
- Facilities for the safe disposal of waste should comply with the current guidelines for holding waste prior to collection/disposal. A separate secure area, inside or outside the operative facility, e.g. a lockable bin, should be provided.
- For mechanical ventilation, 15 air changes per hour, as required for the removal of airborne chemicals/anesthetic gases and a positive pressure differential of 5 Pa between the operating facility and the surrounding area is recommended.
- For mechanically ventilated facilities, temperature should be within the standard range, i.e. 18–22°C with a relative humidity of 20–60%.

A meticulous planning and designing of the operation theatre might seem like an uphill task and may initially be time consuming, but it is extremely important in maintaining a proper functioning of a surgical specialty hospital. A well planned operation theatre, adhering to proper guidelines and recommendations not only helps in preventing adverse events, both for the hospital staff and patients, but is also highly cost-effective in the long run. It is also extremely important that the entire hospital staff understands the importance of the same and strictly adheres to the recommended guidelines.

REFERENCES

1. Gupta SK, Kant S, Chandrashekhar R. Operating unit – planning essentials and design Considerations. Journal of Academy of Hospital Administration. 2005;17:01-12.
2. MaCaulay, HMC and Davies LL. Hospital planning and Administration. WHO; 1966.
3. Rice NS, Harry J. Ophthalmic operating theater design: methods of sterilization. Proceedings of the Royal Society of Medicine. 1969;62(12):1203-4.
4. Harsoor SS, Bhaskar SB. Designing an ideal operating room complex. Indian J Anaesth. 2007;51:193-9
5. Republic of Namibia, Ministry of Health and Social Services, Operation Theater Manual Available from: *http://mhss.gov.na*
6. Humphreys H, Coia JE, Stacey A, et al. Healthcare Infection Society. Guidelines on the facilities required for minor surgical procedures and minimal access interventions. J Hosp Infect. 2012;80(2):103-9.
7. Kelkar U, Kelkar S, Bal AM, et al. Microbiological evaluation of various parameters in ophthalmic operating rooms. The need to establish guidelines. Indian J Ophthalmol. 2003;51(2):171-6.

CHAPTER 3

Air Flow System in Ophthalmic Operation Theatre

Prateek Kakkar, Neelima Aron, Atul Kumar

INTRODUCTION

One of the leading complications in any surgical field in today's scenario is surgical site infection (SSI) and in ocular setups, it amounts to wound infection or endophthalmitis, which can lead to visually devastating outcomes. All possible measures must be taken to reduce the potential of infection during surgeries. Airborne and other sources of infection must be reduced to a minimum to achieve optimal operating theatre conditions.

Studies have shown that an effective airflow and ventilation system helps to reduce the incidence of surgical wound infection.[1-4] Therefore, a knowledge of what makes up the system and its requirements must be known before any operation theatre is established. In India, National Accreditation Board for Hospitals and Healthcare providers (NABH) is the quality control body that provides set guidelines and benchmarks for maintaining a desired level of healthcare facilities in hospitals.

VENTILATION/AIR CONDITIONING

Ventilation is necessary for the regulation of temperature and humidity. It also provides cleaning of fresh air and circulating air.[5] Air handling systems process air through various stages. Air is cooled, moisture is removed and is filtered to remove dust particles, bacteria, viruses; and some air handling systems additionally remove gases, odors and other volatile organic compounds.

Every operation theatre requires a dedicated air handler. It can either be fitted outside operation theatre, normally floor mounted, known as air handling unit, i.e. AHU, or fitted inside on ceiling known as ceiling suspended air handler. The minimum size of the air supply area should be 6′ × 4′ to cover the entire OT table, surgical team and sterile instruments trolley. The air quality at the supply level can be Class 1000/10,000 ISO. Class 1000/10,000 means a cubic foot of air must have no more than 1000/10,000 particles respectively measuring 0.5 microns or larger.

A theatre's air handler must not be linked to air conditioning of any other area.[6] Window or split air conditioners (AC) are not recommended for the same, as they are considered to provide pockets of microbial growth which cannot be sealed. Also the flow system should have a uniform and unidirectional flow and therefore recirculating air conditioning systems like window or split ACs are not preferred. However, every hospital in our country cannot afford a centralized system of air conditioning. Split AC's with portable air cleaners and millipore filters may be a good and cheaper alternative.

Cooling of air is done within the AHU and, therefore, a separate AC is not required in the OT. This provides a good cooling input for smaller OTs with less number of operating tables. For larger setups running multiple tables and multiple operation theatre rooms, a larger water chiller is used. This water chiller works on large air conditioning plants **(Fig. 3.1)** where the water is cooled using heat exchange system with Freon-22 or other gases and the chilled water is supplied to the AHU of the OT.

It is advised that the temperature is maintained at 21°C (Range 18–24°) at all times inside the OT. A relative

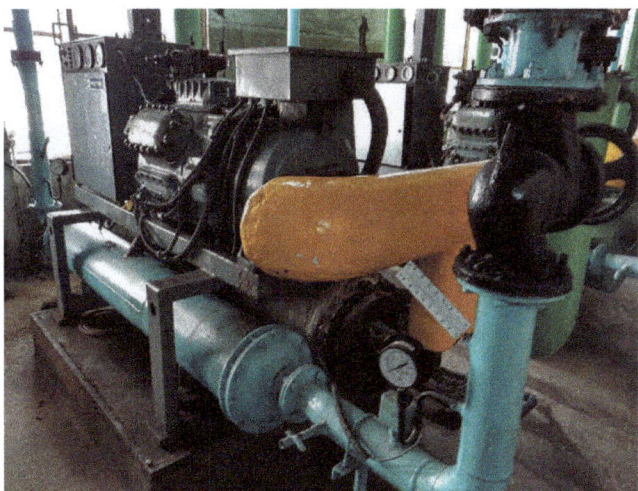

Figure 3.1 The air cooling system with water chiller and pump. This system cools down the temperature of flowing water and pumps it towards the AHU of the concerned OT. This provides cooling for large areas and multiple operation theatres

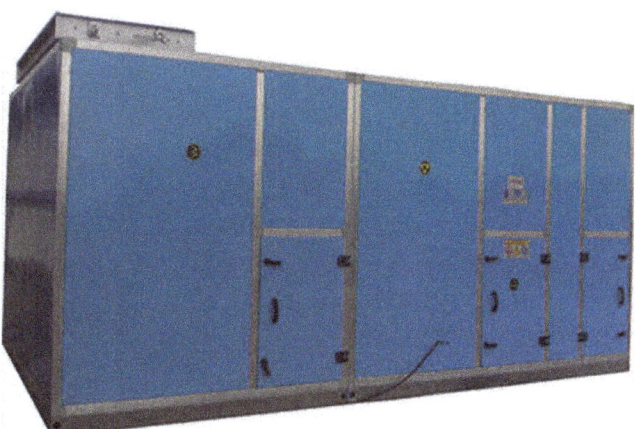

Figure 3.2 An outside view of air handling unit (AHU), having multiple chambers for various kinds of fans and filters

humidity (RH) must be maintained between 20% and 60%. This prevents excessive drying of the surgical field. A constant monitoring of both the parameters is a must and appropriate devices to monitor and display them must be installed. High humidity predisposes for *Pseudomonas aeruginosa* growth while lower humidity favors *Klebsiella pneumoniae* activity.

LAMINAR AIR FLOW

To avoid turbulences, a unidirectional and a uniform flow is necessary. This technique has become popular as the laminar flow technique. Fans are used to generate the air current within the AHU **(Fig. 3.2)**. They should preferably be free-running impeller fans (without fan scroll), which are cleanable. A vibration isolator to eliminate any vibration must also be sought.

The airflow must be a full laminar airflow without any turbulences, i.e. with air flowing in parallel lanes. The airflow from the generation site must be at higher pressure so as maintain a constant current through the filters to the operating site. The direction of the flow should be from the clean area towards the less clean site and finally out of the operating room. There must be no backflow of air into the cleaner area. Preferably, the first zone of air must be the instrument table and the operating field. This helps to carry away the germ-load from the operating field to the outside and prevents recirculation of contaminated air at operating site.

AIR CHANGE PER HOUR

Based on international guidelines, the airflow must be able to replace the total air volume of the operation theatre at least 20 times. It is important and done to ensure removal of less clean air contaminated with pre-existing room air so as to maintain a level of cleanliness and freshness. Therefore, wherever bacterial load is expected to be more, the minimum air changes should be increased accordingly. It is advised that the fresh air replacement must be at least four times out of the 20 total air changes. It has been seen that ten or more total air changes per hour decreases the level of any contamination present in air by about 99%.[5]

AIR VELOCITY

The vertical down flow of air coming out of the diffusers should be able to carry bacteria-carrying particle load away from the operating table.[7] The airflow needs to be unidirectional and downwards on the OT table. The air face velocity of 25–35 FPM (feet per minute) from non-aspirating unidirectional laminar flow diffuser/ceiling array is recommended. Faster air flow is expected to cause excessive drying of surgical site. Slower air velocity shall not be able to carry out the bacterial particle load away from surgical site. It is also necessary to maintain the sterility of the operating field.

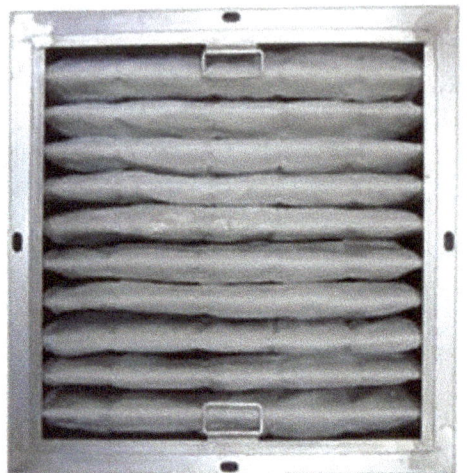
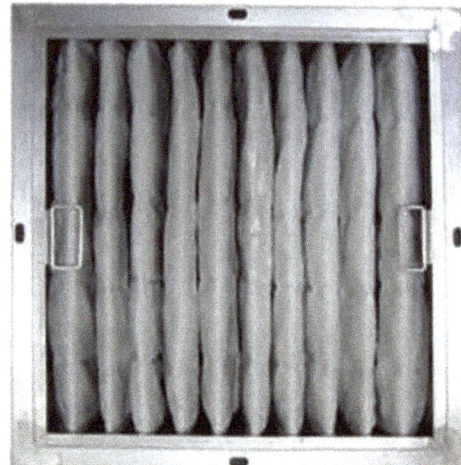

Figure 3.3 Prefilters with surrounding aluminum body

POSITIVE PRESSURE

It is required to maintain positive pressure differential between OT and adjoining areas to prevent outside air entry into OT. It takes fresh air from outside, filters it and continuously blows it in. This system is also called as fresh air system. This pressure gradient is necessary to maintain a laminar unidirectional airflow, right from the operating table to the OT exit. Air outside the OT is warmer than air inside and hence must be cooled again before it can be recirculated inside so as to maintain the pressure gradient. Positive pressure must be maintained in OT at all times (operational and nonoperational hours). The minimum positive pressure recommended is 2.5 Pascal (0.01 inches of water).

AIR FILTRATION

The AHU (i.e. air handling unit) must be an air purification unit and air filtration unit. NABH recommends that there must be two sets of washable flange type filters of efficiency 90% down to 10 microns, known as prefilters **(Fig. 3.3)** and 99% down to 5 microns with aluminum/SS 304 frame within the AHU, called as microfilters. The necessary service panels are to be provided for servicing the filters, motors and blowers. High-efficiency particulate arrestance (HEPA) filters (high efficiency particulate air) of efficiency 99.97% down to 0.3 microns or higher efficiency are preferable **(Fig. 3.4)**. However, in hospitals where its not feasible to install a HEPA filter, the OTs should be well

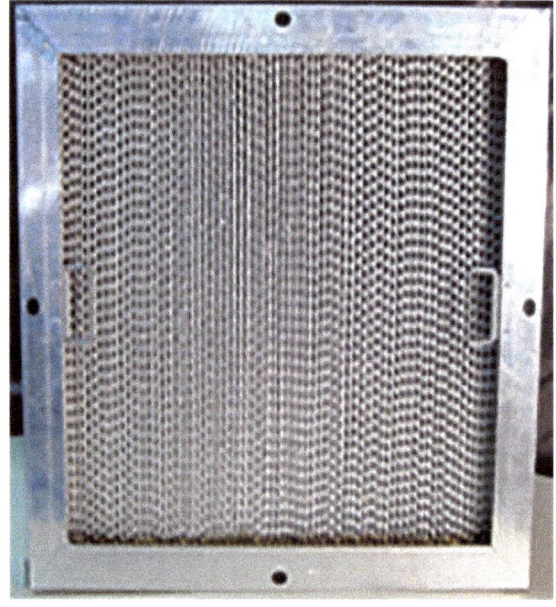

Figure 3.4 High-efficiency particulate arrestance (HEPA) microfilters situated within the air handling unit

ventilated with two levels of filtrations with efficiencies as specified previously (pre- and microfilters).

MAINTENANCE OF AIR FLOW SYSTEM

During the nonfunctional hours, AHU blower must be operational round the clock (may be without temperature control). Variable frequency devices (VFD) may be used to preserve energy. Air changes can be reduced to 25% during nonoperating hours through

VFD provided positive pressure relationship is not disturbed during such period.

Validation of system is to be done as per ISO 14664 standards and should include:
- Temperature and humidity check
- Air particulate count
- Air change rate calculation
- Air velocity at outlet of terminal filtration unit
- Pressure differential levels of the OT with respect to ambient/adjoining areas
- Validation of HEPA filters by appropriate tests like DOP (dispersed oil particulate)/PAO (poly alpha olefin), etc.; repeat after 6 months in case HEPA found healthy.

Preventive maintenance of the system: It is recommended by NABH that periodic preventive maintenance must be carried out in terms of cleaning of prefilters and microfilters at the interval of 15 days. Preventive maintenance of all the parts of the AHU is carried out as per manufacturer recommendations.

REFERENCES

1. Madeo M. The role of air ventilation and air sampling in reducing the incidence of surgical wound infection rates. Br J Theatre Nurs. 1996;6(9):29-32.
2. Dharan S, Pittet D. Environmental controls in operating theatres. J Hosp Infect. 2002;51(2):79-84.
3. Kałuzny J, Muszyński Z, Kałuzny BJ. Ophthalmic operating theatre—chance of limiting contamination and infection risk. Part I. Decontamination of the microbial air pollution. Klin Oczna. 2008;110(1-3):102-7.
4. Talon D, Schoenleber T, Bertrand X, Vichard P. Performances of different types of airflow system in operating theatre. Ann Chir. 2006;131(5):316-21.
5. Lorenz R. Air conditioning systems. Acta Neurotic (Wien). 1980;55(1-2):49-61.
6. American Society of Heating, Refrigerating and Air Conditioning Engineers (ASHRAE) Standards. Ventilation for Indoor Air Quality; 2013
7. National Accreditation Board for Hospitals and Healthcare Providers. Revised guidelines for air conditioning in operation theatres. NABH Guidelines; 2015.

Water Requirement in Ophthalmic Operation Theatre

Mrittika Sen, Neelima Aron, Namrata Sharma, Atul Kumar

INTRODUCTION

Water is an indispensable part of the infrastructure of any operation theatre complex. A continuous supply of clean water is essential for the functioning of an operation theatre (OT), maintenance of sterile environment, disinfection, sterilization of instruments, handwashing and presurgical scrubbing by OT personnel. An ideal operating room complex must have provision for adequate and continuous water supply at the rate of 400 L/bed/day. Apart from this, there should be a separate reserve emergency overhead tank. The chapter describes the water requirements for various activities in an operation theatre.

HANDWASHING

Surgical hand antisepsis with medicated soap or disinfectants requires clean water to rinse the hands. Gloves may prevent but do not eliminate the transmission of microorganisms from the hands of a surgeon to the patient. This is because of the presence of microperforations in the gloves that are present in about 18% cases at the end of the surgery. About 35% of all gloves have punctures after two hours of surgery; and 80% of the times, these punctures are not perceived by the surgeons.[1] Thus, prior preparation of hands is essential for preventing surgical-site infections.

Ohmori et al[2] examined the suitability of tap water for surgical handwashing. The volunteers who participated in the handwashing test using tap water showed immediate, persistent and cumulative bacterial activity within the limits set by the Food and Drug Administration (FDA). They concluded that tap water in their institution was safe for surgical handwash. Furukawa et al[3] conducted another study to examine whether sterile water and brushes are necessary for handwashing before surgery. No difference in bacterial counts was found between tap water and sterile water. However, storage of tap water in reservoir tanks lowers the chloride concentration and increases the chance of bacterial contamination. The concentration of chlorine in water is important for maintaining the microbiological quality. It has been reported that 0.2 mg/L of free chlorine can kill 90% of *Escherichia coli* in water within 2 hours. Hence, it is recommended that presurgical scrubbing should ideally be performed with water purified by reverse osmosis (RO). In hospitals where RO water system is not present, purified filter water can suffice.

INSTRUMENTS

Cleaning of Surgical Instruments

The guidelines for cleaning surgical instruments as provided by the American Operating Room Nursing (AORN)[4] Recommended Practices Committee suggest that the instruments should be washed with sterile distilled cold water to remove protein materials followed by brushing the instruments with special brushes. The instruments are then rinsed in clean water and dried. Mechanical cleaning using an ultrasonic cleaner is preferred as it minimizes handling and exposure to infectious material. Similar to handwashing, RO water is preferred, however, distilled water is sufficient to clean the instruments.

Cox and Stevens recommended use of either rain water or distilled water for cleaning surgical instruments.[5] When neither is available, freshly boiled cooled tap water may be used.

Corrosion and Rust

Corrosion and rust are caused by:
- Inadequate cleaning, rinsing and drying
- Using tap water
- A malfunctioning autoclave.

Most surgical instruments are made of stainless steel and do not usually rust but can corrode if they are washed with saline or left to soak in any liquid for long. Chrome- or nickel-plated instruments commonly get rusted. Once the carbon steel is exposed, it is further corroded by autoclaving and washing. Sodium nitrate is an antirusting agent that can be added to water while washing the instruments.

Autoclaving

Autoclaving is a method of wet sterilization using steam under pressure. The water being used for this purpose will determine the lifespan of the autoclave and the types of load that can be sterilized.

Tap water is a practical source of producing steam. However, if the quality of tap water is not adequate, it can damage the autoclave. This is because tap water contains a number of dissolved minerals and salts depending on the geographic location and source of water, i.e. ground well, lake, river, etc. Hard water can drastically lower the efficiency and functionality of an autoclave. On boiling, hard water is converted to steam while leaving behind salt and mineral deposits within the steam generator, pipes and valves. Over time, these get accumulated in layers and can clog the pipes and valves. It is recommended that any water harder than 85 mg/L should be treated.

Methods to Remove Impurities from Tap Water to Make of it Suitable for Use in an Autoclave[6]

Reverse Osmosis

Osmosis is a process that occurs naturally while reverse osmosis is an active process requiring energy. High pressure is applied on the side which is more hypertonic. The pressure forces the water across a semipermeable membrane while 95–99% of dissolved salts are left behind in the reject stream. Reverse osmosis is capable of removing up to 99% of the dissolved salts (ions), particles, colloids, organic matter, bacteria and pyrogens from the water.

Deionization

Deionization (DI), and continuous electrodeionization (CEDI) are methods of improving the quality of water by removing cations and anions. DI systems have charged resins that require periodic regeneration with an acid and base.

Distillation

Distillation units purify water by thermal vaporization, mist elimination, and water vapor condensation. The water should be treated for hardness and silica impurities should be removed before feeding it in the distilled water systems as these impurities may corrode the heat transfer surfaces. In spite of general perceptions, even the best distillation process cannot afford absolute removal of contaminating ions and endotoxins.

The level of water purity is defined by American Society for Testing and Materials (ASTM) international standards to have characteristics of resistivity, measured in ohm-cm or conductivity measured in μS/cm. Type I water is further defined by its total organic carbons (TOC) purity, measured in parts/billion (ppb).

- *Type I:* Ultrapure, type I water is defined by the ASTM as having a resistivity of >18 MΩ-cm, a conductivity of <0.056 μS/cm and <50 ppb of TOC. Type I water is ultrapure and used in analytical labs, HPLC, cell and tissue culturing, mass spectrometry.
- *Type II:* ASTM defines type II water as having a resistivity of >1 MΩ-cm, a conductivity of <1 μS/cm and <50 ppb of TOCs. Type II water is cleaner than type III/RO water but not ultrapure like type I. Type II water is used to feed clinical analyzers because there is less calcium build-up. It is also used for electrochemistry, radioimmunoassay and media preparation.
- *Type III:* ASTM defines type III water as having a resistivity of >4 MΩ-cm, a conductivity of <0.25 μS/cm and <200 ppb of TOCs. It is less pure than type I and II water. Type III water removes 90–99% of contaminants. It is produced using a reverse osmosis (RO) system directly from tap water, and is the starting point for many laboratory applications such as glassware rinsing, media preparation, and other non-critical laboratory applications. It is also

a source of feed water for systems producing type I ultrapure water.
- *Type IV:* ASTM defines type IV water as having a resistivity of 200 KΩ-cm and a conductivity of <5 µS/cm. Type IV water is most generally produced by RO and is used as feed water to a type I or type II deionized (DI) system.

The easiest and the least expensive method of treating tap water for use in an autoclave is to install a type III RO filter in the water line and an 'Automatic generator blowdown' feature in the steam generator. The RO filter retains majority of the contaminants while the blow down feature flushes away any minerals that make it through.

Recommended Quality of Water

Water between 0.1 MΩ-cm and 1.0 MΩ-cm is considered appropriate for majority of the items that need to be sterilized for research work, biohazardous waste, clothing, glassware, media and instruments. This level of purity is achieved with type III RO filter. One must remember that highly pure water which lacks ions or minerals will try to leach impurities from everything it touches like glass, steel and copper. This could result in corrosion. Hence, high purity water should only be used in autoclaves constructed from stainless steel.

Water is the lifeline of an operation theatre and its supply is essential for all activities from the time the doors of the OT are opened in the morning till last of the instruments are put back in their respective containers. Hence, appropriate measures should be taken to ensure a high quality water supply in the operation theatre to prevent ocular infections.

REFERENCES

1. Gonçalves Kde J, Graziano KU, Kawagoe JY. A systematic review of surgical hand antisepsis utilizing an alcohol preparation compared to traditional products. Rev Esc Enferm USP. 2012;46:1484-93.
2. Ohmori Y, Tonouchi H, Mohri Y, Kobayashi M, Kusunoki M. Evaluation of tap water for surgical handwashing. Surg Today. 2006;36(2):119-24.
3. Furukawa K, Tajiri T, Suzuki H, Norose Y. Are sterile water and brushes necessary for handwashing before surgery in Japan. Journal of Nippon Medical School. 2005;72(3):149-54.
4. Recommended practices for the care and cleaning of surgical instruments and powered equipment. AORN Journal. 1997;6:124-8.
5. Cox I, Stevens S. Care of ophthalmic surgical instruments. Community Eye Health. 2000;13(35):40-1.
6. US Pharmacopeia. Water for pharmaceutical purposes. *www.pharmacopeia.cn/v29240/usp29nf24s0_c1231.*

CHAPTER 5

Operation Theatre List and Record Maintenance

Pranita Sahay, Srikant Kumar Padhy, Neelima Aron

Most of the ophthalmic surgeries are elective cases with few exceptions like post-traumatic open globe injuries, perforated cornea ulcer, endophthalmitis, orbital cellulitis, acute angle closure glaucoma and fresh rhegmatogenous retinal detachment (RRD) with macula attached which require urgent intervention. The operation theatre list prepared for elective and emergency surgeries holds an area of prime importance. This enables the nursing staff to prepare the operation theatre (OT) for the next day surgery and to avoid last minute confusions in the OT.

THE OPERATION THEATRE LIST

To prepare for the surgical procedures, it is important to provide the nursing staff in advance with a meticulous operation theatre (OT) list which gives the following details:

- Date of the surgery
- *Patient details:* Name/Age/Sex/Contact Number/Ward and bed number of the patient
- Diagnosis of both the eyes
- Systemic illness (if any) such as diabetes mellitus, hypertension, asthma, coronary artery disease, etc.
- Need for oxygen supplementation
- Presence of high risk factors such as HIV/HbsAg/HCV
- *Surgical plan:* A clear description of the type of operation to be performed and the eye to be operated. This is important to prevent an operation being performed on the wrong side or the wrong operation.
- *Surgeon details:* Name of the operating surgeon and assistant
- Any investigation which needs to be checked on the day of surgery
- The scheduled time for the operation should also appear on the list. If the surgeon decides to do a patient earlier or later on the scheduled list or cancel an operation, the OT nurse must inform the nurse in the particular ward of the change on the operating list immediately.
- *Mode of anesthesia:* Local anesthesia/Topical anesthesia/Cardiac monitoring/General anesthesia.

These details enable the nursing staff to be prepared well in advance both for the routine surgery as well as the anticipated complications by the information from the OT list. A specimen OT list is shown in **Figure 5.1**.

RECOMMENDATIONS

- The operation list should preferably be sent at least 12 hours before the day of surgery.
- The operation list should be handed in person or by fax or email and not telephonically.
- The name and contact details of the doctor/nurse who compiled the theatre list should be clearly indicated.
- The surgeon should discuss the operation list in co-operation with the OT nurse-in-charge.
- The operation list must not exceed the permitted time allocated to it. This does not refer to the time during an operation of an individual patient.

Ocular Infections: Prophylaxis and Management

Figure 5.1 A representative operation theatre list showing the date of surgery, the sequence of operations planned, the identification details of the patient, diagnosis, surgical plan and eye to be operated, the operating surgeon and assistant and the type of anesthesia

- The operation list should preferably be put on a notice board near the patient's admission/ entrance to the OT.

SPECIAL CONSIDERATIONS WHILE PREPARING AN OPERATION THEATRE LIST

- *Age of the patient*—infants and children below 6 years of age are posted at the beginning of the OT list with the cases being arranged in the chronological order of age.
- *Types of surgery*—major operations are always booked at the beginning of the OT list, e.g. orbitotomies, keratoplasty etc.
- Patients with active eye infection such as infective keratitis, endophthalmitis, panophthalmitis, etc should be posted at the end of the OT list to avoid cross infection. A prehand information of the infected cases enables the nursing staff of the OT to keep the instruments tray for septic OT ready.
- Patients with positive serology such as HIV, HbsAg and HCV should be placed at the end of the list. A clear mention of the serology status of the patient enables the nursing staff to keep the things ready for sterilization and disinfection of the OT thereafter.
- Patients with diabetes mellitus must not be starved for long periods as there is risk of hypoglycemia and hence should be placed in the beginning of the OT list schedule.
- Patients with cardiac or any other systemic illness should also be posted early and should be put in the beginning of the list.
- Abbreviations should never be used as it may cause confusion.

DISTRIBUTION OF THE OPERATION THEATRE LIST

It is pertinent that the operation theatre (OT) list is first checked and signed by a resident before distribution to avoid any hassles in the OT. A copy of the complete list is then distributed to the following:
- *The nursing staff* of respective wards from where the patients are posted—this helps the ward nursing staff to prepare and counsel the patients in advance for the surgery.
- *The operating surgeon* and assistants—so that they are aware of their respective cases and are on time in the OT. This avoids wastage of the precious OT time.
- *The anesthetist*—so that they can do a proper pre-anesthetic check-up and advise the necessary investigations when required, a day prior to the surgery. This avoids unnecessary cancellation of cases on the day of surgery and keeping nil per oral of patients who are not fit for anesthesia.
- *The nursing staff of OT*—so that they can sterilize and prepare the set of instruments in advance that will be required on the day of surgery.
- *The day care facility*—so that they are aware of the number of patients posted on the coming day.

RECORD MAINTENANCE IN OPERATION THEATRE

Different registers are used in the OT, namely:
- Operation registers
- Daily register
- Sterilization register
- Temperature and humidity control register
- Microbiology register
- Water analysis and culture register
- Instrument register
- Central sterile supply department register (CSSD)
- Linen stock register
- Complaints register

Operation Register

Every operation done in the OT, whether under general or local anesthesia, must be recorded in the operation register.

The operation register is a legal document which must be stored in the records section for enquiry as well as statistical purposes for at least five years. All the information and particulars of the patient must be complete:
- The patient's full name, age and sex
- Registration number
- Ward in which the patient is admitted
- Full description of the surgery performed
- Name of anesthesiologist
- Name of the operating surgeon and assistant
- Anesthetic agent used for anesthesia
- Name of the scrubbed nurses
- Name of the OT assistant
- Operation theatre table on which the patient was operated
- Indicate whether the patient underwent major or minor surgery
- Duration of the operation

Daily Register

It is a detailed record regarding the infection control activities of OT. It mentions the following:
- Name of the concerned cleaning staff on duty
- Assessment of temperature control
- Samples sent from the OT for microbiological tests
- Biomedical waste management
- The fumigation details of the OT with the name of chemical reagent used.

Sterilization Register

It mentions the following details:
- The number of instrument sets that are sterilized along with the method of sterilization. Specific indicators are placed on all the instrument boxes to indicate the method of sterilization (Plasma, ETO, Autoclave). A change in color is noted in these indicators if proper sterilization has been done.
- The total time taken for sterilization along with its starting and ending time is also documented.
- The nursing staff responsible for sterilization is documented.
- The various files for maintaining records are steam sterilization indicator file, steam autoclave receiving and issued record, high speed autoclave indicator file, chemical integrator file, biological indicator file, Bowie Dick test file and ETO things receiving and issued record, fumigation record and autoclave maintenance record.

Temperature and Humidity Control Register

The temperature and humidity of the OT is checked every 2 hours and documented. If any deviation from the ideal temperature is noted then immediate action is taken.

Microbiology Register

Samples are sent from every new batch of ringer lactate and viscoelastic before it is used. Samples are sent from various areas of the OT every week for both fungal and bacterial culture. Samples are also sent from the air conditioning system ducts. The microbiology report of these is attached in the register.

Water Analysis and Culture Register

Water samples for microbiological tests are sent from various areas of the OT like scrub room and sterilization room and a record of the same is maintained.

Instrument Register

It mentions the total number of instrument sets that are used in a single day in the various OTs. This helps in keeping track of the OT instruments to prevent loss of instruments.

Biomedical Waste Management Register

This includes the record maintenance of proper waste disposal from OT along with date and time.

Central Sterile Supply Department Register

It mentions the details of the quantity of linen sent for sterilization and received after the sterilization procedure is over.

Linen Stock Register

It mentions in detail the linen type and quantity that the OT has, like bed sheets, towels, gowns, eye towels, trolley covers, etc.

Complaints Register

All complaints for the OT are recorded in this register and necessary action is taken accordingly by the OT in-charge.

CHAPTER 6

Pre-operative Patient Preparation

Mukesh Patil, Neelima Aron, Namrata Sharma, Atul Kumar

INTRODUCTION

Adequate measures should be taken before any ocular surgery for the preparation of the patient to reduce perioperative morbidity and hasten the process of post-operative recovery. This aims at minimizing the risk of contamination or hospital acquired infection to the patient. Pre-operative preparation starts right from patient admission to the hospital (in-patient cases) till the commencement of surgery. It includes the following things: baseline investigations, maintenance of hygiene, ruling out pre-existing infections, clean operation theatre (OT) dress, aseptic precautions in the perioperative period including cleaning of the surgical area, and surgical preparation of the patient. Each one of these would be discussed separately.

PRE-OPERATIVE MEASURES

Patients undergoing surgery should preferably be admitted a day prior to the surgery for detailed evaluation and perioperative preparation. Patients being operated on day care basis should be evaluated well in advance and properly instructed. Detail history of ocular as well as any systemic problems should be taken like previous history of ocular surgery, systemic illness like diabetes mellitus, hypertension, heart disease, asthma, neurological problems, arthritis and dental caries. Fasting blood sugar levels and blood pressure measurement should be done in all patients above 40 years of age which would help to know the systemic status and sometimes can detect underlying hidden illness. It is desirable to have random blood sugars less than 200 mg/dL. However, no studies have correlated blood sugar levels with ocular infection. Rather, a rapid reduction in blood sugar has been implicated to cause endophthalmitis.

All the necessary clearance for systemic problems should be taken from the specialist prior to surgery. Blood hemoglobin levels and urine examination for culture and microscopy should be sent for all pediatric cases. In patients who are at risk of perioperative blood loss like in orbit surgeries, cross matching for blood group should be done as well as bleeding and clotting time should be evaluated.

Topical broad spectrum antibiotics (preferably fluoroquinolones) should be started four times a day at least three days prior to surgery to decrease conjunctival bacterial flora. There is no role of systemic antibiotics in prophylaxis. Patients requiring dilatation should be advised to use tropicamide drops three to four times, every 10 minutes before surgery. Avoid phenylephrine in dilating eye drops in hypertensive and cardiac patients.

All patients should be subjected to slit lamp examination to rule out any infectious foci in the eyelids or adnexa. In the presence of any ocular, adnexal as well as systemic infection, surgery should be postponed. Trimming of eye lashes is no longer considered necessary before intraocular surgery with no demonstrable effect in decreasing endophthalmitis.[1,2] However, it should be made sure that the eyelashes are well covered with the surgical drape. A pre-operative regurgitation on pressure over the lacrimal sac (ROPLAS) test is mandatory for all patients one day before surgery.

Lacrimal sac syringing is desirable but not mandatory for all cases. Avoid syringing on or one day before the surgery since it causes washing-off of the bacteria from the lacrimal sac to the conjunctival sac thus increasing the chances of contamination. In case of a positive regurgitation test, intraocular surgery should be postponed and the patient should be subjected to dacryocystorhinostomy or dacryocystectomy. A minimum gap of 2 weeks is recommended before undertaking any intraocular surgery after the sac surgery.

Avoid any contact procedure on the day of surgery. A-scan biometry for axial length measurement should be performed at least one day prior to the surgery followed by instillation of an antibiotic to prevent infection. In case of one eyed patients, a conjunctival swab collection is preferable from both eyes and surgery should be performed only after negative or insignificant culture reports.

All patients should preferably take bath on the day of surgery or at least cleaning of face with soap and water is a must. The patients should be given clean clothes to be worn on the day of the surgery.

OPERATION THEATRE ATTIRE

The main aim of operation theatre attire is to achieve a sense of discipline amidst the personnel and patients in the operation theatre, to identify theatre as a clean and separate area, and also to ensure the prevention of spread of harmful organisms during surgery.

The components of OT attire are a specific means of preventing contamination and the risk of infection to the patient. For the patient, it includes the armamentarium of body cover, head cover and shoe cover **(Fig. 6.1)**.

Head covers are made up of soft, lint free, cloth like material and should fit well to serve the purpose of confining microorganisms. All hair must be covered inside the operation theatre.

Body covers are usually made of cotton as it can be easily washed at high temperature and allows easy breaths. The body cover should preferably be designed in a wraparound style for ease of removal. Shirts should be tucked well inside the lowers so as to avoid touching the sterile areas.

The patients should be given shoe covers that cover the feet entirely to prevent contamination. This should be worn at all times till the patient is inside the OT premises **(Fig. 6.2)**.

Apart from these, it is important to remove all the jewellery (including rings, and piercings etc.), glasses, contact lenses, or any other prosthesis. If it is not possible to remove certain valuables, they should be either taped or tied to prevent any loss. Nail polish is to be removed from the fingers and toes to allow for observation of the color of the nail bed, which is an indication of circulation as well as oxygenation.

MARKING AND CLEANING OF THE SURGICAL AREA

It is indeed very important to prepare the surgical area well in advance of the surgery so as to avoid any

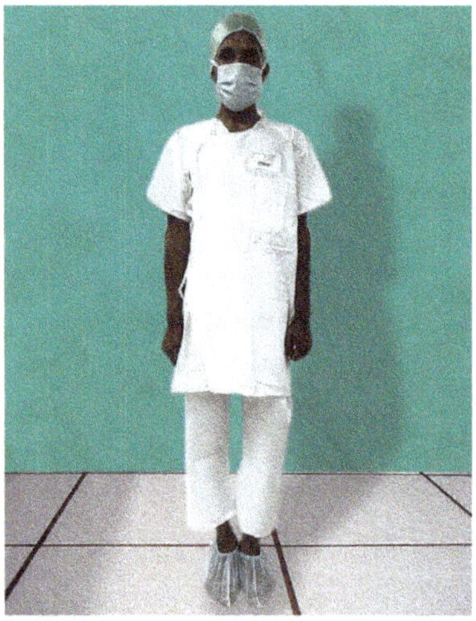

Figure 6.1 A patient with body cover, head cover, face mask and shoe cover in the recovery room before surgery

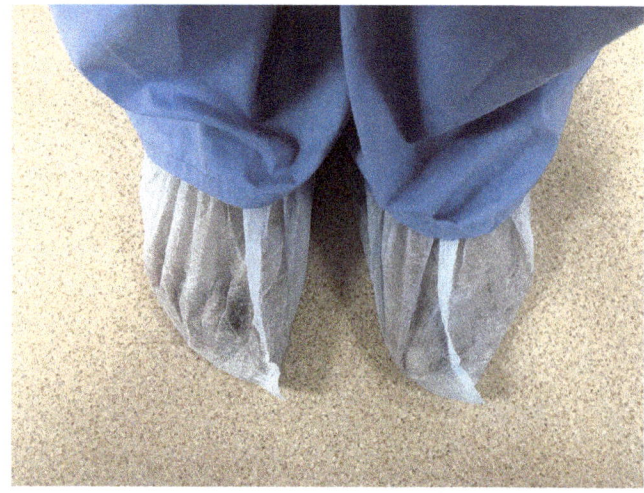

Figure 6.2 Shoe covers should snugly fit the feet covering them adequately

contamination in the perioperative period. The need for marking the correct eye for surgery before shifting the patient to the OT is unprecedented. In the pre-operative waiting area, the periocular skin is cleaned with 10% povidone iodine solution before giving any local block **(Fig. 6.3)**. The eye to be operated is marked with a cross over the forehead above **(Fig. 6.4)**. An identification wrist band may be tied on to the patient's hand on the side of the eye to be operated. Further, the patient's name with hospital ID should be stuck in the form of a badge to prevent interchange of patients with the same name **(Fig. 6.5)**. If necessary, pre-operative dilatation of the eye should be started in the ward

DR. RAJENDRA PRASAD CENTRE FOR OPHTHALMIC SCIENCES	
UHID: 102377389	Date: 21/11/2016 11:02:06 AM
CR No. : R-037511-16	Ward Name: Bed No:
Name: XYZ	RPC Day Care. 68
Age: 25 Y 0M 2 D/M	Unit In-charge: Mr SR RPC
S/O:KUWER SAIN	Unit-III

Figure 6.5 Identification badge of the patient to confirm the patient identity before shifting to the operation theatre

(in-patients) by instillation of tropicamide every 15 minutes. This should be continued in OT taking care to use separate bottles for each patient to avoid cross infection.

SHIFTING THE PATIENT TO OPERATION THEATRE

The patient should be shifted to the operation theatre on a patient trolley/chair. He/she should be accompanied by the porter and an attendant. The patient should be received by the OT nurse in a polite and friendly manner at the OT reception area. Thereafter, the receiving nurse should be quite vigilant about checking the patient particulars especially the patient identification and the type of surgery. It is also imperative to ask for any long-term illnesses such as hypertension and diabetes mellitus and whether the patient has taken any medications for the same. The receiving nurse should ensure that the vitals are checked before coming to the operation theatre. Check if the patient has maintained the pre-operative dietary and fluid restrictions, if any. It is also the responsibility of OT nurse to ensure that the patient has been previously explained about the surgical procedure and associated risks and benefits by the doctor and has signed the consent form for the same. The consent form should be completed correctly and signed by the patient, parent or guardian, two witnesses, and the surgeon. It is also to be checked if the patient has received the topical antibiotics as mandated.

SURGICAL PREPARATION

It is important to pay attention to the allergies or any other untoward reactions to the anaesthetic agents before administering any form of topical, local, or general anesthesia and in case of any known allergies, the agent should be avoided and replaced by another

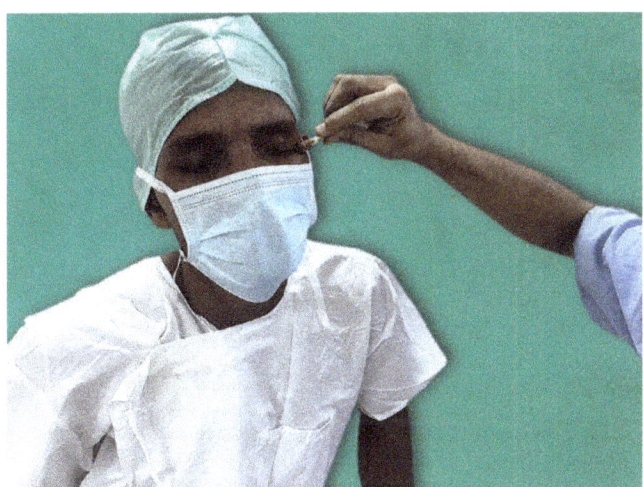

Figure 6.3 Periocular cleaning of the left eye with povidone iodine 10% in the waiting area before shifting the patient to operation theatre

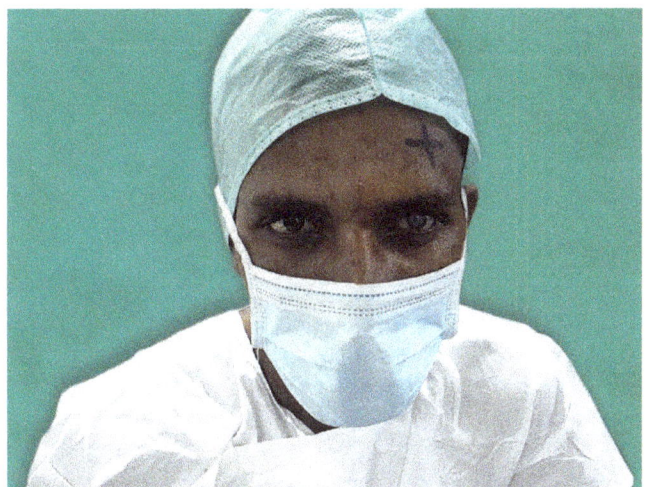

Figure 6.4 Identification mark in the form of cross on the forehead on the side of the eye to be operated

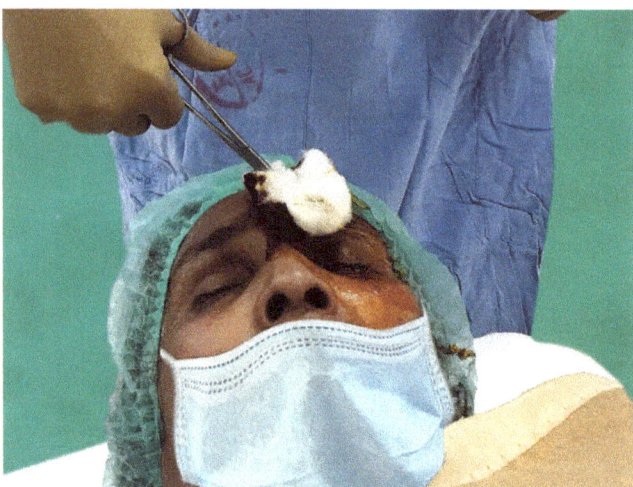

Figure 6.6 Periocular cleaning of the left eye with artery forceps using povidone Iodine 10% on the operation theatre table after shifting the patient

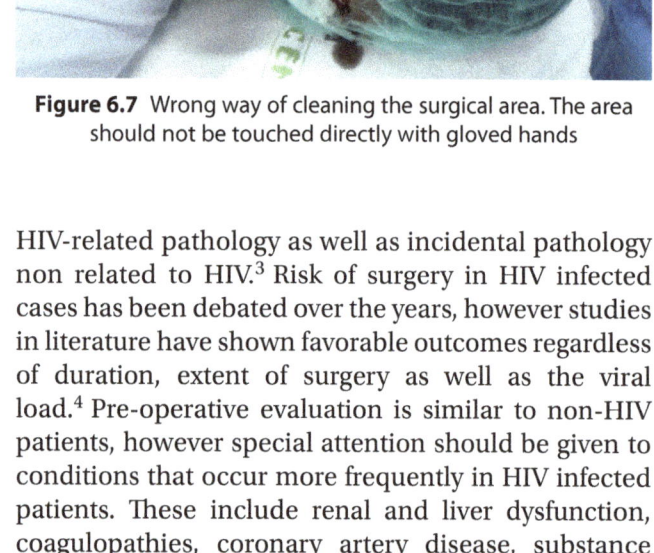

Figure 6.7 Wrong way of cleaning the surgical area. The area should not be touched directly with gloved hands

anesthetic agent. The antidote should be kept handy for quick administration in case of any allergic reactions. The patient's anxiety level is to be checked and premedication is to be administered accordingly. After shifting the patient to the operation theatre room, the cul de sac is instilled with a 5% povidone iodine solution which is kept for atleast 3 minutes. The periocular area is again cleaned using a 10% povidone iodine solution with an artery forceps before placing the sterile linen and plastic eye drape over the eye **(Fig. 6.6)**. Avoid touching the patient's skin directly with gloved hands **(Fig. 6.7)**. The speculum is then placed so as to keep the eyelashes away from the surgical field. The eye is to be washed with balanced salt solution or ringer lactate before starting the surgery to remove all the povidone iodine and prevent its entry inside the eye.

HIGH RISK: HIV, HBsAg, HCV

Patients suffering from HIV, HbsAg and HCV fall in the high risk category for elective as well as emergency cases that require special attention. This section addresses pre-operative preparation of HIV infected, HBV and HCV positive patients.

The prevalence of human immunodeficiency virus (HIV) infection is increasing and drug therapies available nowadays are prolonging the survival of patients with HIV infection which indirectly increases the chance of performing surgery on these patients. About 25% of the patients with HIV require surgery for HIV-related pathology as well as incidental pathology non related to HIV.[3] Risk of surgery in HIV infected cases has been debated over the years, however studies in literature have shown favorable outcomes regardless of duration, extent of surgery as well as the viral load.[4] Pre-operative evaluation is similar to non-HIV patients, however special attention should be given to conditions that occur more frequently in HIV infected patients. These include renal and liver dysfunction, coagulopathies, coronary artery disease, substance abuse like alcohol and drugs, history of infection especially with methicillin resistant *Staphylococcus aureus* (MRSA) and drug allergies. In case of confirmed or suspected substance abuse, elective surgery should be deferred till urine toxicology report is obtained.

Antiretroviral therapy (ART) should be continued in the perioperative period. ART is effective against hepatitis-B virus (HBV) and should be continued in HBV co-infected patients. When ART interruption is required due to unavoidable reasons, the help of clinicians expert in managing ART treatment should be sought. Vancomycin should be given in place of cefazolin for prophylaxis in HIV infected patients with a history of MRSA infection. Potential drug interactions risk should be ruled out before starting a new drug. Sedatives/hypnotics and anxiolytics may show interaction with protease inhibitors, so better avoided. Commonly used sedative midazolam is contraindicated with ritonavir while antacids like H2 blockers and proton pump inhibitors severely affect absorption of atazanavir.

Patients with HBV and HCV are known to have chronic hepatitis and they are at high risk of morbidity and mortality due to general anesthesia and stress of surgery. General anesthesia decreases the blood flow to liver which can precipitate total liver necrosis to already compromised liver. Elective surgeries are safe in patients with asymptomatic mild chronic hepatitis.[5]

Hepatitis-B virus (HBV) is considered more transmissible than HIV. However, there has been no evidence to support that either HBV or HIV can be transmitted from contact lenses, tears, or patient contact but there is a theoretical risk of transmission of virus through the mucous membranes as it may be present in tears of infected individuals, and reasonable precautions should be taken.[6]

It has been suggested that 70% isopropyl alcohol is quite effective against HIV, therefore cleaning tonometer tips with 70% isopropyl alcohol provides protection against HIV. The entire tip should be cleaned immediately after use by immersing it in a solution of 70% isopropyl or ethyl alcohol for a period of 5 minutes and allowing it to dry for at least a period of 1–2 minutes. This ensures that no alcohol is transferred to the ocular surface on using the tip again. Alternatively, 3% hydrogen peroxide may also be used for disinfection and it is recommended to change this solution at least twice daily.[7] For disinfecting the diagnostic lenses such as gonio lens or macular lens, the lens should be placed inverted and then wiped with alcohol sponge ensuring that the contact surface is adequately cleaned. For further protection, a 1: 100 diluted solution of household bleach may be used.[7,8] Similarly, the tip of ultrasound probe for axial length measurement should be cleaned with 70% isopropyl alcohol/ethyl alcohol or alcohol sponges for 5 minutes and allowed to dry before using for next patient.

CONCLUSION

The importance of knowing the various steps to be followed in the pre-operative period is to ensure strict asepsis and prevention of contamination and infection. As there are multiple sources of contamination, precautions have to be taken at each step to prevent ocular morbidity and complications, and to ensure early visual recovery.

REFERENCES

1. Kelkar A, Kelkar J, Amuaku W, Kelkar U, Shaikh A. How to prevent endophthalmitis in cataract surgeries? Indian Journal of Ophthalmology. 2008;56(5):403-7.
2. Schmitz S, Dick HB, Krummenauer F, Pfeiffer N. Endophthalmitis in cataract surgery: results of a German survey. Ophthalmology. 1999;106(10):1869-77.
3. Madiba TE, Muckart DJ, Thomson SR. Human immunodeficiency disease: how should it affect surgical decision making? World J Surg. 2009;33(5):899-909.
4. Guth AA, Hofstetter SR, Pachter HL. Human immunodeficiency virus and the trauma patient: Factors influencing post operative infectious complications. J Trauma. 1996;41:251-5.
5. Runyon BA. Surgical procedures are well tolerated by patients with asymptomatic chronic hepatitis. J Clin Gastroenterol. 1986;8:542-44.
6. Yhurst KN, Hettler DL. Infection control guidelines—an update for the optometric practice. Optometry. 2009;80(11):613-20.
7. Pepose J, Linette G, Lee SF, et al. Disinfection of Goldmann tonometers against human immunodeficiency virus type I. Arch Ophthalmol. 1989;107:983-5.
8. Centers for Disease Control: Universal precautions for prevention of transmission of human immunodeficiency virus, hepatitis B virus and other blood-borne pathogens in health-care settings. MMWR. 1988;37:377-8.

CHAPTER 7

Pre-operative Preparation of Operation Theatre Personnel

Archita Singh, Sagnik Sen, Ankit Singh Tomar, Neelima Aron

In the present day scenario where large number of surgeries are being carried out in theatres on daily basis, it is important to improve the efficiency and performance. The patients especially presenting to tertiary care centres expect high level quality care. Guidelines should thus, be formulated for operation theatre (OT) personnel in terms of occupancy, attire, working policy and functioning thus, allowing for smooth running of the operation theatre right from patient entry into the preparation room to the OT table and final shift to the recovery room post-surgery.

OPERATION THEATRE OCCUPANCY

The number of people in the OT should always be limited to a fixed number so as to decrease the risk of cross-infections. The personnel occupying the OT include:
- *The operating surgeon*: The primary surgeon performing the surgery.
- *Assisting surgeon(s)*: Other surgeons apart from the primary surgeon.
- *Anesthesiologists*: The team of anesthetists.
- *Technicians:* Group of people employed by the hospital authorities to help in functioning of the OT. They help in shifting patients, preparation of machines, opening of sterile packages from the outer unsterile covers, tying of gowns, and arranging additional supplies.
- *Nursing staff*: It refers to the sister in-charge of the OT, the unscrubbed nurses and the scrubbed nurses for assisting the surgeons. The unscrubbed nursing staff includes the nurses in pre-operative room, recovery room, day-care and in the sterile room for distribution of sterile instruments to the surgical tables.
- *Visitors to the OT*: This group of personnel includes the students who visit the OT in the academic institutes as a part of their curriculum, medical representatives for demonstration of ophthalmic equipment and attendants of patients who require general anesthesia for the surgical procedure.

The maximum number of OT personnel recommended is 5-8 people in a single OT (180 sq feet) at a given time to prevent the transmission of infection to the patient.

OPERATION THEATRE ATTIRE

The OT attire forms an important component of safe OT practices. An appropriate OT attire as per the specifications acts as an effective barrier to prevent perioperative infections. Below we discuss in detail about the OT attire, its components, the right method of adorning it, safe sterilization and disposal practices.

The OT attire refers to the clothing worn by the OT personnel. The aim is to minimize the shedding of microorganisms that normally harbor the human body. Suitable surgical attire helps decrease the risk of perioperative infections by preventing the transmission of microorganisms from the OT staff. Also, proper surgical attire decreases the risk of transmission of infection to the healthcare personnel who in turn are also at a high risk due to a persistent exposure to infectious and hazardous agents.

Pre-operative Preparation of Operation Theatre Personnel

There are strict guidelines regarding the OT attire that need to be adhered to while in the pre-operative patient preparation room, the operation theatre and the recovery room.

Before entering the OT, all persons need to change into a clean linen dress in place of street attire. OT clothes are to be worn in a changing room meant specifically for this purpose. Along with the linen, caps and masks, proper footwear should also be worn. Generally, changing rooms are kept separate for the staff and the patients. After removing all outside clothes and jewellery everyone needs to be 'bare below the elbow', wash hands, cover hair with cap, wear mask and don clean theatre footwear.

COMPONENTS OF THE ATTIRE

Body Cover

Surgical scrubs are the preferred OT attire. "Scrub" refers to a set of a short sleeved top and a pant. Wearing surgical scrubs in the restricted areas of the hospital helps to prevent cross-infections as the skin of the healthcare personnel tends to be another major source of microbial contamination along with patient's own endogenous flora.[1]

The ideal material for the scrubs is a woven fabric made of microbial-resistant material. As recommended by the Association of Perioperative Registered Nurses (AORN), the material used for scrubs should be tightly woven, durable and stain resistant fabric.[2] The scrubs should be tailored to size so that they are not ill-fitted or loose. The ends of the pants should not sweep the floor and the sleeves of the top should be adjusted above the elbow to prevent wetting while scrubbing. Tucking in of the top is a preferred practice so as to decrease the chance of contamination. The preferred colors for surgical scrubs are shades of green and blue.

It is advised that the scrubs are worn in the OT area only and not outside. They should be changed in the designated changing rooms before entering the theatre area. The personnel should also change the scrubs every time they have been out of the restricted area before entering back in the OT room. Use of cover gowns while outside the OT premises for brief periods of time is not routinely advised.

Reusable scrubs should be laundered after every use only in the OT–specific laundry facility. They should be stored and maintained within the surgical theatre premises and not be taken out for personal use.

Surgical Mask

The surgical mask is an essential component and should be worn at all times while in the restricted and semirestricted areas. The mask should be worn in such a fashion that both the mouth and nose are completely covered **(Figs 7.1 and 7.2)**. It should preferably be made up of disposable material with a high microbial filtering efficiency. It usually has three pleats which allow expansion in size while covering the nostrils and mouth up to the chin. The flexible plastic or metal strip at the top allows it to be contoured to the shape of the nose for comfortable fitting. This not only prevents the slipping of the mask but also fogging of surgeons' spectacles or eye-protection goggles. They should be secured properly with no venting, so that any dispersion of pathogens from the healthcare personnel is decreased. The surgical mask should be worn by all the OT staff in close association of the sterile area (3 meters) including the anesthetist at all times.[3] They should never be allowed to hang loosely around the neck. The once used masks should not be put in

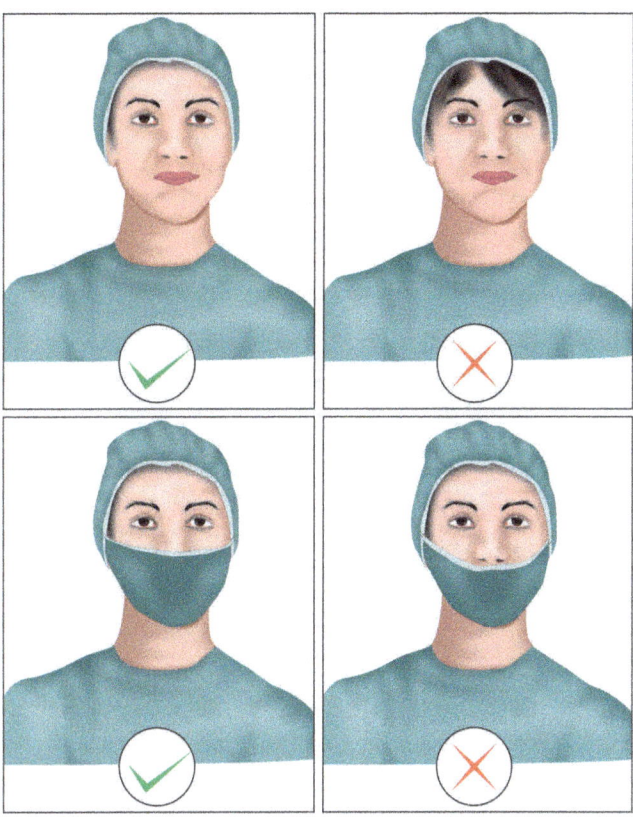

Figure 7.1 Correct method of wearing cap and mask inside the operation theatre

pockets of the scrubs for re-use but should be disposed adequately. Whenever taken off, they should never be held at the centre pleated area but the tapes or strings at the ends should be handled while disposing.

The different methods of securing the surgical mask include the following:
- *Ear loop type:* Where the sides of mask have elastic loops to be secured behind the ear
- *Tie-on type:* The four corners of the mask have strings attached which are tied behind the head
- *Head band type:* An elastic band around the head is required to hold the mask in place
- No straps or adhesive types

Masks also protect the user against blood and body fluid splashes and protective face shields must be used whenever there is a risk of splash of any body solution.

Head Cover

It is an essential part of the OT attire and should be donned at all times while in the OT premises. It should neatly and snugly cover the head and the hair **(Figs 7.1 and 7.2)**. It has been advised that head cover should be the first component of the surgical attire that should be worn first to prevent bacterial contamination of the scrubs.[4]

They can be of two types, bouffant surgical cap or the bonnet like wrap. The bouffant-type tends to be used commonly as it completely covers the head and secures the hair inside.

They are made of disposable, water resistant and light air permeable spun bond PP fabric, the main purpose being to prevent any contamination of the surgical field by hair strands, dandruff and resident bacterial flora. The reusable type of head covers are not recommended but if used should be washed and autoclaved after every use.

Eye Protection Goggles

The eye protection goggles protect the eyes from exposure to any form of splashed blood or body fluids while working in the surgical fields. It particularly becomes essential in cases where the patient is HIV/HBsAg positive as a part of the universal precautions.

Room Shoe and Shoe Covers

The footwear for use in OT should not be used outside at any times. Preferred ones are the closed leather or rubber boots so as to protect exposure to infectious agents and body fluids. They should be water-proof, light weight and comfortable to wear. The OT footwear should be regularly cleaned and stored within the OT complex. Separate slippers should be designated for use in the outer zone and for toilet use.

Shoe covers do not tend to decrease the spread of infection but in turn prevent exposure of healthcare personnel to body fluids and other potential sources of infection.[5] They may be avoided and instead closed shoes may be worn for this purpose.

Surgical Gowns

Gowns are one of the most important components of the theatre attire. They not only prevent contamination of the surgical field by bacterial flora of the healthcare personnel but also protect the staff from exposure to potential sources of infection.[6] The gowns can either be disposable or reusable. Based on the permeability, they may be permeable like cotton gowns or impermeable which have special coating on them. On comparison of the disposable gowns with the permeable cotton gowns, it was seen that the disposable gowns tend to significantly decrease the risk of infections.[7] The disposable gowns are usually made of non-woven material with additional plastic coating making them impermeable to fluids. The impermeable gowns tend to be better as compared to the permeable gowns in terms of prevention of transmission of the microbial flora. The reusable gowns are also laundered at the

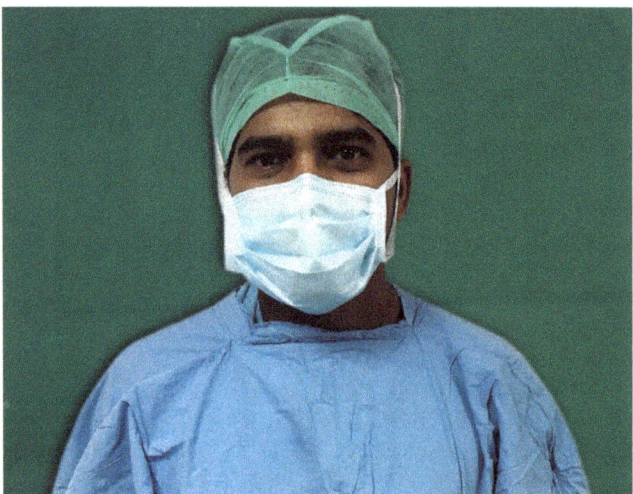

Figure 7.2 Head cover and face mask donned by the surgeon with the hair tucked inside and nose fully covered

in-house laundry service in the OT. They are washed first followed by autoclaving and packed into sterile bundles. The gowns are always packed with the inside of the gown out, so that the surgeon does not touch the outside of the gown at any time before gowning and gloving.

Surgical Gloves

Surgical gloves are a special pair of hand gloves donned by the surgical staff to prevent exchange of infectious agents between them and the patient. They are usually made of latex, other materials being vinyl, nitrile rubber, or neoprene. Different sizes are available to ensure snugly fitting comfortable gloves.

The gloves of appropriate size should be worn after adequately scrubbing and drying the hands. Dexterity should be kept in mind when wearing the gloves. They are for one time use and should be removed and appropriately disposed after every surgical procedure. Sometimes one may require a change of gloves during the surgical procedure. This may be due to inadvertent tearing or contamination of the gloves.[4] The gloves available are either powdered or unpowdered. Previously the gloves had powder in them so that they could be worn easily but the powder may increase the chance of inflammation and delay healing in case it contaminates the surgical field. Further, it increases the chances of toxic anterior segment syndrome. As of March 2016, the use of powdered gloves has been banned by the Food and Drug Administration (FDA).[8]

SPECIAL CASES: HIV, HEPATITIS B AND C

The risk of transmission of the infection from an HIV positive patient following a hollow needle stick injury was found to be 0.3%.[9-11] This risk further increases with the higher viral titres of the patient and advanced stages of acquired immunodeficiency syndrome (AIDS).

Though oral zidovudine decreases the risk of infection post-exposure by 80%,[12] safe surgical practices should be strictly adhered to avoid undue exposure.

Exposure to blood and other body fluids should be avoided at all times. Even minimal exposure is not acceptable. Intra-operatively sharp instruments should be passed across in trays and not directly hand to hand.

The risk of transmission of hepatitis B infection following percutaneous exposure is significantly higher than HIV being 30%.[13] The risk of seroconversion following needle stick injury from hepatitis C virus (HCV) positive patient is around 1.8%.[14-17]

Surgical Attire in Special Cases

It is important to follow set protocols for universal precautions while operating such patients. These cases should be done as the last case of the day and the OT personnel should be kept to a minimum to prevent unnecessary exposure. All the OT personnel who are directly or indirectly in contact with the patient should adorn protective gear which includes disposable protective eye cover, face shield, head cover, disposable impermeable gowns, waterproof aprons, shoe covers and gloves **(Fig. 7.3)**. Double glove wearing is advised which further decreases the chances of infection getting transferred from the patient to the surgeon. All the scrubbing solutions and sterile drapes for the preparation of the patient should be kept separate and disposed properly after use.

During the procedure REMEMBER:
- Minimum instrumentation.
- Do not recap, bend or break used needles. Dispose them immediately after use in puncture proof containers.
- Keep minimum sharps on surgical table.
- All linen should be marked separately as infected before sending for laundry.
- Keep adequate hypochlorite solution available.

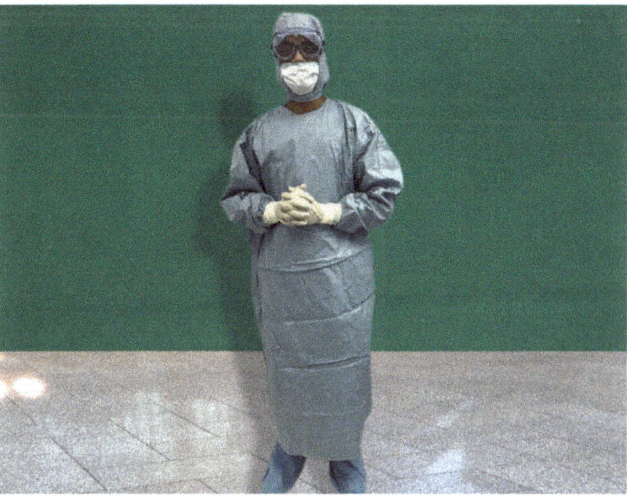

Figure 7.3 Surgical attire in special cases such as HIV, HBSAg and HCV: Disposable impermeable body cover, eye protection goggles, double gloving, shoe covers and arm covers

- In case of any exposure to body fluids immediate measures should be taken and exposure should always be reported.

Precautions to Prevent Transmission of Infection

The Centers for Disease Control and Prevention (CDC)[18,19] stresses on the use of "Universal Precautions" for all patients, especially cases that are operated as emergency[20] since a full blood workup is not always possible. These include:
- Ensure use of proper surgical attire and gloves while in contact with tissues and body fluids. Change gloves after every patient contact.
- In case of any contact with blood or body fluids, wash the hands immediately. Also hands should be washed thoroughly after removal of gloves.
- Prevent injury from sharps by careful handling. One such practice is to avoid recapping of used needles.
- Health personnel with open wounds or exudative lesions should refrain from patient contact directly.
- Pregnant healthcare workers have increased susceptibility to infections and therefore should take extra care.

SURGICAL SCRUBBING

Preparation of Scrubbing

Personal hygiene and cleanliness is of utmost importance. The healthcare personnel should avoid OT in case of any open wounds, lesions or rash. The fingernails should be trimmed and nail polish should be avoided. All pieces of jewellery such as rings, watches and bracelets should be removed before scrubbing. The practice of "bare below the elbow" should be practiced. After wearing a head cover, scrubs, OT shoes and face mask the individual should head towards the scrub room.

A scrub room is essentially an area of washing used by the surgeons and nursing staff involved in surgical procedures. It should open directly into the operating room. The scrub room has a series of basins which are deep enough to prevent splashing of water on the scrubs. The water temperature may be adjusted before starting the scrubbing procedure. The levers for water supply should ideally be controlled by foot to prevent any contamination. Stop watch may be placed in OT to keep track of the scrubbing time. The minimum recommended time for hand scrubbing is 5 minutes with at least 3 washes before gowning. It is preferable to use povidone iodine 7.5% scrub for hand wash. In case of allergy, chlorhexidine 2% is a good alternative. Use of soap and water is avoided.

Surgical scrubbing is done with solutions containing povidone iodine/chlorhexidine as they are nonirritant to the skin, have high and prolonged antimicrobial action, lather easily and are required in small amounts. The surgeon should scrub before the start of every case, and at any time of the day in case of contamination.

Scrubbing Procedure

The aim of surgical scrubbing is to control and decrease the microbial flora on the skin of the surgeon and surgical staff. Ayeliffe has laid down protocols for surgical scrubbing prior to surgery.

The procedure is as follows **(Figs 7.4A to H)**:
- Adjust the water temperature to a comfortable level.
- A hand scrub brush can be opened before starting with scrubbing, however it is not mandatory.
- Wet the hands and arms. Apply small amount of antiseptic solution and lather up. Rinse two inches above the elbow.
- The flow of water should always be directed from the hands to the elbow with the elbow in flexed position. Let the water drip down. Shaking of hands should be avoided.
- Using the sterile file, fingertips and spaces underneath are cleaned under running water.
- The sponge side of brush is used to lather at the fingertips first following which the bristle side is used to clean under the nails with 30 circular strokes.
- Then scrub on four side of each finger with atleast 20 strokes each.
- Similarly, scrub the palm, heel and back of the hand and space between the thumb and index finger.

> **REMEMBER**
> - Posture while scrubbing—hold the body away from the sink and slightly bend forward. The hands are kept above the waist with the elbows flexed.
> - The direction of scrubbing should always be from fingertips towards elbow.
> - One forearm/arm should be scrubbed completely before starting with the other.
> - Rinsing should always be done in the direction of fingertips to elbow. No retracing is allowed.
> - Anytime while scrubbing if there is contamination the entire scrub process should be started from the beginning.
> - Duration of surgical scrubbing varies from 5–7 minutes.

Pre-operative Preparation of Operation Theatre Personnel

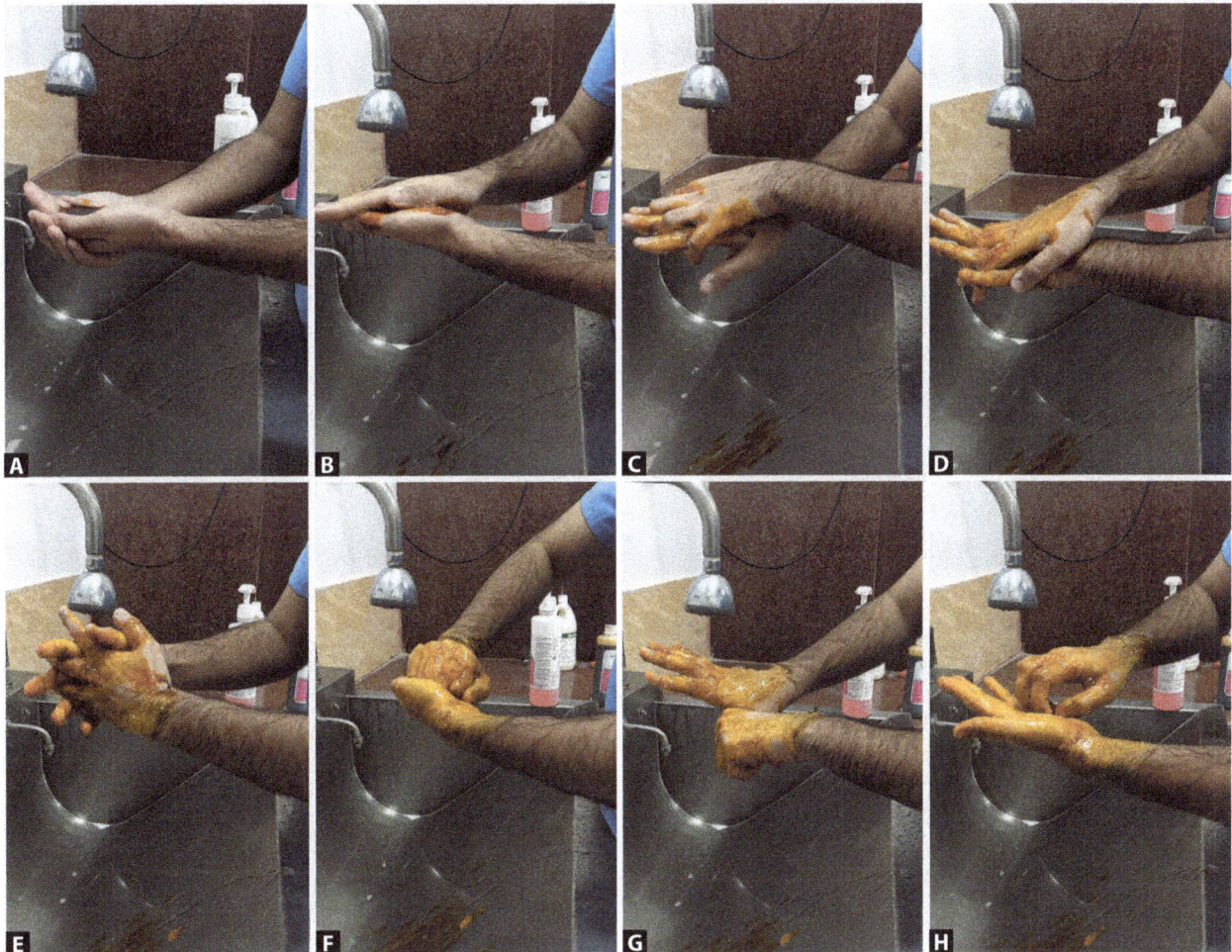

Figures 7.4A to H The hand scrubbing technique. (A) Take adequate amount of scrubbing agent in the palm of one hand and then follow the steps for surgical scrubbing in a specified manner (as per the Ayliffe Protocols) as shown in the figure; (B) Palm to palm; (C and D) Palm of one hand over the dorsum of the other; (E) Interlacing of fingers; (F) Back of fingers towards opposite palm with fingers interlocked; (G) Scrubbing of thumb in a rotational movement; (H) Rubbing the fingertips over palm of opposite hand in a rotational movement. Repeat steps F, G, H for both hands

- The forearm should now be scrubbed with twenty circular strokes on all four sides up to two inches above the elbow.
- Repeat for the other arm.
- Rinse thoroughly and allow water to drip down.
- A towel folded to double its length is used to dry the hands in rotational and blotting motions. Always dry in the direction of fingers to elbow ensuring the spaces between the fingertips are dried. One side of the towel is used for one arm and the other side for the other arm.
- Discard the towel appropriately.
- Once fully dried, the surgeon is ready to don the gown and the gloves.

The hand cleaning technique as per the guidelines of the Ayliffe protocol has been described step-by-step in **Figures 7.4A to H**.

GOWNING AND GLOVING

Gowning

The surgeon should always hold the gown for wearing from the inside part. The surgeon should hold the gown at the neck and allow it to open with the arm holes facing him/her. The arms are then slid into the sleeves. Area from fingertips to two inches above the elbows and from the scrubbed personnel's chest to the operation table or the draped patient is defined the sterile area and hence, hands should not be kept below the waist line, near one's neck/shoulder, touch the axillary area or the back of the gown. At all times the hands should be kept at a level above the waist preferably the shoulders. The techniques for donning a gown include closed cuff method and open cuff method.

- *Closed cuff technique:* The hands and fingertips are not exposed outside after donning the gown. This is done by grasping the inside of the sleeve-cuff juncture between the thumb and index finger. The assistant then ties the gown at the level of the neck and waist **(Figs 7.5A to D)**.
- *Open cuff technique:* In this, the sleeve is not grasped from inside allowing fingers and hand to get exposed. The assistant can pull from the inside of the shoulders to adjust the sleeves accordingly.

Gloving

The process of donning the gloves is known as gloving. The gloves are packed in a manner, so that during the process of gloving, the bare hands of the surgeon do not come in contact with the outer surface of gloves.

Procedure

- *Closed cuff method:* The glove is picked up by holding at the folded cuff edge with sleeve covered hand. The glove is then put on the closed sleeve till the rolled edge reached the cuff sleeve junction keeping in mind the correct orientation and dexterity. With the other hand under the sleeve, this edge of the glove is unrolled and stretched. The glove should be pulled on till the fingers are snugly fitted. Repeat the same procedure for other hand.

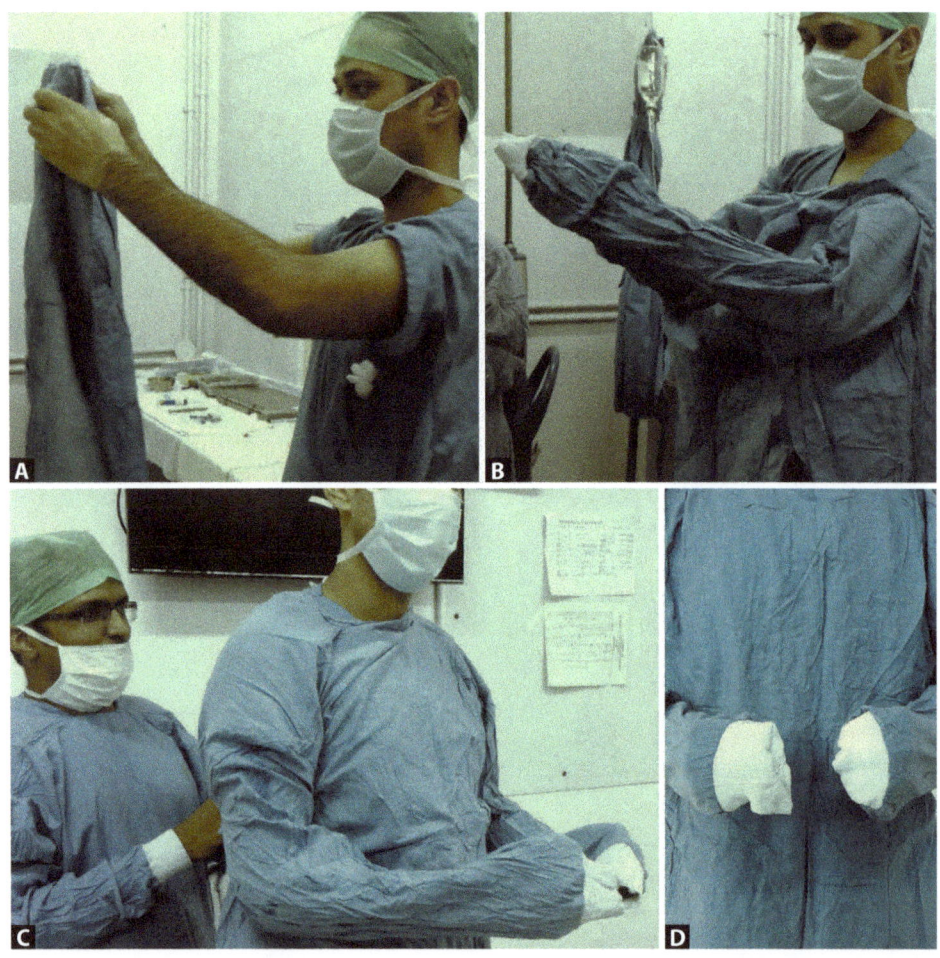

Figures 7.5A to D The gowning technique. (A) Hold the gown from the inside with the armholes facing the surgeon; (B) Slide the arms inside one by one and at all times keep the hands above waist level; (C) An assistant should always help tie the gown without touching the sterile part of the gown; (D) The closed cuff technique without exposure of hands and fingertips

Pre-operative Preparation of Operation Theatre Personnel

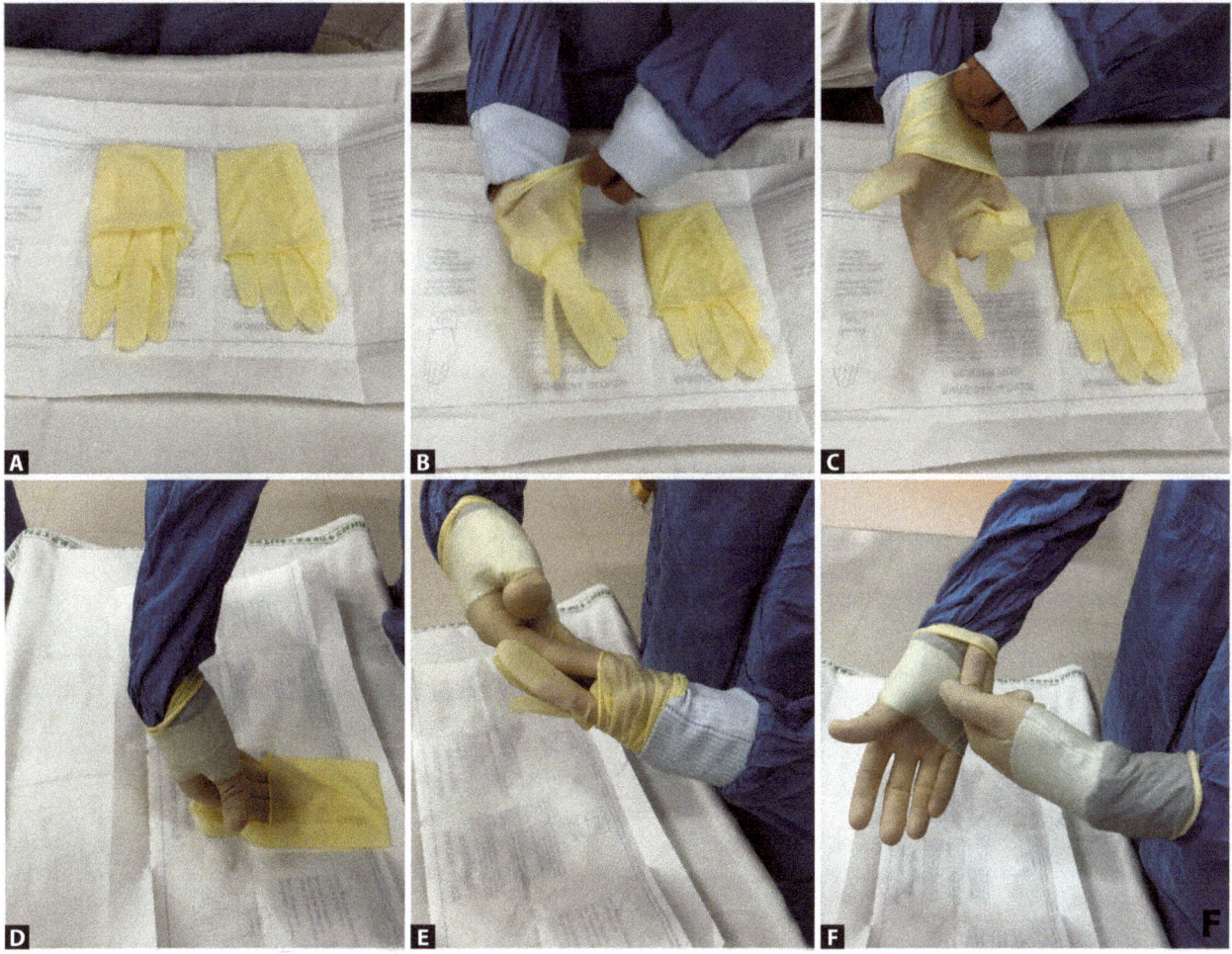

Figures 7.6A to F The gloving technique. (A) A pair of appropriately sized non-powdered gloves should be opened on the sterile table; (B to F) Steps of gloving by open-cuff method have been shown. The steps are as described in the text

- *Open cuff method:* In this case, the fingers and hands are exposed. The right sided glove is picked up by the left hand at the level of the folded cuff. The right hand is then slid in and the left hand fingers are used to unroll the cuff and pull the glove proximally for better fitting. Repeat the same procedure for the other hand but this time, the gloved right hand will hold the glove for left hand from the outer edge of the folded cuff **(Figs 7.6A to F)**.

The preparation of the OT personnel is one of the most crucial things before any surgery to prevent the transmission of any infection to the patient due to the surgeon per se. Proper method of scrubbing, gloving and gowning can greatly reduce the risk of post-operative infection translating into excellent post-operative outcomes.

REFERENCES

1. Braswell ML, Spruce L. Implementing AORN recommended practices for surgical attire. AORN J. 2012; 95(1):122.
2. Recommended practices for surgical attire. AORN J. 2005;81(2):413e20.
3. Centers for Disease Control (CDC). Guideline for isolation precautions: preventing transmission of infectious agents in healthcare settings. Available at http://www.cdc.gov/ncidod/dhqp/pdf/isolation. 2007; 52.
4. Hughey M. Scrub Gown and Glove Procedures, 2008 [online]
5. Humphreys H, Marshall RJ, Ricketts VE, et al. Theatre overshoes do not reduce operating theatre floor bacterial counts. Journal of Hospital Infection. 1991;17:117-23.
6. Woodhead K, Taylor EW, Bannister G, et al. Behaviours and rituals in the operating theatre. A report from

the Hospital Infection Society Working Party on Infection Control in Operating Theatres. J Hosp Infect. 2002;51(4):241e55.
7. Moylan JA, Fitzpatrick KT, Davenport KE. Reducing wound infections. Improved gown and drape barrier performance. Arch Surg. 1987;122(2):152-7.
8. "FDA proposes ban on most powdered medical gloves". FDA. March 21, 2016.
9. Henderson DK, Saah AJ, Zak BJ, et al. Risk of nosocomial infection with human T-cell lymphotropic virus type III/lymphadenopathy-associated virus in a large cohort of intensively exposed health care workers. Ann Intern Med. 1986;104(5):644-7.
10. Gerberding JL, Bryant-LeBlanc CE, Nelson K, et al. Risk of transmitting the human immunodeficiency virus, cytomegalovirus, and hepatitis B virus to health care workers exposed to patients with AIDS and AIDS-related conditions. J Infect Dis. 1987;156(1):1-8.
11. Update: acquired immunodeficiency syndrome and human immunodeficiency virus infection among health-care workers. MMWR Morb Mortal Wkly Rep. 1988;37(15):229-34, 239.
12. Case-control study of HIV seroconversion in health-care workers after percutaneous exposure to HIV-infected blood--France, United Kingdom, and United States, January 1988-August 1994. MMWR Morb Mortal Wkly Rep. 1995;44(50):929-33.
13. Gerberding JL, Bryant-LeBlanc CE, Nelson K, et al. Risk of transmitting the human immunodeficiency virus, cytomegalovirus, and hepatitis B virus to health-care workers exposed to patients with AIDS and AIDS-related conditions. J Infect Dis. 1987;156:1-8.
14. Alter MJ. Occupational exposure to hepatitis C virus: a dilemma. Infect Control Hosp Epidemiol. 1994;15: 742-4.
15. Lanphear BP, Linnemann CC Jr, Cannon CG et al. Hepatitis C virus infection in healthcare workers: risk of exposure and infection. Infect Control Hosp Epidemiol. 1994;15:745-50.
16. Puro V, Petrosillo N, Ippolito G. Italian Study Group on Occupational Risk of HIV and Other Bloodborne Infections. Risk of hepatitis C seroconversion after occupational exposures in health care workers. Am J Infect Control. 1995;23:273-7.
17. Mitsui T, Iwano K, Masuko K, et al. Hepatitis C virus infection in medical personnel after needlestick accident. Hepatology. 1992;16:1109-14.
18. CDC. Recommendations for preventing transmission of infection with human T-lymphotropic virus type III/lymphadenopathy-associated virus in the workplace. MMWR. 1985;34:681-6, 691-5.
19. CDC. Recommendations for preventing transmission of infection with human T-lymphotropic virus type III/lymphadenopathy-associated virus during invasive procedures. MMWR. 1986;35:221-3.
20. Baker JL, Kelen GD, Sivertson KT, et al. Unsuspected human immuno-deficiency virus in critically ill emergency patients. JAMA. 1987;257:2609-11.

CHAPTER 8

OT Protocol: Codes of Conduct

Sagnik Sen, Neelima Aron, Vaishali, Namrata Sharma

INTRODUCTION

Modern ophthalmic operation theatres (OT) have to maintain the strictest of sterility standards in order to deliver aseptic surgeries to the patient and thereby avoid unnecessary hospital-borne infections. The degree of bacterial colonization of the wound is the major risk factor for post-operative infection. The only way to reduce bacterial contamination inside the OT is disinfection and sterilization and adjunct to this is maintenance of a set of etiquettes and infection prevention practices by the OT personnel, which apply to all patients regardless of their infective status.

Skill of a surgeon lies in his/her maintenance of the aseptic conditions during the surgery and awareness of reduction of bacterial contamination of the surgical wound. All of the scrubbed-in surgical team members must adhere to strict asepsis techniques themselves and encourage others in the OT environment to do the same.

GENERAL CONSIDERATIONS

Almost 10% of infections in healthcare setup come from the OT and one of the most important sources is the healthcare worker himself. Another important aspect is airborne dispersion. The most common source of bacterial contamination inside the OT comes from the skin of the OT personnel. Staff with infected lesions of the skin or bacterial infections of the upper respiratory system should not participate in any procedure done under aseptic precautions.

Segregation of patients into "**clean**" and "**infected**" has been a traditional practice and it helps the OT staff to be more alert about maintaining sterilization. Undoubtedly, the maintenance of the same set of standards and practices for sterilization should be looked after each subsequent case in order to obtain the best quality assurance.

The codes of conduct of various personnel in and around the OT have been laid down to help in proper maintenance of asepsis standards for better management of patients. The aseptic technique of scrubbing, gowning and gloving has already been explained in detail in the previous chapter. This chapter highlights the important points to be kept in mind while in OT to prevent the transmission of infection and contamination.

SCRUBBED SURGEON AND ASSISTANT

- The surgeon should never wear the gown on his own as the back of the gown, the area below the waist, armpit and around neck are considered unsterile.
- Gloved hands are always kept above the waist and folded in front **(Fig. 8.1)**. Hands should not touch the back or the sides of the gown **(Fig. 8.2)**. Bare hands should only touch the insides of the gown and the gloves.
- When changing places, the surgeon should always turn back to back.
- The surgeon should clean the surgical area with a single use antiseptic solution in a concentric fashion moving out of the surgical field to the periphery. Sufficient waiting period is given for the combustible materials in the antiseptic to dry. After this, proper draping of the surgical area is done with clean linen and plastic drapes preferably **(Fig. 8.3)**.

Ocular Infections: Prophylaxis and Management

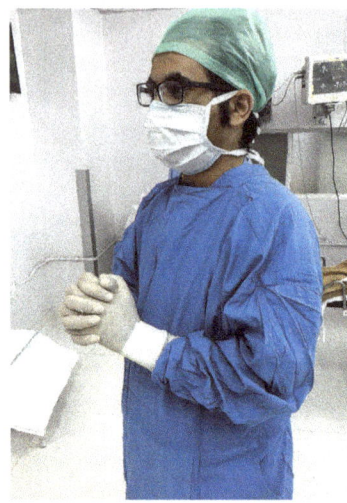

Figure 8.1 A scrubbed surgeon with hands folded in front to avoid glove contamination

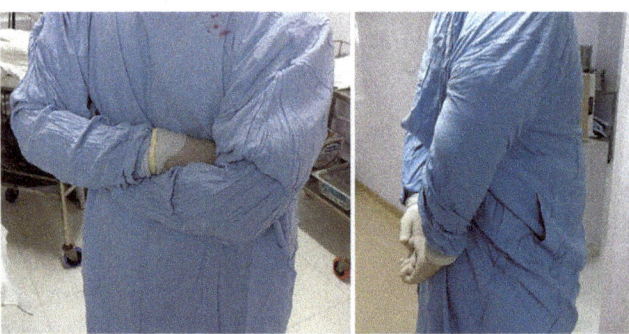

Figure 8.2 Wrong ways of keeping hands after getting scrubbed

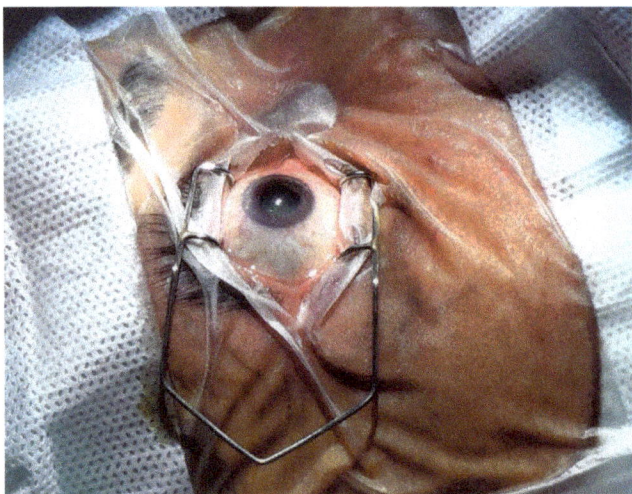

Figure 8.3 Plastic surgical drape over the eye covering all eyelashes to maintain a sterile field for surgery

- Use of cell phones within the OT should be avoided as they are an important source of microbial organisms and distraction.
- The unsterile portion of the microscope should not be touched with gloved hands.
- In between two cases, the surgeon should change the gloves and should not move with hands folded onto armpit or inside gown pocket as both the areas are unsterile.
- An alcohol wash must be taken in the hand and allowed to dry in between subsequent surgeries for at least 30 seconds.
- On suspicion of puncture of gloves, they should be discarded and changed immediately.

NURSING STAFF

- Scrubbed-in nursing staff should stay within the sterile boundaries maintaining a wide and safe distance from unscrubbed personnel.
- Sterile fields and trolley should be prepared as close as possible to the time of use and should be continuously monitored to rule out any compromise of sterility **(Fig. 8.4)**.[1]
- The scrubbed nurse should move draped sterile trolleys by holding the horizontal surfaces only.

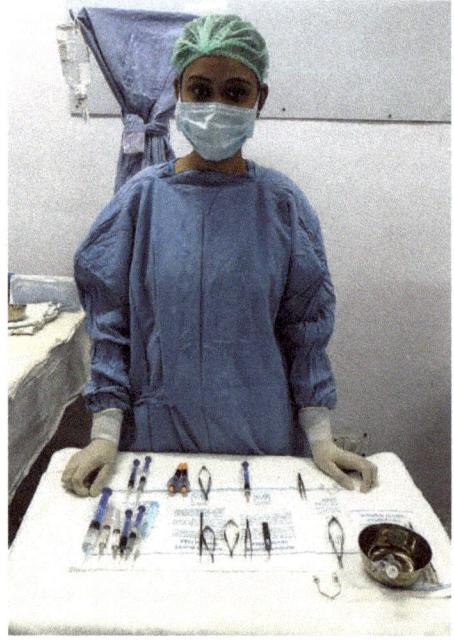

Figure 8.4 A scrubbed OT nurse with neatly arranged trolley for surgery

OT Protocol: Codes of Conduct

- The scrubbed nurse should not cross the sterile field while handing the instruments to the surgeon. Sharps and heavy items must be presented to the scrubbed surgeon to avoid penetration of the sterile field.
- They should also not lean across a sterile field to avoid clothing to touch the sterile field.

Opening Packages

- The nursing staff and OT assistants should have received proper training regarding differences between sterile and non-sterile objects and must be able to make sure that the sterility of the pack of instruments and expiry date is ascertained before opening **(Fig. 8.5)**.
- A sterile package is to be opened on a flat surface away from the body and always kept covered if it is not used immediately. It is not to be tossed on to the sterile field as objects may roll away or displace other items into unsterile fields.
- Packages are never to be passed above the sterile field. While opening the wrapper, the farthest end is opened first, followed by the sides and the end closest to the nurse is opened last.

Pouring Sterile Solution

- Considering the outer surface of the bottle unsterile and the inside area and the solution sterile, the nurse should pour the sterile liquid into a sterile container with the container held 6 inches above the sterile field, in a slow and controlled manner to prevent splashing and contamination of the sterile field. The total amount is to be poured in a continuous manner and not stopped in between, as this disrupts the sterile continuity.
- Previously opened containers are considered unsterile and such solutions should not be poured again onto the sterile field.
- Betadine solutions must be discarded at the end of the day.

OPERATION THEATRE ASSISTANT

- The OT assistant is in charge of shifting the patients in and out of the OT, properly laying him/her down on the table and taking care of the belongings **(Fig. 8.6)**.
- He will also make sure that the patient does not touch or keep the operation materials on any part of the sterile area.
- The assistant will also be responsible for putting in proper drops into the eye when the patient is on the OT table and for the final pad and bandaging of the patient's eye after the surgery is over.
- It is the duty of the OT assistant to tie the surgeon's gown before surgery and untie it at the end of the surgery.
- The wound dressings from the patient should be carefully removed in order to avoid contamination. It is better done by an OT assistant wearing gloves.

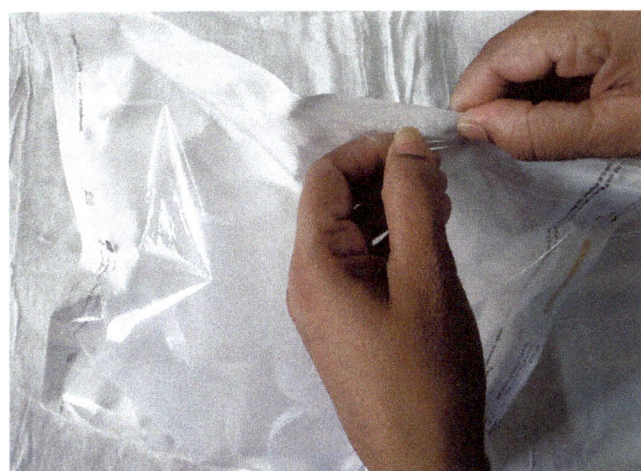

Figure 8.5 Proper method of opening of packages with sterile trays/instruments inside

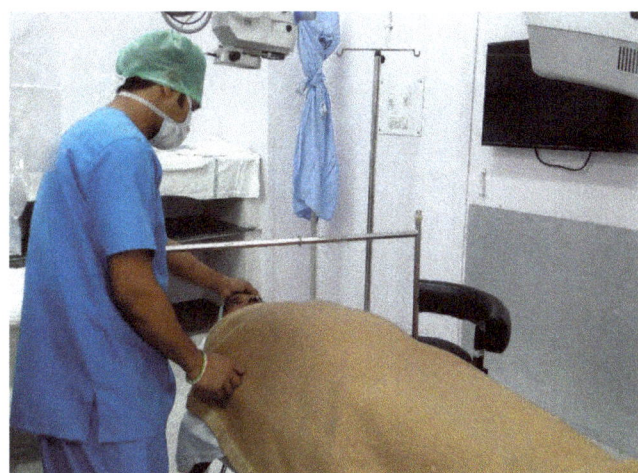

Figure 8.6 OT assistant helping the patient to lie down on the OT table

OBSERVER IN THE OPERATION THEATRE

- Observers inside the OT arena may include medical students, interns, trainees, lab technicians, surgical company representatives, engineers, etc. Entry of casual observers is to be strictly discouraged inside the OT.
- Students and trainees may observe surgeries from a distance on the television.
  The following set of rules is to be maintained:
  - Hands should be kept behind the back as this would reduce the temptation to reach out and contaminate the sterile areas.
  - Leaning over on to the aseptic field of surgery is strictly to be avoided.
  - Maintain at least a 1 foot clearance distance from the sterile area.
  - Hands should not cross or touch any sterile object/person.
  - Excessive coughing/sneezing should be avoided to prevent aerosolized spread of infective particulate matter. In case of emergency coughing, the person should leave the OT.
  - Clothes made of wool are not to be allowed inside the OT as it may harbor carriage of more microorganisms.

VISITORS IN THE OPERATION THEATRE

- Visitors include relatives of the patients posted for surgery and medical representatives.
- Apart from maintaining proper decorum outside the OT premises, relatives are supposed to wait patiently outside and not enter the sterile area of the OT without proper changing of clothes and taking sterile precautions.
- Medical representatives are not to be allowed free access inside the OT and should take appropriate permissions for the same. They may be requested to enter the OT in times of specific needs such as when information regarding intraocular lens or machine is required.

INTRA-OPERATIVE AND POST-OPERATIVE PRACTICES[2]

- Good intra-operative practices are always welcome as the surgery itself is the most common method of spreading infection inside the eye and in spite of extremely good techniques used in the surgery if one is not careful about maintenance of asepsis, then the outcome of the surgery becomes extremely risky.
- Apart from the preparation of the sterile field before surgery with povidone iodine solution, the sterile area is covered with adhesive drapes and strict asepsis is maintained during handling of tissues.
- Tissue handling is reduced to a minimum and instruments to be used on the outside of the eye are never used inside.
- Suture materials should not touch the eyelid margins. Also the used and unused instruments are kept separated to avoid mixing and contamination.
- At the end of surgery, a meticulous search for any wick of cotton fiber or any foreign body inside the eye is carried out.
- Instillation of a drop of antibiotic and/or a drop of 5% povidone-iodine into the conjunctival cul-de-sac at the end of surgery is a routine practice. Intracameral antibiotics (vancomycin, cefuroxime) maybe used but is not preferred as a routine practice to avoid emergence of antibiotic resistance. Subconjunctival antibiotics do not have much role in prevention of ocular infections.
- Post-operatively, topical antibiotics are to be continued for a minimum period of 7–10 days routinely along with moderate potency topical steroids. Systemic antibiotics are to be given only if adnexal infections are present otherwise they have no benefit over topical therapy. Short acting mydriatic agents may be continued till 2 weeks to avoid synechiae formation due to inflammation.
- The preferred follow-up schedule in post-operative period is Day 1, 1 week and 1 month after the surgery. Visual acuity record, slit lamp examination and fundus examination should be done on each follow-up to rule out any evidence of endophthalmitis, retinal detachment and cystoid macular edema.
- The gap between the other eye surgery should be at least 2 weeks.
- After 2–3 weeks of follow-up and after stopping mydriatic agents, the final refraction with near correction can be done for the patient.
- During the follow-up, post-operative advice should be given in the patient's vernacular language to ascertain better compliance.
- Water should not be allowed to enter the eye for at least 2 weeks following phacoemulsification and 4 weeks after SICS surgery.

- The eye should be cleaned with boiled water from the outside and bathing below the neck is advised. The eye should be kept covered with protective goggles with side covers whenever travelling outside and the patient should avoid dust, smoke and sunlight.
- The topical medications should be carried with the patient wherever he is travelling outside as no dose should be missed in the early post-operative period.
- The danger signs of any infection or retinal detachment are explained to the patient and they are asked to follow-up then on an emergency basis.

PRACTICES IN THE USE OF INTRA-OPERATIVE ADJUNCTS

Various assistive aids are used intra-operatively which are essential during phacoemulsification and other intraocular surgeries. Various points should be kept in mind for their use.

Irrigating Solutions

Irrigating solutions constitute one of the most important causes of cluster endophthalmitis.
- It is preferable to use smaller volume packs which can be discarded after each case. However, one bottle can be used for 2-3 patients.
- Always check for floating particles in the irrigating fluid bottles before use.
- Autoclaving of irrigating bottles is preferable but not essential. The irrigating solutions may be exposed to ultraviolet light for 2-4 hours when the lights are kept on during operation theatre sterilization.
- The irrigating solutions can be used in a glass bottle or a flexible plastic bag. Avoid rigid plastic non-transparent containers.
- All solutions which have been opened should be discarded at the end of the day.
- Infusion of antibiotics in the irrigating solution for maintaining sterility is not necessary.

Ophthalmic Viscoelastic Devices

- Viscoelastics should preferably be packaged in glass syringes. Plastic syringes should be avoided in view of high incidence of post-operative sterile reaction in the eye.
- The cannula of the ophthalmic viscoelastic devices (OVD) should be changed if the same syringe is being used for more than one patient.
- The left over viscoelastic solutions should be discarded at the end of the day and not reused for the next day surgery.

Phacoemulsification Instruments

- It is desirable to change the phaco handpiece tip and sleeve after every case. However, it may also be changed after every 5 cases.
- Phaco tubings should be changed after very 5 cases when they are discarded.
- A minimum of 60-100 mL distilled water should be used for flushing the handpiece. 60-100 mL air should be flushed after this.
- Do not use formalin to sterilize the tips.
- Do not use saline since it causes corrosion.
- Keratomes should not be reused before sterilization.

To conclude, it is the responsibility of all OT personnel to follow the above OT etiquettes intra-operatively and also ascertain a proper follow-up of patients post-operatively to prevent OT infections.

REFERENCES

1. Pereira LJ, Lee GM, Wade KJ. The effect of surgical hand washing routines on the microbial counts of operating room nurses. Am J Infect Control. 1990;18:354-64.
2. AfPP Principles of Safe Practice in the Perioperative Environment 2011.

CHAPTER 9

Operation Theatre Sterilization

Ruchita Falera, Sagnik Sen, Neelima Aron

An Operation theatre (OT) complex is the heart of any surgical hospital.[1] Good surgical skills have to be backed by scientific design of OT for optimizing the outcomes. A thorough knowledge and implementation of OT hygiene and asepsis is of paramount importance in order to ensure best surgical results and reduce the incidence of post-operative infections and in this regard, cleaning, disinfection and sterilization are the cornerstones in ensuring operation room (OR) asepsis.

It is believed, that people rather than objects are the principal concern in control of surgical infection. However, lay out of a surgical theatre does affect utilization patterns and traffic in and around the suite.[2] Hence configuration of an OR complex can indirectly affect the incidence of surgical infections.[3] The OR complex should be away from the crowded areas of the hospital. It is generally located on the top floor of the building, such that the OR premises are traversed only by the patients and OT personnel, thus minimizing the infective load being carried into the operation theatre.[4]

OPERATION THEATRE CLEANING

Cleaning is a form of decontamination. It mainly involves the removal of visible dirt and organic matter from the surface of objects, which may interfere with the action of the disinfectant. It also helps reduce the bacterial load on such surfaces. Cleaning mainly involves friction to remove foreign material and fluids to rinse away contamination. Failure to adequately clean results in higher bioburden and protein load which will decrease the efficiency of the sterilization procedure.[5]

Use of water and a simple detergent for cleaning reduces flora by 80%, the efficacy of which increases to 95% by the use of disinfectants. Floors should be cleaned with vacuum cleaners or wet mops **(Fig. 9.1)**. Walls should be washed with water and disinfectant weekly. Open shelves should be cleaned daily using detergent. Closed cabinets may be cleaned once in a week.[6]

At the end of the day, all the table tops sinks and door handles should be thoroughly cleaned using detergent/low level of disinfectant. Floors should first be cleaned with detergents mixed with warm water and then mopped with disinfectant like phenol in the concentration of 1: 10. Nowadays more potent commercially available disinfectants like Ecoshield are

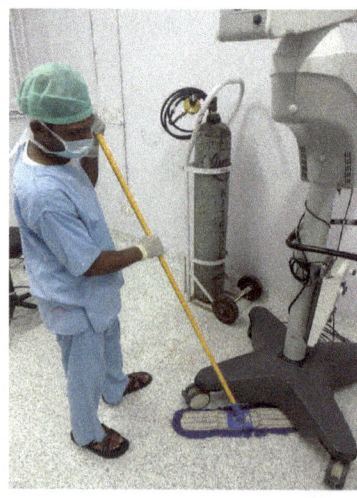

Figure 9.1 Mopping of floor by the operation theatre worker

being widely used as disinfectants. The air-conditioning (AC) ducts should be cleaned using machines, wet vacuum with detergent or approved disinfectants.

OPERATION THEATRE DISINFECTION AND STERILIZATION

Disinfection is defined as thermal or chemical destruction of pathogenic and other types of microorganisms. Sterilization is a validated process used to render a product free of all forms of viable microorganisms including spores. Disinfection is less lethal than sterilization because it destroys most recognized pathogenic microorganisms but not necessarily all microbial forms (e.g. bacterial spores).[5]

Surfaces may contribute to transmission of a number of microbes (e.g. vancomycin-resistant enterococci, methicillin-resistant *S. aureus*, viruses) and hence disinfectants are needed for surfaces contaminated by blood and other potentially infective material. Disinfectants are more effective than detergents in reducing microbial load as detergents can get contaminated and result in seeding the patient's environment with bacteria, thus causing a lapse in sepsis. A single product can be used for decontamination of noncritical surfaces, both floors and equipment.

Environment Protection Agency (EPA) approved the use of disinfectants or chemical sterilants for regular cleaning of the OT table, floor and wall.[7]

Chemical Disinfection

- *Phenol (Carbolic acid 2%):* Phenol is routinely used as a disinfectant in OT setups. These chemicals have carbolic acid base, derived from coal tar. Chlorinated fraction and petroleum residues are added to improve their cleansing and physical properties. These are irritant to skin and mucosal surfaces and corrosive to metal surface. White fluids are emulsified suspensions which precipitate on surface making subsequent cleaning difficult. It is used for washing floor every day after surgery, mopping of OT walls, OT tables, mats, instrument trolleys, stools, etc. This is followed by a wipe done with 70% alcohol.
- *Formaldehyde fumigation:* Formaldehyde is commonly used to sterilize the OT and other rooms. The room to be fumigated is prepared by sealing the windows and switching off fans and AC. Formaldehyde gas is then generated by adding 150 g of $KMnO_4$ to 280 mL of formalin for every 1000 cubic feet (28.3 cu mm) of room volume. Alternatively, a fumigator can also be used for the same. When formalin vapor is formed, doors should be sealed and left unopened overnight for at least 6 hours. The next day morning, 300 mL of 10% ammonia solution is kept for 2–3 hours to neutralize formalin vapors. It is recommended that fumigation should be carried out on weekly basis.

Formaldehyde inactivates microorganisms by alkylating the amino acid and sulfhydryl groups of proteins and ring nitrogen atoms of purine bases.

However, Occupational Safety and Health Administration (OSHA) states that formaldehyde should be handled in workplace as a potential carcinogen and fumigation of OT using formalin is not recommended by the Center for Disease Control and Prevention (CDC).[7,8]

- *Bacillocid rasant:* Bacillocid rasant is a newer commercially available compound used for surface and environmental decontamination **(Fig. 9.2)**. It has excellent cleansing properties with bactericidal, virucidal, sporicidal and fungicidal activity. It contains glutaraldehyde, benzyl-C12-18-alkyldimethyl ammonium chloride and didecyl dimethyl ammonium chloride as the active ingredients. Complete asepsis is achieved within 30–60 minutes and cleaning with detergent or carbolic acid not required. Moreover, the OT need not be shut down for 24 hours.

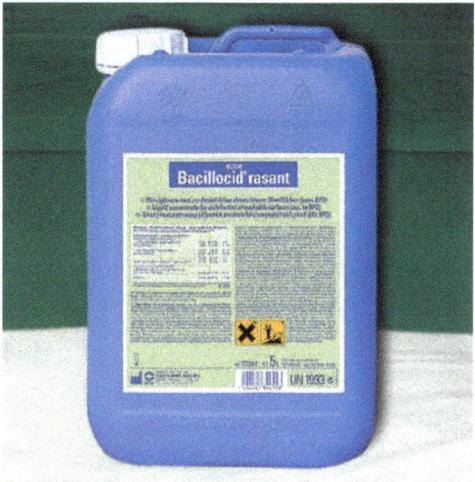

Figure 9.2 Chemical disinfectant: Bacillocid rasant

- *Ecoshield:* It is 11% w/v stabilized hydrogen peroxide and 0.01% w/v diluted silver nitrate solution **(Fig. 9.3)**. It can be used for routine mopping of floors and cleaning of OT equipment. It is also used in the form of hydrogen peroxide vapors (fogging) in the disinfection of OT at the end of routine cases, as well as infected cases.
- *Aldekol:* This solution contains 6% formaldehyde, 6% glutaraldehyde and 5% benzalkonium chloride as active ingredients and the OT needs to be closed for 3 hours **(Fig. 9.4)**.

These disinfectants are sprayed with the help of a disinfectant spraying machine as shown in **Figure 9.5**.

Fogging Method

Fogging involves nebulization of a disinfectant in a room until all surfaces are wet, followed by wiping off residual fluid from surfaces by masked and gowned personnel. It is not commonly used in recent times. Earlier fogging was carried out using formaldehyde. However due to its carcinogenic effects it is now seldom used. Commercially available disinfectants like Ecoshield are now used for fogging. The disinfectant is put in a fogger machine and the machine is switched on for 45 minutes in the sealed OT following which the room is kept sealed for another 45 minutes **(Fig. 9.6)**.

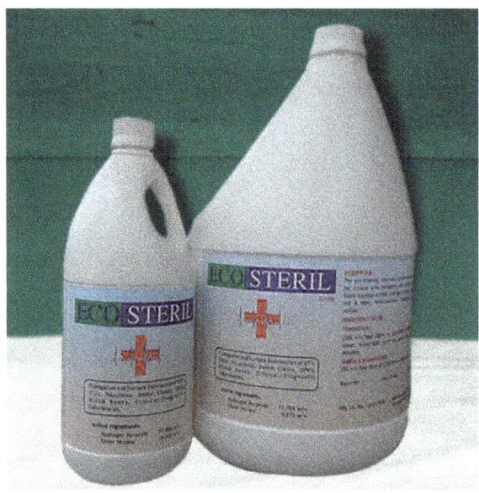

Figure 9.3 Chemical disinfectant: Ecoshield

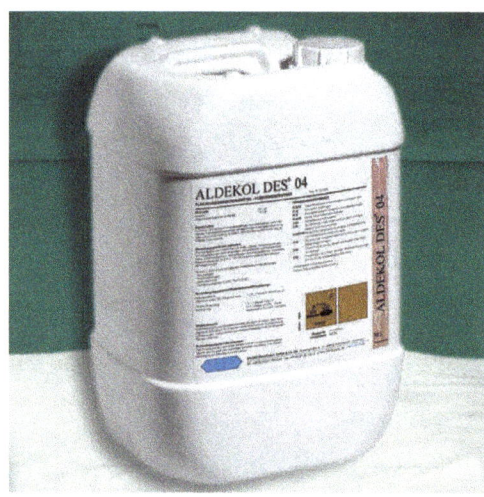

Figure 9.4 Chemical disinfectant: Aldekol

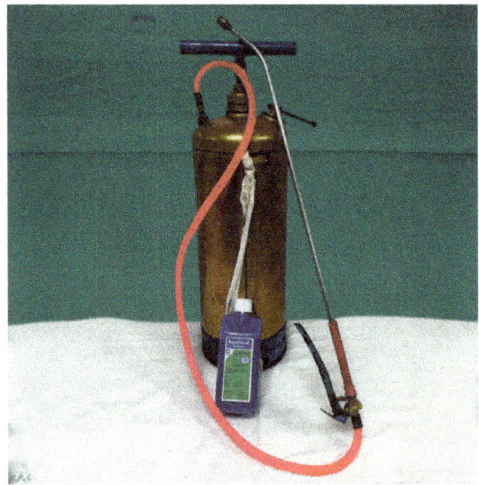

Figure 9.5 Disinfectant spraying machine used to spray over the OT surfaces

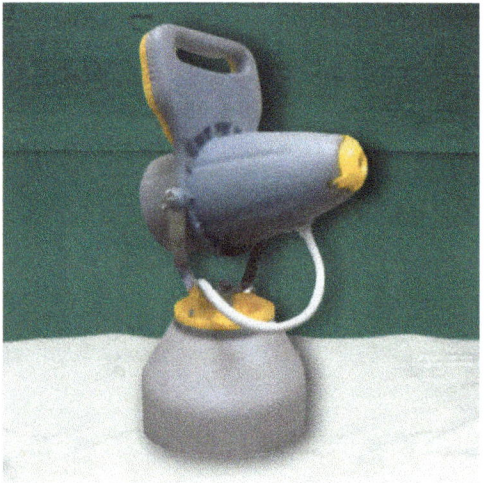

Figure 9.6 Fogger machine used in operation theatre for fumigation

Hydrogen peroxide has the advantage of being safer, less irritating, and has shorter cycle times compared with formalin fumigation.[9]

Ultraviolet Rays

This can be done by daily UV irradiation for 12–16 hours and is to be switched off 2 hours before starting OT.

CLEANING SCHEDULE

Before Surgery

- Wet mopping must be done in the morning.
- The OT is cleaned with 0.5% chlorine solution. Commercially available disinfectants like Baccillocid are more potent and are commonly used.
- All equipment, OT tables, walls and floors have to be cleaned and sterilized using appropriate methods.

Between Operative Procedures

- Cleaning of operation tables and theatre equipment with disinfectant solution is recommended.
- The sterile sheets laid on the OT table and instrument trolley should be changed between consecutive procedures.
- In case of spillage of blood/body fluids, decontamination with chlorine solution should be done.
- Ideally the floor should be cleaned using wet mop after each surgical procedure.
- Wastes should be discarded in recommended color coded plastic bags.
- Soiled gowns must not be disposed inside the operation theatre.

After Surgery

- Linen and waste material is collected in color-coded bags according to hospital waste disposal protocol.
- Soiled linen is collected separately outside the OT and taken to the dirty utility room, where it is disinfected by soaking in clean water with 0.5% bleaching powder solution for 30 minutes before being dispatched to the laundry facility.
- Sharps are separately disposed in puncture proof containers.
- The OT table is cleaned with water and then carbonized with 0.5% chlorine/70% isopropyl alcohol.
- Equipment including foot switches are first cleaned with a wet cloth and then disinfected by wiping with 70% isopropyl alcohol.

SEPTIC OPERATION THEATRE

Septic Operation theatre is one where infected cases are operated such as evisceration, abscess drainage, dacryocystectomy, dacryocystorhinostomy, therapeutic keratoplasty, endophthalmitis vitrectomy, etc. It is very important to plan and organize the septic OT in order to prevent added intra-operative and post-operative infections. Higher level of caution needs to be taken in maintenance of asepsis in these cases.

The septic OT should ideally be located away from the main OT. Patients should have minimal access to the OT, however the patients should be easily transferable. The OT should be provided with a separate changing and scrubbing room. The instruments and eye towels should be sterilized separately in order to avoid infections. In recent times, functional separation of septic and aseptic surgery is more commonly carried out. Functional separation means that septic procedures are performed at the end of aseptic operations instead of having two separate OT's in two different locations.[10]

Setup of Septic Operation Theatre

- Laminar air flow, within the OT will ensure clean area about the operation table and instruments within 2 minutes, thereby enabling reuse of the theatre within five minutes of disinfection.
- An effective disinfectant should be used to clean the OT table in between procedures, and the time interval between reuse of the operation theatre should be according to the minimum exposure time.
- All potentially contaminated areas near and away from the patient need to be wiped and disinfected with disinfectant, allowing for adequate contact time.
- All equipment used and clothes worn in the OT need to be discarded separately
- All team members (i.e. nurses, surgeons, anesthesiologists) should change clothes and shoes inside the OT, before leaving the area.

Sterilization of Septic Operation Theatre

The OT is sprayed with commercially available disinfectant like 1% Baccillocid and sealed for 6 hours. It is then fogged using hydrogen peroxide vapor (Ecoshield) for one hour with a contact time of an additional 45 minutes. Fumigation using formaldehyde can alternatively be carried out. Before using the OT for the next procedure, it is wet mopped using water and appropriate disinfectant.

SPECIAL CASES: HIV, HEPATITIS B, HEPATITIS C

The CDC recommends high level of disinfection of OT in cases of HIV, Hepatitis B and Hepatitis C positive patients. Special precautions need to be taken in the preparation of the OT prior to surgery, intra-operatively as well as post-surgery in order to prevent transmission of the disease.

Setup of Operation Theatre

- The OT table and instrument trolley are covered with disposable covering sheets.
- Any blood spill during the surgery should be dealt with utmost caution. The blood is first absorbed using a good absorbent material. Appropriate disinfectant like sodium hypochlorite is then poured over the absorbent material for ten minutes. The whole spill is then wiped off with a fresh absorbent material, which is then disposed separately. The surface is again cleaned using a low-intermediate level disinfectant.[9]
- After the surgery, the OT doors are closed and OT is sprayed with 2% Bacillocid. The OT is kept sealed for six hours, following which fogging using hydrogen peroxide vapors or fumigation is carried out allowing adequate contact time.
- Prior to subsequent use, the OT as well as the equipment is wet mopped using low level disinfectants.

In a nutshell, the operation theatre is a crucial area in ophthalmic practice. An incidence of infection can ruin the results of a well done surgery. A thorough knowledge of OT hygiene and sterilization can reduce the chances of infection and thus ensure optimal surgical outcomes.

REFERENCES

1. Dorsch JA, Dorsch SE. Operating room design and equipment selection. Understanding Anaesthesia Equipment, 4th edition; Williams and Wilkins; 1999. pp. 1015-6.
2. Laufman H. The operating room. Hospital Infections, In: Bennett JV, Brachman PS (Eds). Little Brown & Co., Boston; 1986. pp. 315-24.
3. Laufman H. Surgical hazard control: Effect of architecture and engineering. Arch Surg. 1973;107:552.
4. Sharma S, Bansal AK, Gyanchand R. Asepsis in ophthalmic operating room. Indian J Ophthalmol. 1996; 44:173-7.
5. Rutala WA, Weber DJ and the Healthcare Infection Control Practices Advisory Committee (HICPAC). Guideline for Disinfection and Sterilization in Healthcare Facilities, 2008.
6. Kabbin JS, Shwetha JV, Sathyanarayan MS, Nagarathnamma T. Disinfection and Sterilization techniques of operation theatre: a review. International Journal of Current Research. 2014;6(5):6622-6.
7. Sapna, Majumdar S, Venkatesh P. The operation theatre: basic architecture. Delhi Journal of Ophthalmology. 2011;21(3):9-14.
8. Ananthanarayan R, Paniker CKJ. Sterilisation and Disinfection. In: Kapil A (Ed). Textbook of Microbiology, 9th edition. Hyderabad: Universities Press; 2013. pp. 334-5.
9. Taneja N, Biswal M, Kumar A, Edwin A, Sunita T, Emmanuel R, Gupta AK, Sharma M. Hydrogen peroxide vapour for decontaminating air-conditioning ducts and rooms of an emergency complex in northern India: time to move on. J Hosp Infect. 2011;78(3):200-3.
10. Kramer A, Assadian O, Wendt M, Stengel D, Seifer J. Functional separation of septic and aseptic surgical procedures. GMS Krankenhaushygiene Interdisziplinär 2011;6(1):ISSN 1863-5245.

CHAPTER 10

Ophthalmic Instrument Sterilization

Nishat Hussain Ahmed, Manthan Chaniyara, Sagnik Sen, Neelima Aron, Gita Satpathy

Sterilization is a term referring to any process that eliminates (removes) or kills (deactivates) all forms of life and other biological agents such as fungi, bacteria, viruses, prions, spore forms, unicellular eukaryotic organisms like *Plasmodium*, etc. present in a specified region, such as a surface, volume of fluid, medication, or biological culture media.[1] However, disinfection describes a process that eliminates many or all-pathogenic microorganisms, except bacterial spores, on inanimate objects.[2] The instruments go through a phase of cleaning, packaging, disinfection and sterilization before intraocular use **(Fig. 10.1)**.

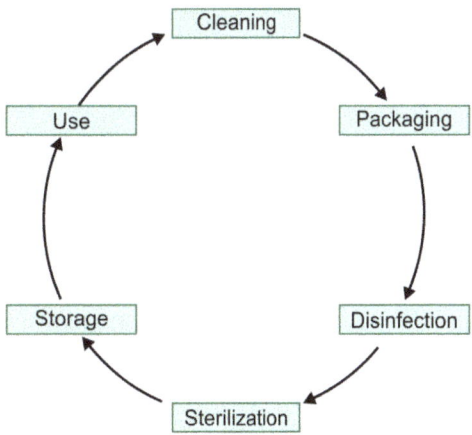

Figure 10.1 Cycle of sterilization

INSTRUMENT PROCESSING

Cleaning of Instruments

Cleaning is a process, usually involving the use of water with detergents or enzymatic products that remove foreign material (organic and inorganic) from an object. It is the most essential step in reprocessing instruments and equipment before high-level disinfection and sterilization because inorganic and organic materials that remain on the surfaces of instruments interfere with the effectiveness of these processes.

Cleaning consists of the steps of mechanical scrubbing wherever applicable, rinsing and drying. It may be of two types[2]: manual **(Figs 10.2A to C)** and mechanical/automated cleaning **(Fig. 10.3)**, which may be washer-sterilizers, ultrasonic cleaners or washer-decontaminators. Studies have shown that manual and mechanical cleaning results in significant reduction of contaminating organisms.[3] In manual cleaning, removal of the matter is done manually. Two key components of manual cleaning are friction (to remove foreign matter with the help of brush) and fluidics (use of fluid under pressure to rinse away contamination after brushing or when the design of instrument does not allow passage of brush).[4] Mechanical scrubbing loosens the organic matter and debris, which is followed by rinsing which is the most important part of the cleaning and flushes the loosened debris and organic matter. Distilled or demineralized water should be used for the final rinse to prevent the accumulation of mineral deposits and to reduce the potential for pyrogens.

Automated instrument rinsing systems may be used as per availability. They have the advantage of standardized protocol being used for the items and are especially helpful to facilitate thorough rinsing of tiny cannulas. All instruments should be cleaned with

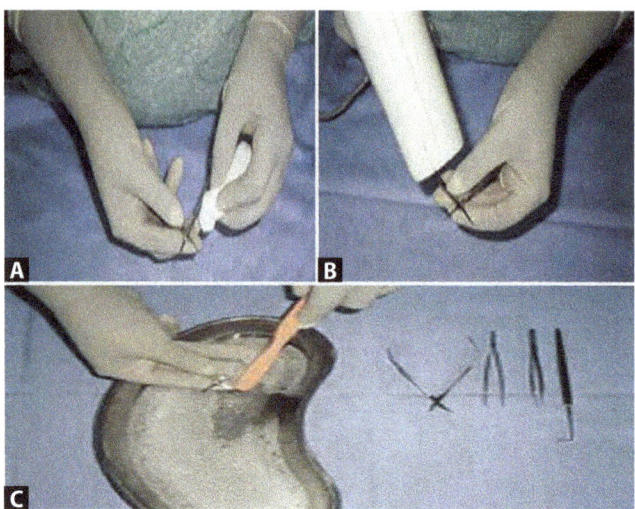

Figures 10.2A to C Method of manual cleaning

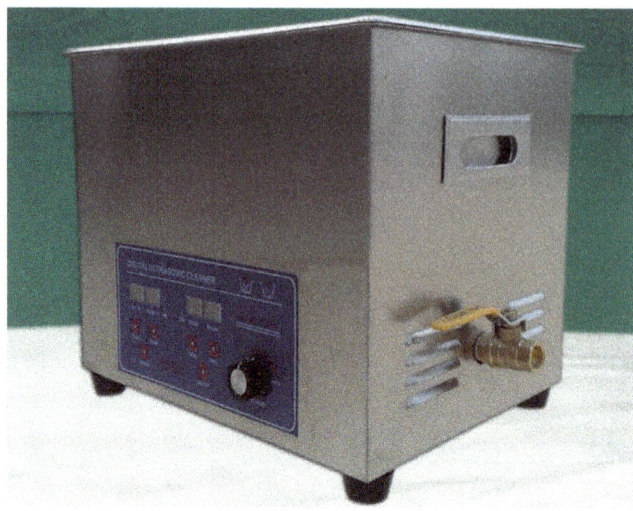

Figure 10.3 Mechanical method of cleaning: ultrasonic cleaner

ultrasonic cleaner at least once a week. Cannulated instruments need to be cleaned every day. The cycle time should be 30 minutes.

Drying should follow rinsing. It reduces the risk of re-contamination during inspection and assembly of instruments, and minimizes rusting and staining. Residual moisture interferes with the sterilization process and can damage instruments. With a particle-free cloth or an air-drying machine, drying of instruments should be done. After all the steps of cleaning are over, articles are visually inspected for removal of organic matter and debris, removal of moisture, proper functioning and alignment, corrosion, pitting, nicks, and cracks and dullness of cutting edges. After ensuring the quality of cleaning, the articles are sent for sterilization or disinfection depending on the category they are falling in as per their intended use.

Packaging of Instruments

Once items are cleaned, dried, and inspected, those requiring sterilization must be wrapped or placed in rigid containers and should be arranged in instrument trays/baskets. Hinged instruments should be opened, items with removable parts disassembled, complex instruments prepared and sterilized according to device manufacturer's instructions and test data, devices with concave surfaces positioned to facilitate drainage of water, and heavy items positioned not to damage delicate items.

There are several choices in methods of wrapping and packaging, including rigid containers, peel-open pouches, roll stock or reels (paper-plastic combinations of tubing designed to allow the user to cut and seal the ends to form a pouch) and sterilization wraps (woven and nonwoven).

A *rigid container* may be of tray type, case type or roll type. In tray type, each individual slot holds single instruments which must not touch each other. A case may be made up of metal or plastic containing a protective silicone mat and this can be used for storage, transportation and during sterilization procedure. Rolls are made up of strong fabric material which are inexpensive and each pocket holds a single instrument.

Peel pouch (**Fig. 10.4**) is flexible for packaging materials. It combines a paper or synthetic barrier material and a transparent plastic film. It is designed for individual, lightweight devices and as a means to separate dissimilar metals or surgeon specific instruments from rest of all.

Woven fabric (**Fig. 10.5**) is made of natural cotton or linen fibers or synthetic materials, such as polyester. It provides the least effective sterile barrier. *Nonwoven* fabric is disposable, single use fabric wrap and resists tear and punctures.

The packaging material must allow penetration of the sterilant, provide protection against contact contamination during handling, provide an effective barrier to microbial penetration, and maintain the

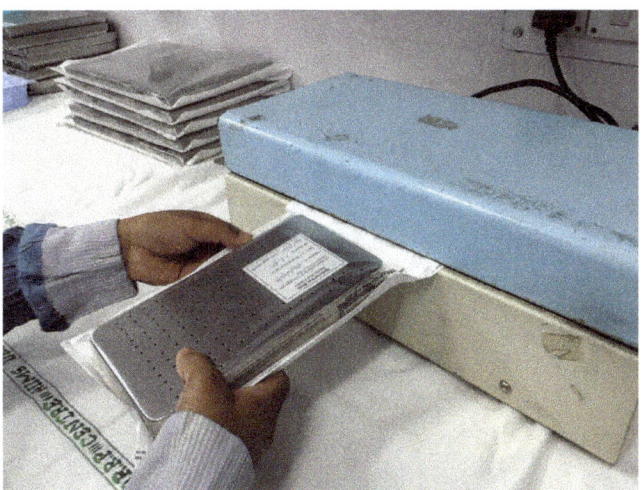

Figure 10.4 Peel pouch packaging

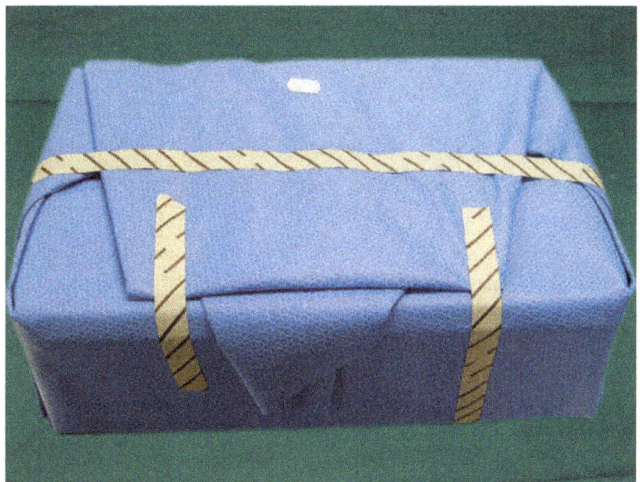

Figure 10.5 Woven fabric/linen packaging

sterility of the processed item after sterilization. Also, the packaging should be easy to use, puncture resistant, nontoxic, odorless and easily disposable.

Prior to sterilization, each package is labeled which lists the package contents, lot control number, initials of the person processing the item, and the date of sterilization. Sterilized items also should have load control identification indicating the sterilizer used, the cycle or load number, and the date of sterilization.

Loading

All items to be sterilized should be arranged so that all surfaces are directly exposed to the sterilizing agent. Thus, loading procedures must allow for free circulation of the sterilant around each item. Perforated trays should be placed so that the tray is parallel to the shelf, non-perforated containers should be placed on their edge (e.g. basins), small items should be loosely placed in wire baskets, and peel packs should be placed on edge in perforated or mesh bottom racks or baskets.

Storage

Sterilized articles remain sterile for varying periods depending on the type of material used to wrap the trays. Safe storage times for sterile packs vary with the porosity of the wrapper and storage conditions. Some hospitals date every sterilized product and use the time-related shelf-life as an indicator of sterility of the item; some others use event-related shelf-life practice. According to event-related shelf-life practice, a product should remain sterile until some event causes it to become contaminated (e.g. tear in packaging, packaging becomes wet, seal is broken). Thus, any item that has been sterilized should not be used after the expiration date has been exceeded and/or if the sterilized package is wet, torn, or punctured. Sterile supplies should be stored far enough from the floor, the ceiling and the outside walls to allow for adequate air circulation, ease of cleaning, and compliance with local fire codes. Items should not be stored under sinks or in other locations where they can become wet.

Handling

Post-sterilization, instruments must be handled using aseptic technique in order to prevent contamination. Any package that has fallen or been dropped on the floor must be inspected for damage to the packaging and contents (if the items are breakable). If the package is heat-sealed in impervious plastic and the seal is still intact, the package should be considered not contaminated. If undamaged, items packaged in plastic need not be reprocessed.

STERILIZATION

There are many methods of instrument sterilization. Routinely used methods for ophthalmic instrument sterilization are autoclaving (high temperature sterilization), low temperature sterilization like ethylene oxide gas sterilization and hydrogen peroxide gas plasma sterilization, and chemical sterilization.

The methods of sterilization (and disinfection) can be physical or chemical methods. An understanding of different sterilizing agents is vital in applying them for different categories of patient care items and areas. They can be classified grossly into:

- *Physical agents*
  - Sunlight
  - Dry and moist heat
  - Ionizing and nonionizing radiation
- *Chemical agents*
  - Ethylene oxide
  - Hydrogen peroxide
  - Peracetic acid

Heat

Heat is a powerful sterilizing agent and should be the method of choice unless there is a contraindication. Heat can be used in different manners depending on the article to be sterilized and the intended purpose. **Table 10.1** enumerates the advantages and disadvantages of heat method of sterilization.

Steam Under Pressure/Moist Heat (Autoclave) (Fig. 10.6)

Of all the methods available for sterilization, moist heat in the form of saturated steam under pressure is the most widely used and the most dependable. It is a nontoxic, inexpensive, and rapidly microbicidal and sporicidal method.

Principle: Each item is exposed to direct steam contact at the required temperature and pressure for the specified time. Thus, there are four parameters of steam sterilization—steam, pressure, temperature, and time. Pressure serves as a means to obtain the high temperatures necessary to quickly kill microorganisms. Moist heat destroys microorganisms by the irreversible coagulation and denaturation of enzymes and structural proteins. Specific temperatures must be obtained to ensure the microbicidal activity.

Types of autoclaves: Two basic types of autoclaves are the *gravity displacement autoclave* and the *high-speed prevacuum sterilizer*.[5,6] In the former, steam is allowed to enter from the top or the sides of the sterilizing chamber and, because the steam is lighter than air, forces air out of the bottom of the chamber through the drain vent. The penetration time into porous items is prolonged because of incomplete air elimination, the entrapped air retards steam permeation and heating efficiency. The high-speed prevacuum sterilizers are equipped with a vacuum pump to ensure air removal from the sterilizing chamber and load before the steam is admitted. The advantage of using a vacuum pump is that there is nearly instantaneous steam penetration even into porous loads.

Time of sterilization: The two common steam-sterilizing temperatures are 121°C and 132°C. The temperature must be maintained for a minimal specified time to kill microorganisms. Recognized minimum exposure periods for sterilization of wrapped healthcare supplies are 30 minutes at 121°C in a gravity displacement sterilizer or 4 minutes at 132°C in a prevacuum sterilizer. At a given temperature, sterilization times vary depending on the type of item (e.g. metal versus rubber, plastic, items with lumens), whether the item is wrapped or unwrapped, and the sterilizer type. Some objects and their optimum timing for autoclaving is shown in **Table 10.2**.

Considerations

- Autoclaved instruments should not be used beyond 24 hours after sterilization.
- The outer and inner surfaces of the autoclave should be cleaned regularly.
- The water should be drained out fortnightly to avoid salt settling on the instruments.

Dry Heat (Hot Air Oven)

Dry heat sterilizers (hot air ovens) should be used only for materials that are likely to be damaged or are impenetrable to moist heat (e.g. powders, petroleum products, sharp instruments). It is a nontoxic method of sterilization, is easy to install and has relatively low operating costs; it penetrates materials; and is noncorrosive for metal and sharp instruments. The disadvantages include the slow rate of heat penetration

Table 10.1 Advantages and disadvantages of heat method

Advantages	Disadvantages
• Nontoxic	• Not useful for heat sensitive instruments
• Rapidly acting	• May damage instrument
• Least affected by organic/inorganic soil	• Potential for burns
• Can be used to sterilize liquids	• Needs maintenance
	• Does not sterilize powders, ointments or oils

Ophthalmic Instrument Sterilization

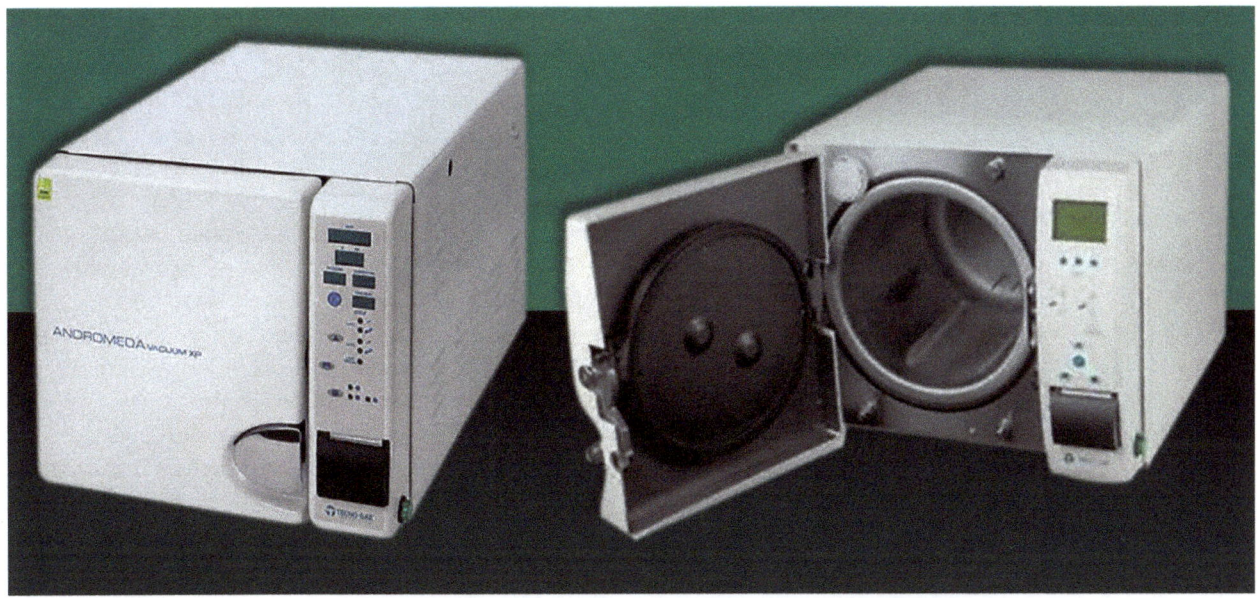

Figure 10.6 Moist heat method of sterilization (Autoclaves)

Table 10.2 Nature of objects with optimum time of autoclaving				
Type of sterilization	Item	Exposure time at 121°C	Exposure time at 132°C	Drying time
Gravity displacement	Wrapped instrument	30 minutes	15 minutes	15–30 minutes
	Textile packs	30 minutes	25 minutes	15 minutes
Pre-vacuum	Wrapped instrument		4 minutes	20–30 minutes
	Textile packs		4 minutes	20 minutes

and microbial killing, thus prolonging the time of sterilization. In addition, the high temperatures are not suitable for many materials.

Principle: Temperature and time are the two important parameters of sterilization by dry heat. The lethal effect is because of protein denaturation, oxidation of cell constituents and toxic effect of elevated levels of electrolytes.

Time of sterilization: The most common time-temperature relationships for sterilization with hot air sterilizers are 170°C for 60 minutes, 160°C for 120 minutes, and 150°C for 150 minutes.

Types of hot air ovens: There are two types of hot air ovens—the *static-air type* and the *forced-air type*. The static-air type has heating coils at the bottom, which cause the hot air to rise inside the chamber via gravity convection. It is much slower in heating, requires longer time to reach sterilizing temperature, and is less uniform in temperature control throughout the chamber. The forced-air or mechanical convection sterilizer is equipped with a motor-driven blower that circulates heated air throughout the chamber at a high velocity, permitting a more rapid and uniform transfer of energy from the air to the instruments.

Flash Sterilization[7]

Flash steam sterilization was originally defined as sterilization of unwrapped objects at 132°C for 3 minutes at 27–28 lbs. of pressure in a gravity displacement autoclave. It is thus a modification of conventional steam sterilization in which the flashed item is placed in an open tray or is placed in a specially designed, covered, rigid container to allow for rapid penetration of steam. It has quick sterilization cycle. The time required depends on the type of sterilizer and the type of item. Although the wrapped method of sterilization is preferred, correctly performed flash sterilization is an effective process for the sterilization of critical medical devices when it is in close proximity to the area of usage, e.g. operating rooms. It is not recommended as routine sterilization method but used only when there is insufficient time to sterilize the instruments such as in between cases.

Ethylene Oxide Method[8-11] (Fig. 10.7)

Ethylene oxide (EtO) is a colorless gas that is flammable and explosive. It has been widely used as a low-temperature sterilant since the 1950s and is one of the most commonly used processes for sterilizing temperature and moisture sensitive patient care items, without deleterious effects on the material used in the item. The main disadvantages associated with EtO are the lengthy cycle time, the cost, and its potential hazards to patients and staff. Other than the mild and moderate reactions and conditions like neuropathies, cataracts and abortions identified with the chronic exposure to EtO; it is also considered a known human carcinogen. EtO is absorbed by many materials and considering the toxicity of the gas, it is important that following sterilization the item must undergo aeration to remove residual EtO.

Principle

The four essential parameters are gas concentration (450–1000 mg/L), temperature (37–63°C), relative humidity (40–80%) as the water molecules carry EtO to reactive sites and exposure time (1–6 hours). It causes alkylation of protein, DNA, and RNA. Alkylation, or the replacement of a hydrogen atom with an alkyl group within cells prevents normal cellular metabolism and replication.[12]

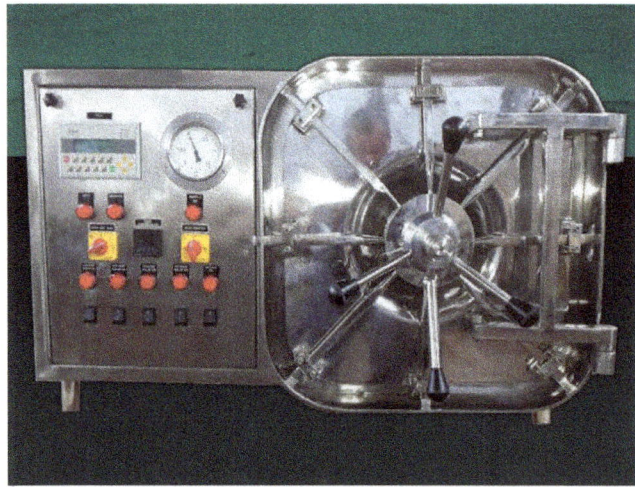

Figure 10.7 Ethylene oxide sterilization

Time of Sterilization

The basic EtO sterilization cycle consists of five stages, i.e. preconditioning and humidification, gas introduction, exposure, evacuation, and air washes. Excluding aeration time, the cycle takes approximately 3–9 hours depending on exposure time. Mechanical aeration for 8–12 hours at 50–60°C allows desorption of the toxic EtO residual contained in exposed absorbent materials. Thus, the total time of sterilization is 11–21 hours. Within certain limitations, an increase in gas concentration and temperature may shorten the time necessary for achieving sterilization. Two types of EtO sterilizers are available, mixed gas and 100% EtO. Until 1995, ethylene oxide sterilizers combined EtO with a chloroflourocarbon (CFC) stabilizing agent, most commonly in a ratio of 12% EtO mixed with 88% CFC (referred to as 12/88 EtO). More recently, 100% EtO is also being used for healthcare items. Alternative technologies to EtO with CFC that are currently available and cleared by the FDA for medical equipment include EtO with a different stabilizing gas, such as carbon dioxide or hydrochlorofluorocarbons (HCFC); immersion in peracetic acid; hydrogen peroxide gas plasma; and ozone.[12] Technologies under development for use in healthcare facilities, but not cleared by the FDA, include vaporized hydrogen peroxide, vapor phase peracetic acid, gaseous chlorine dioxide, ionizing radiation, or pulsed light.[13]

Hydrogen Peroxide Gas Plasma Method[14,15] (Fig. 10.8)

This is a new sterilization technology and gas plasmas have been referred to as the fourth state of matter (i.e. liquids, solids, gases, and gas plasmas). Gas plasmas are generated in a closed chamber under deep vacuum using radiofrequency or microwave energy to excite the gas molecules and produce charged particles, many of which are in the form of free radicals. A free radical is an atom with an unpaired electron and is a highly reactive species.

Hydrogen peroxide gas plasma system consists of a sterilization chamber which is evacuated and hydrogen peroxide solution is injected from a cassette and is vaporized in the sterilization chamber to a concentration of 6 mg/L. The hydrogen peroxide vapor diffuses through the chamber and comes in contact of all surfaces of the load. An electrical field created by a radiofrequency is applied to the chamber to create gas

Ophthalmic Instrument Sterilization

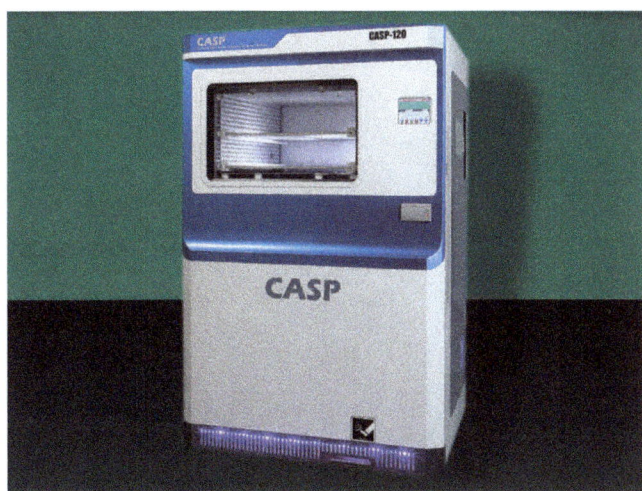

Figure 10.8 Gas plasma sterilization

plasma. Microbicidal free radicals (e.g. hydroxyl and hydroperoxyl) are generated in the plasma.

The steps in plasma sterilization are:
- Vacuum phase
- Injection phase
- Diffusion phase
- Plasma phase
- Vent phase

The excess gas is removed and in the final stage (i.e. vent) of the process the sterilization chamber is returned to atmospheric pressure by introduction of high-efficiency filtered air. If any moisture is present on the objects, the vacuum will not be achieved and the cycle aborts. The by-products of the cycle (e.g. water vapor, oxygen) are nontoxic and thus, the sterilized materials can be handled safely, either for immediate use or storage. This method may have advantages over the other alternatives, which have been depicted in **Table 10.3**.

Principle
It inactivates microorganisms primarily by the combined use of hydrogen peroxide gas and the generation of free radicals during the plasma phase of the cycle.

Time of Sterilization
The process operates in the range of 37–44°C and has a cycle time of 75 minutes. Newer versions with modifications in cycle time have sterilization time as short as 52 minutes and 38 minutes.

Table 10.3 Advantages and disadvantages of gas plasma method

Advantages	Disadvantages
• Safe for environment	• Paper, linen and liquids cannot be used
• Leave no toxic residuals	• Relatively large instrument
• Less cycle time	• Expensive
• No aeration required	
• Useful for heat sensitive material	

Peracetic Acid Method[14,16]

Peracetic acid is a highly biocidal oxidizer that maintains its efficacy in the presence of organic soil. It was introduced for use in patient care in 1988 in United States.

Principle
The proposed mechanism is as an oxidizing agent, i.e. it denatures proteins, disrupts cell wall permeability, and oxidizes sulfhydral and sulfur bonds in proteins, enzymes, and other metabolites.

Time of sterilization: 30–45 minutes

Ionising Radiation[17]

Sterilization by ionizing radiation, primarily by cobalt 60 gamma rays or electron accelerators, is a low-temperature sterilization method that has been used for a number of medical products (e.g. tissue for transplantation, pharmaceuticals, medical devices). There are no FDA-cleared ionizing radiation sterilization processes for use in healthcare facilities. Because of high sterilization costs, this method is an unfavorable alternative to EtO and plasma sterilization in healthcare set-ups. It is, however, suitable for large-scale sterilization. It is associated with deleterious effects on some patient-care equipment.

Other Methods

Ozone[18]
Ozone is produced when O_2 is energized and split into two monatomic (O_1) molecules. The monatomic oxygen molecules then collide with O_2 molecules to form ozone, which is O_3. Thus, ozone consists of O_2 with a loosely bound third oxygen atom that is readily available to attach to, and oxidize other molecules. This additional oxygen atom makes ozone a powerful oxidant that destroys microorganisms but is highly unstable, with

half-life of 22 minutes at room temperature. It has been used for years as a drinking water disinfectant. The use of ozone as a sterilant was cleared by FDA in August 2003 for processing reusable medical devices. The duration of the sterilization cycle is about 4 h and 15 m, and it occurs at 30–35°C. The process is considered to be safe for use by the operator because there is no handling of the sterilant, no toxic emissions, no residue to aerate, and low operating temperature means there is no danger of an accidental burn.

Microwave[8,19-21]

Microwaves are radiofrequency waves, which are usually used at a frequency of 2450 MHz. The microwaves produce friction of water molecules in an alternating electrical field. The intermolecular friction derived from the vibrations generates heat and some authors believe that the effect of microwaves depends on the heat produced while others postulate a non-thermal lethal effect. Microwaves used for sterilization of medical devices have not been FDA cleared.

Vaporized Hydrogen Peroxide[22,23]

Vaporized hydrogen peroxide (VHP) as a sterilant was considered in mid-1980s. It offers advantages like rapid cycle time (e.g. 30–45 minutes), low temperature, environmentally safe by-products, good material compatibility; and ease of operation, installation and monitoring. It has limitations including less penetration and deleterious effects on some materials like cellulose and nylon. VHP has not been cleared by FDA for sterilization of medical devices in healthcare facilities.

Formaldehyde Steam[24]

Low-temperature steam with formaldehyde is used as a low-temperature sterilization method in some countries. The process involves the use of formalin, which is vaporized into a formaldehyde gas that is admitted into the sterilization chamber. A formaldehyde concentration of 8–16 mg/L is generated at an operating temperature of 70–75°C. The sterilization cycle consists of a series of stages that include an initial vacuum to remove air from the chamber and load, followed by steam admission to the chamber with the vacuum pump running to purge the chamber of air and to heat the load, followed by a series of pulses of formaldehyde gas, followed by steam. Formaldehyde is removed from the sterilizer and load by repeated alternate evacuations and flushing with steam and air.

This system has some advantages, e.g. the cycle time for formaldehyde gas is faster than that for EtO and the cost per cycle is relatively low. However, it is less penetrating and operates at higher temperatures than other low temperature strerilizing methods.

Performic Acid

Performic acid is a fast-acting sporicide. However, systems using performic acid are not currently FDA cleared.

A summary of commonly used sterilization technologies is given in **Table 10.4**.

INSTRUMENT STERILIZATION IN OPHTHALMIC OT

- Vitrectomy cutters, cautery wires, cryoprobes and retinal instruments should only be autoclaved. The alternative method is EtO sterilization. They should be totally dry and packaged in polythene bags with indicator tapes inside.
- Suture material should ideally be disposed off and should not be reused after sterilization.
- OT clothing should be thoroughly washed with detergent and dried. They are then neatly folded and packed for autoclaving with the indicator tape on the outside. Disposable caps and masks are preferred for use which are not sterilized. In hospitals where linen cap is used, the same method of sterilization as OT clothing is followed.
- Sterilization of irrigating solutions is carried out at many places by autoclaving. However, this may be omitted in sealed glass bottles with clear solution. Exposure to ultraviolet light may be carried out for 2–4 hours before use.
- Chemical sterilization of instruments should be avoided. Inadequate wash off of the chemical can lead to *toxic anterior segment syndrome.*
- *Sterilization of sharp instruments:* The preferred method of sterilization is autoclave with the alternative method being EtO sterilization.
- Sutures, keratomes and viscoelastics should ideally be used in a single setting. They should be discarded after single use and should not be reused after sterilization. **Table 10.5** shows few common objects used inside the ophthalmic OT and their preferred method of sterilization.

It is not necessary to have all the facilities in your operation theatre for sterilization of instruments.

Table 10.4 Summary of commonly used sterilization technologies

Sterilization method	Advantages	Disadvantages	Uses
Steam under pressure (Autoclave)	• Nontoxic to patient, staff and environment • Rapidly microbicidal and sporicidal • Rapid cycle time • Minimally affected by organic/inorganic soils • Penetrates medical packing, device lumens • Cycle easy to control and monitor • Inexpensive	• Deleterious for heat and moisture sensitive instruments • Microsurgical instruments damaged by repeated exposure • May leave instruments wet, causing them to rust • Potential for burns	• Most efficient and reliable method of sterilization • Used for all heat and moisture resistant critical and semi-critical items, e.g. surgical instruments, drapes, dressings, etc.
Dry heat (Hot air oven)	• Nontoxic to patient, staff and environment • Cycle easy to control and monitor • Inexpensive • Noncorrosive	• Uneven penetration due to non-uniform flow • Time consuming • Deleterious for heat and moisture sensitive instruments • Potential for burns	• Used only on heat resistant, moisture sensitive/impermeable items, e.g. sharp instruments, glassware, powders, etc.
Flash sterilization	• Rapid sterilization • Useful if kept at the point of use of sterilized items	• Prone to contamination as packing not done • Potential for burns	• Used for heat resistant, critical and semicritical medical devices, for immediate use
Ethylene oxide (EtO)	• Penetrates packaging materials, device lumens • Simple to operate and monitor • Compatible with most medical materials	• Requires aeration time to remove EtO residue, thus time consuming • EtO is toxic, a carcinogen, and flammable • Costly	• Used for heat and moisture sensitive critical and semicritical items
Hydrogen Peroxide Gas Plasma	• Safe for the environment • Leaves no toxic residuals • Cycle time is less, 28–75 minutes (varies with model type) and no aeration necessary • Simple to operate, install and monitor • Compatible with most medical devices • Good material compatibility	• Cellulose (paper), linens and liquids cannot be processed • Some endoscopes or medical devices with long or narrow lumens cannot be processed • Requires synthetic packaging (polypropylene wraps, polyolefin pouches) and special container tray • Hydrogen peroxide may be toxic at levels greater than 1 ppmTWA • Moisture interferes with the performance • Costly	• Used for heat- and moisture-sensitive items since process temperature <50°C
Peracetic acid	• Rapid cycle time (30–45 minutes) • Environmental friendly by-products • Sterilant flows through endoscope which facilitates salt, protein and microbe removal • Compatible with wide variety of instruments and materials	• Point-of-use system, no sterile storage • Biological indicator may not be suitable for routine monitoring • Used for immersible instruments only • Some material incompatibility (e.g. aluminum anodized coating becomes dull) • Potential for serious eye and skin damage with contact • Relatively costly	• Mostly advocated for sterilization of endoscopes

Table 10.5 Few common objects used in the OT with their respective methods of sterilization

Article to be sterilized	Sterilizing method
Linen	Autoclaving
Glassware	Autoclaving/Dry heat
Metal instrument-heat labile	Ethylene oxide/dry heat/plasma sterilization
Metal instrument-heat resistant	Autoclaving
Plastic instrument	Ethylene oxide/plasma sterilization
Vitrectomy cutters	Autoclaving/ethylene oxide
Sharp-edge instrument	Autoclaving/ethylene oxide/plasma sterilization
Intraocular lenses	Ethylene oxide
Sutures	Autoclaving/ethylene oxide
Diathermy/cautery electrodes	Autoclaving/ethylene oxide
Endoilluminators	Ethylene oxide
Buckles/Sponges	Autoclaving

(Adapted from Gajiwala UR. Journal of Clinical Ophthalmology and Research)

A vertical autoclave can be used for sterilization of almost all instruments except for cannulated instruments such as tubings which require a horizontal autoclave. To conclude, a comprehensive understanding of cleaning, sterilization and disinfection of operation theatres and patient care articles in operating rooms is as valuable as expertize in surgical procedures and other interventions, for a favorable outcome of ophthalmic surgeries and interventions.

REFERENCES

1. WHO Glossary.
2. http://www.cdc.gov/hicpac/pdf/guidelines/disinfection_nov_2008.pdf
3. Roberts CG. Studies on the bioburden on medical devices and the importance of cleaning. In: Rutala WA, Ed. Disinfection, sterilization and antisepsis: principles and practices in healthcare facilities. Washington, DC: Association for Professional in Infection Control and Epidemiology; 2001. pp. 63-9.
4. Reichert M. Preparation of supplies for terminal sterilization. In: Reichert M, Young JH (Eds). Sterilization technology for the health care facility. Gaithersburg, MD: Aspen Publication; 1997. pp. 36-50.
5. Joslyn L. Sterilization by heat. In: Block SS (Ed). Disinfection, sterilization, and preservation. Philadelphia: Lippincott Williams & Wilkins; 2001. pp. 695-728.
6. Agalloco JP, Akers JE, Madsen RE. Moist heat sterilization--myths and realities. PDA J. Pharmaceutical Sci. Technol. 1998;52:346-50.
7. Rutala WA. Disinfection and flash sterilization in the operating room. J Ophthal Nurs Technol. 1991;10: 106-15.
8. Association for the Advancement of Medical Instrumentation. Ethylene oxide sterilization in health care facilities: Safety and effectiveness. AAMI. Arlington, VA, 1999.
9. Occupational Safety and Health Administration. Ethylene Oxide: OSHA Fact Sheet: Occupational Safety and Health Administration, 2002.
10. Lindbohm ML, Hemminki K, Bonhomme MG, et al. Effects of paternal occupational exposure on spontaneous abortions. Am J Public Health. 1991;81:1029-33.
11. Parisi AN, Young WE. Sterilization with ethylene oxide and other gases. In: Block SS (Ed). Disinfection, sterilization, and preservation. Philadelphia: Lea & Febiger; 1991. pp. 580-95.
12. Schneider PM. New technologies for disinfection and sterilization. In: Rutala WA (Ed). Disinfection, sterilization and antisepsis: Principles, practices, challenges, and new research. Washington DC: Association for Professionals in Infection Control and Epidemiology; 2004. pp. 127-39.
13. Schneider PM. Emerging low temperature sterilization technologies (non-FDA approved). In: Rutala WA (Ed). Disinfection, sterilization, and antisepsis in healthcare. Champlain, New York: Polyscience Publications; 1998. pp. 79-92.
14. Rutala WA, Gergen MF, Weber DJ. Comparative evaluation of the sporicidal activity of new low-temperature sterilization technologies: ethylene oxide, 2 plasma sterilization systems, and liquid peracetic acid. Am J Infect. Control. 1998;26:393-8.
15. Jacobs PT, Lin SM. Sterilization processes utilizing low-temperature plasma. In: Block SS (Ed). Disinfection, sterilization, and preservation. Philadelphia: Lippincott Williams & Wilkins; 2001. pp. 747-63.
16. Block SS. Peroxygen compounds. In: Block SS (Ed). Disinfection, sterilization, and preservation. Philadelphia: Lippincott Williams & Wilkins; 2001. pp. 185-204.
17. Russell AD. Ionizing radiation. In: Russell AD, Hugo WB, Ayliffe GAJ (Eds). Principles and practices of disinfection, preservation and sterilization. Oxford: Blackwell Science; 1999. pp. 675-87.
18. Berrington AW, Pedler SJ. Investigation of gaseous ozone for MRSA decontamination of hospital side-rooms. J Hosp Infect. 1998;40:61-5.

19. Rohrer MD, Bulard RA. Microwave sterilization. J Am Dent Assoc. 1985;110:194-8.
20. Rohrer MD, Terry MA, Bulard RA, Graves DC, Taylor EM. Microwave sterilization of hydrophilic contact lenses. Am J Ophthalmol. 1986;101:49-57.
21. Najdovski L, Dragas AZ, Kotnik V. The killing activity of microwaves on some nonsporogenic and sporogenic medically important bacterial strains. J Hosp Infect. 1991;19:239-47.
22. Bates CJ, Pearse R. Use of hydrogen peroxide vapour for environmental control during a *Serratia* outbreak in a neonatal intensive care unit. J Hosp Infect. 2005;61:364-6.
23. Boyce JM, Havill NL, Otter JA, et al. Impact of hydrogen peroxide vapor room bio-decontamination on environmental contamination and nosocomial transmission of *Clostridium difficile*. The Society of Healthcare Epidemiology of America, 2006; Abstract 155:109.
24. Petrocci AN. Surface active agents: quaternary ammonium compounds. In: Block SS (Ed). Disinfection, sterilization, and preservation. Philadelphia: Lea & Febiger; 1983. pp. 309-29.

CHAPTER 11

Waste Disposal in Ophthalmic Operation Theatre

Reena Singh, Rajesh Sinha

INTRODUCTION

Any healthcare facility can produce enormous amount of waste that can be both hazardous and non-hazardous in nature. Proper disposal of healthcare waste is immensely important for infection control in hospitals and also for the environment. The National Accreditation Board for Hospitals and Healthcare Providers (NABH) has defined the standards for infection control in hospitals enlisted in **Table 11.1**.[1] The waste generated in healthcare facilities can be infectious or noninfectious. The biomedical wastes include the waste that is potentially infectious. These can be solid or liquid. The sharps are included in biomedical waste whether they are infected or not, since they have the possibility of being contaminated with blood and have a propensity to cause injury when not properly contained and disposed off.

In India, the management laws for handling these wastes were passed in 1998. Further amendments were done on 28th March 2016. These rules were notified by the central government. The states have been given the responsibility for implementing these rules.[2] Even though the Government of India has established laws for waste management, however, most of the establishments lack in implementing them. This improper management can be hazardous for the environment, in which we have to live.

Proper waste management in ophthalmology OT includes various steps before final disposal of wastes. These steps include:
- Categorization of waste in OT
- Segregation and accumulation of categorized waste
- Packaging of segregated wastes
- Transportation of packed wastes from OT to final site of treatment or disposal
- Treatment of waste.

Table 11.1	NABH guidelines for setting standards for management for infection control including hospital waste management
HIC 1	Hospital should have properly designed and coordinated hospital infection prevention and control for patients, visitors and also for health care providers
HIC 2	Infection control manual should be implemented in all areas of hospital
HIC 3	Surveillance and monitoring of infection control should be done by the hospital organization
HIC 4	Hospital should take action to prevent and control healthcare associated infections (HAI) in patients
HIC 5	Hospital should provides adequate resources for prevention and control of healthcare associated infections (HAI)
HIC 6	The hospital should identify and properly control the outbreaks of infections
HIC 7	There should be documented policies and procedures for sterilization activities in the organization
HIC 8	**Biomedical waste (BMW) should be handled appropriately and safely**
HIC 9	The infection control program should be supported by the management and include the training of staff

Abbreviations: HIC, Hospital Infection Control; NABH, National Accreditation Board of Hospitals and Healthcare Providers

CATEGORIZATION OF WASTE IN OPERATION THEATRE

The term "medical waste" covers all wastes produced in healthcare or diagnostic activities. 75–90% of hospital wastes are similar to household refuse or municipal waste and do not entail any particular hazard. The other 10–25% is called hazardous medical waste or special waste. This type of waste entails health risks. It can be divided into five categories according to the risks involved. **Table 11.2** gives a description of these various categories and their sub-groups. The various kinds of waste that can be expected to be generated in ophthalmic OT are paper, clothes, linen, polybags, plastic, glasses, sharp waste (needles, scalpels, keratomes, clear knives, crescents, etc.), blood and body fluid spillage (including urine, vomitus), pathological waste, anatomical waste, chemical and pharmaceutical waste. All the staff including doctors, nursing staff, OT assistants and sweepers should have been properly trained and informed about the type of wastes generated in OT.

SEGREGATION AND ACCUMULATION OF CATEGORIZED WASTE

Best way of segregation is to encourage all the OT personnel to put the waste in color coded bags/containers designated for that specific types of waste **(Fig. 11.1)**. Simply throwing the wastes in these appropriate bags or containers will be of immense help to the cleaning staff at the end of the OT day for segregation, packaging and transportation of wastes for adequate disposal. Worldwide, there are specific colored bags, bins and labels that are recommended for each type of waste **(Table 11.3)**. The bags can be made of polyethylene of specific colors. The bags must be placed either in rigid containers or on castor-fitted stands. In certain circumstances, if no plastic bags are available, the containers must first be emptied, then washed and disinfected with 5% active chlorine solution before reusing them. Sharps should be accumulated and put in puncture proof containers with lid with proper indicators/labels **(Fig. 11.2)**. Do not bend, recap,

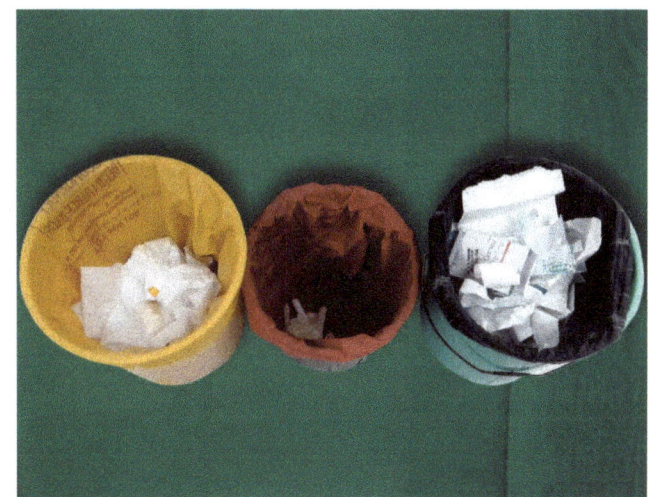

Figure 11.1 Different colors of bags fitted in plastic containers

Table 11.2 International Committee of the Red Cross (ICRS) classification of hazardous medical waste	
1. Sharps	• Waste entailing risk of injury
2. a. Waste entailing risk of contamination b. Anatomical waste c. Infectious wastes	• Waste containing blood, secretions or excreta entailing a risk of contamination. • Body parts, tissue entailing a risk of contamination • Waste with possible risk of propagating infectious agents (cultures of infectious agents, waste from infectious patients placed in isolation wards)
3. a. Pharmaceutical waste b. Cytotoxic waste c. Waste containing heavy metals d. Chemical waste	• Spilled/unused medicines, expired drugs and used medication receptacles. • Expired or leftover cytotoxic drugs, equipment • Mercury waste (broken thermometers or manometers, compact fluorescent light tubes, batteries) • Chemical substances: leftover laboratory solvents, disinfectants, photographic developers and fixers
4. Pressurized containers	• Gas cylinders, aerosol cans
5. Radioactive waste	• Waste containing radioactive substances: radionuclides used in laboratories or nuclear medicine, urine or excreta of patients treated

Ocular Infections: Prophylaxis and Management

Table 11.3 Specific color bags/bins that are recommended for different types of waste

Waste type	Classification	Color	Description of wastes
Municipal waste	Nonhazardous	(Black)	Includes the domestic type wastes like residual food, food packaging paper/magazines that cannot be recycled
Pharmacological wastes, drugs and tubing	Nonhazardous waste medicines, out of date medicines, denatured drugs which requires disposal by incineration	(Blue)	Saline bottles, intravenous tubing sets, pharmalogical wastes, drugs tablets in container, blister packs, liquid bottles, inhaler cartridge and droplet bottles with pipettes
Clinical/highly infectious waste	Hazardous, highly infectious waste which requires disposal by incineration	(Yellow)	Test vials, anatomical waste, reagents, wipes, gloves, dressings, bandages, aprons, disposable garments soiled with infectious body fluids
Potentially infectious waste	Hazardous/Nonhazardous	(Red)	Includes residual autoclave waste, laboratory wastes, blood-contaminated dressings, contaminated disposable gowns, clinical gloves, swabs, saliva-contaminated items from known infectious patients or where medical history is not available
Cytotoxic/Cytostatic waste	Hazardous	(Purple)	Blister packs, tablets in container, unopened medicines, patches, gloves, gowns, aprons, wipes contaminated with cytotoxic and/or cytostatic medicine
Clinical/infectious waste	Hazardous/Nonhazardous	(Orange)	Wipes, gloves, dressings, bandages, aprons

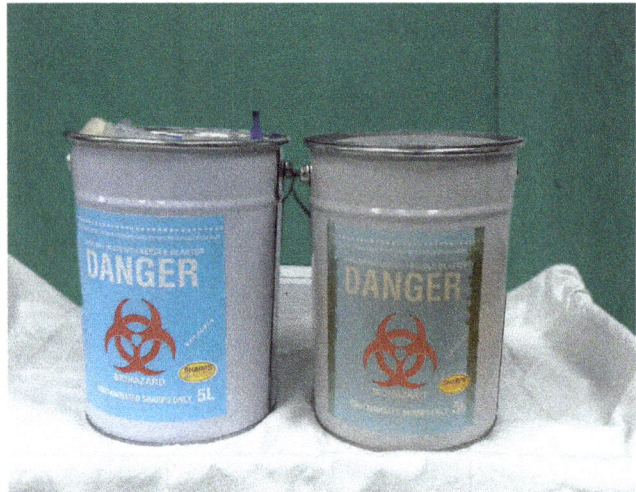

Figure 11.2 Metal puncture proof containers in OT for on-site disposal of sharps

or break used syringe needles before discarding them into a container. Used gowns and towels are collected in large buckets. There should be a separate sorting and cleaning of gowns and linen used for routine cases from those that have been worn for infective cases and soiled with blood or other infective materials spillage.

PACKAGING OF SEGREGATED WASTES

At the end of each day of operation theatre, the waste generated at various sites in OT is aggregated by the cleaning staff **(Figs 11.3A and B)**. Appropriate personal protective measures should be used by all the OT staff handling these wastes. The type of packaging used will vary depending upon the type of waste produced. If the waste consists of sharps, it should only be placed in a sharps receptacle that includes puncture proof containers with lids. Liquids or containers with free liquids (e.g. a partially-discharged syringe body) should be placed in rigid leak proof plastic drums. All other waste may be packaged in flexible bags (infectious or offensive waste bags). The staff handling these wastes should use protective gloves, masks, gowns and protective goggles if needed. The bags of wastes should be only $2/3^{rd}$ filled and should be held carefully on the

Waste Disposal in Ophthalmic Operation Theatre

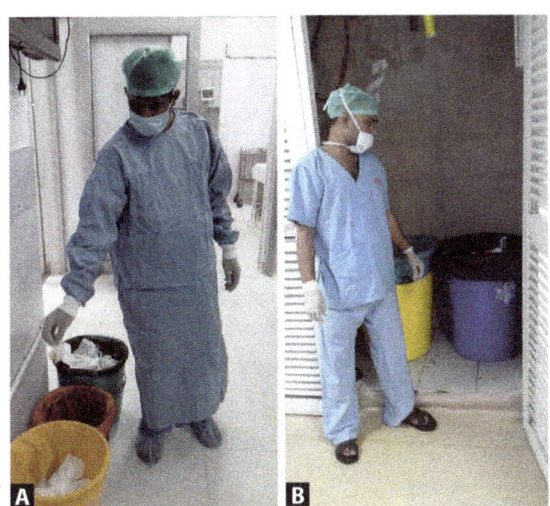

Figures 11.3A and B Waste storage inside the OT at the site of generation (A) and aggregation at a temporary storage site in the OT premises (B)

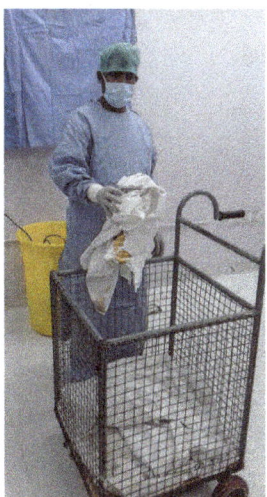

Figure 11.4 On-site mode of transport of disposable gowns, linen and towels inside OT for disposal

upper part of bag while transferring it to main storage site for aggregation.

TRANSPORTATION OF PACKED WASTES FROM OT TO FINAL SITE OF TREATMENT OR DISPOSAL

After collection and packaging of wastes in OT, transportation of wastes depends upon whether the final treatment of wastes are planned on-site inside the hospital premises or off-site at distance places. The on-site involves different type of conveyance like containers on wheel, carts, etc. **(Fig. 11.4)**. Off-site treatment and disposal involves a team of waste disposal services, those who are trained for collecting and handling the biomedical wastes. The wastes are loaded inside cardboard boxes, reusable plastic bins and covered puncture proof containers as required. The vehicles involved for transportation should be properly covered in a secured manner and properly labelled for such transportation.

TREATMENT OF WASTE

The purpose of biomedical waste treatment is to make it safe by reducing the actual amount, eliminating its infectious potential and if possible to make it unrecognizable. Treatment should render the waste safe for subsequent handling and disposal. As mentioned, waste treatment can be done on-site inside the hospital premises or off-site at some distant place outside the site of its generation. However, all the healthcare establishments do not have on-site treatment facilities as it involves a lot of space, labor and budget for such equipment and management, that is why most of the hospitals have the off-site disposal arrangements.

There are various methods of final disposition of waste including landfill, incineration/combustion, recovery and recycling, plasma gasification and composting. Hospitals should develop at least some facilities for inactivation of infectious wastes to reduce the infectious waste load by an approved inactivation method (e.g. autoclaving) before transporting for disposal. There are various treatment methods that can be used for different types of wastes inside and outside the hospital premises. The autoclaving uses steam at high pressure for sterilizing the waste or to decrease the infectious load of wastes to a point at which it may be safely disposed. For sharps, a sharp blaster/needle shredder may be used as a final treatment step to render the waste unrecognizable. Incineration can be another effective method for destroying the pathogens and changing it to non-recognizable ash leading to a decrease in the quantity of waste. For liquids and small quantity waste, the disinfectant solutions like 1–10% bleach and sodium hydroxide can be used. Local draining sanitary sewers can be used for safe disposal of blood, suctioned fluids, ground tissues, excretions and secretions. The government has given permission for this disposal if it is not leading to environment hazards.

TRAINING OF STAFF HANDLING WASTE DISPOSAL IN OPERATION THEATRE

The policy of waste management will only be effective if it is properly supervised and monitored. These policies should be consistently applied in all areas of the hospital and concerned healthcare staff should be properly trained. The staff should be aware of their job related responsibilities. Ideally, targeted training sessions should be arranged for different staff groups. The training should involve the following staff:

- Doctors
- Nursing staff
- Infection control staff
- Healthcare managers
- Administrative staff responsible for implementing regulations on healthcare waste management
- Cleaners, porters, auxiliary staff and waste handlers

The training should be done in a simple, understandable language. The training should focus on different aspects of waste management like identifying the different types of waste, sorting of wastes and identifying hazardous and non-hazardous wastes. The training should be scheduled on a routine basis and repeated regularly.

REFERENCES

1. Guide Book to Accreditation Standards for Hospitals. 4th edn. National Accreditation Board for Hospitals and Healthcare Providers: December 2015.
2. Disposal of medical waste. Press Information Bureau. 25 July 2014. Retrieved 25 July 2014.

CHAPTER 12

Quality Control and Surveillance

Nishat Hussain Ahmed, Gita Satpathy, Neelima Aron

INTRODUCTION

Quality control and surveillance of cleaning, sterilization and disinfection of operation theatres and treatment of patient care articles are of paramount importance. The quality control acts as a check for the correctness of the procedures employed for rendering the patient care articles and space, safe for invasive interventions. Along with quality control and surveillance of the procedures—stringent adherence to sterilization and disinfection guidelines, use of personal protective equipment, maintenance of code of conduct during the treatment of OT and patient care articles, proper storage and transport of the articles, compliance with operation theatre discipline and infection control measures; all are essential to minimize the ingress of infective agents during the intervention.

QUALITY CONTROL

For quality control of a procedure undertaken for sterilization or disinfection, certain indicators are used. Indicators are signature parameters, which specify whether or not a particular end result has been achieved in the procedure employed. The indicators thus vary with the type of procedure employed, the time of performing the procedure, the article or space which has been treated in the procedure and the intended use of the treated article or space. Routinely, combinations of mechanical, chemical, and biological indicators are used to evaluate the sterilization/disinfection conditions and indirectly the microbiologic status of the processed items/treated space.

A sterilization process should be verified before it is put into use in healthcare settings. All sterilizers are first tested mechanically for the required mechanical parameters. The parameters are matched with the standard for treatment of specific articles as per the guidelines or manufacturer's instructions. The sterilizers are also tested with biological and chemical indicators upon installation, when the sterilizer is relocated, redesigned, after major repair and after sterilization failure has occurred; to ensure proper functioning before treating the patient care articles. Three consecutive empty cycles are run with a biological and chemical indicator in an appropriate test package, placed in the core position of the machine. The sterilizer is not put into use until all biological indicators are negative and chemical indicators show a correct end-point response.[1-4]

Along with monitoring of mechanical parameters with each run of the sterilizer, biological and chemical indicator testing is also done for ongoing quality assurance testing of representative samples of actual products being sterilized and product testing when major changes are made in packaging, wraps, or load configuration. Biological and chemical indicators are placed in products, which are processed in a full load. When three consecutive cycles show negative biological indicators and chemical indicators with a correct end-point response, the change made can be put into routine use. Items processed in those three cycles should be quarantined until the test results are negative.[1-4] **Table 12.1** shows the quality control of different sterilization procedures for monitoring the safety of the treated patient-care articles.

Table 12.1 Quality control of different sterilization procedures

Sterilization Procedure	Mechanical monitoring	Chemical monitoring	Biological monitoring
Steam under pressure (Autoclave)	Pressure, temperature and time to be monitored and documented with each cycle	• Internal and external indicator strips to be put in each article with each cycle • Bowie Dick test to be done daily for vacuum sterilizer	• *Geobacillus stearothermophilus* spores (10^5) to be used at least weekly • If several loads are run per day or implantable devices are processed, biological monitoring to be done daily • Loads containing implantable devices to be ideally quarantined till results of biological indicators are available
Dry-Heat (Hot air oven)	Temperature and time to be monitored and documented with each cycle	Internal and external indicator strips to be put in each article with each cycle	• *Bacillus atrophaeus* spores (10^6) to be used at least weekly • If several loads are run per day or implantable devices are processed, biological monitoring to be done daily • Loads containing implantable devices to be ideally quarantined till results of biological indicators are available
Flash sterilization	Pressure, temperature and time to be monitored and documented with each cycle	As articles are not packed, indicator strips cannot be put on individual items, however, chemical monitoring of each cycle should be done	• Conventional biological indicators are not suitable • Rapid-readout biological indicator containing *Geobacillus stearothermophilus* spores can be used once weekly
Ethylene oxide (Eto)	• Pressure, temperature and time to be monitored and documented with each cycle • Gas concentration and humidity cannot be mechanically monitored in healthcare EtO sterilizers	Internal and external indicator strips to be put in each article with each cycle	• *Bacillus atrophaeus* spores (10^6) to be used at least weekly • If several loads are run per day or implantable devices are processed, biological monitoring to be done daily • Loads containing implantable devices to be ideally quarantined till results of biological indicators are available • Rapid-readout biological indicator containing *Bacillus atrophaeus* spores can also be used
Hydrogen peroxide gas plasma	Mechanical and chemical monitoring is inbuilt. It records the concentration of active ingredients and contact time with each cycle		*Geobacillus stearothermophilus* spores (10^5) to be used at least weekly
Peracetic acid	Time to be monitored and documented with each cycle	Chemical monitoring strips which detect the concentration of active ingredient	*Geobacillus stearothermophilus* spores (10^5) to be used at least weekly

Periodic infection control rounds to areas using sterilizers are essential to standardize the use of the sterilizer and supervise operator competence. Documentation of sterilization records, including mechanical, chemical and biological indicator test results, sterilizer maintenance and wrapping, and load numbering of packs is equally significant. Supervision and documentation are imperative to ensure correctness of the procedures, to identify areas of improvement and to ensure that operators are adhering to the established standards.[1,5]

Mechanical Indicators

Mechanical indicators include the physical parameters, such as cycle time, temperature, pressure, concentration of sterilant, relative humidity, vacuum generation, etc.

The mechanical monitors for steam sterilization include the daily assessment of cycle time and temperature by examining the temperature record chart or computer printout of the same, and an assessment of pressure via the pressure gauge. The mechanical monitors for EtO include time, temperature, and

Quality Control and Surveillance

pressure recorders that provide information via computer printouts, gauges, and/or displays. Generally, two important elements for ethylene oxide (EtO) sterilization (i.e. the gas concentration and humidity) cannot be mechanically monitored in healthcare EtO sterilizers.[3]

At some places, biological monitors are not used routinely to monitor the sterilization procedure. Instead, release of sterilizer items is based on monitoring the physical conditions of the sterilization process that is termed 'parametric release.' Parametric release requires that there is a defined quality system in place at the facility performing the sterilization and that the sterilization process be validated for the items being sterilized. 'Parametric release' is, at present, accepted in Europe for steam, dry heat, and ionizing radiation processes, as the physical conditions are understood and can be monitored directly. For example, in steam sterilizers the load could be monitored with probes that would yield data on temperature, time, and humidity at representative locations in the chamber and compared to the specifications developed during the validation process.[1,6]

Chemical Indicators

Chemical indicators are sterilization process monitoring devices designed to respond with a chemical or physical change in the form of change in color to one or more of the physical conditions within the sterilizing chamber. They are often used to detect sterilizer malfunction/failures resulting from improper loading of the sterilizer, faulty packaging, inadequacy of the sterilizing agent, or malfunction of the sterilizer itself.[7] Chemical indicators are convenient, are inexpensive, and indicate whether the item has been exposed to the sterilization process in a satisfactory manner or not. Chemical indicators should be used in conjunction with biological indicators, but should not replace them because only a biological indicator consisting of resistant spores can measure the microbial killing power of the sterilization process.[8]

Types of Chemical Indicators

External indicators: They are affixed outside of each pack and verify that the package has simply been exposed to the sterilization process, but these indicators do not prove that sterilization has been achieved, e.g. steam indicator tape (autoclave tape).

Internal indicators: They are placed in every sterilization package to ensure the sterilization agent has penetrated the packaging material and actually reached the instruments inside.

Chemical indicators usually are either heat- or chemical-sensitive inks that change color when one or more sterilization parameters (e.g. steam-time, temperature, and/or saturated steam; EtO-time, temperature, relative humidity and/or EtO concentration) are present **(Figs 12.1 to 12.4)**. If the indicator suggests inadequate processing, the item should not be used.[1-5]

Chemical indicators have been grouped into five classes based on their ability to monitor one or multiple sterilization parameters.[7]

Process indicators (Class 1): The most basic of chemical indicators, they are also known as throughput indicators. They are intended for use with individual items to be sterilized and demonstrate that the item has been exposed to a sterilization process; thus distinguishing between processed and non-processed items.

Indicators for use in specific tests (Class 2): Also known as specialty indicators, they are designed for use in specific test procedures as defined by relevant

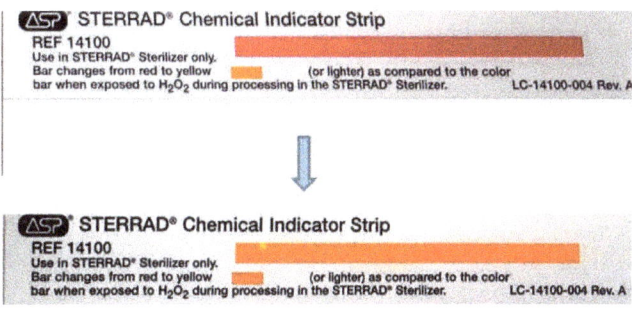

Figure 12.1 Chemical indicator strips suggestive of adequate sterilization by change of color at the end of procedure. Note the color change to orange/yellow when exposed to hydrogen peroxide

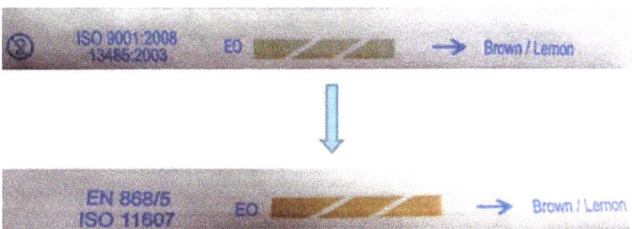

Figure 12.2 Chemical indicator strips suggestive of color change from brown to lemon at the end of sterilization process

sterilization standards. Example of Class 2 indicators is the Bowie-Dick test used in steam sterilizers. Bowie-Dick test is explained in more detail below.

Single-parameter indicators (Class 3): These indicators react to one of the critical process parameters of sterilization indicating exposure to a sterilization cycle at stated values of the chosen parameter. Critical parameters typically chosen for steam sterilization processes, are time or temperature.

Multi-parameter indicators (Class 4): These indicators are more accurate by design than Class 3 indicators.

They react to two or more critical parameters of the sterilization process and indicate exposure to the sterilization cycle at stated values of the chosen parameters. Time and temperature are chosen for steam sterilization parameters, and time and concentration of ethylene oxide (EtO) sterilization.

Integrating Indicators (Class 5): These indicators, known as "integrators," are designed to react to all critical parameters over a specified range of sterilization cycles. Their performance has been correlated to the performance of biological indicators.

Bowie-Dick test: In pre-vacuum steam sterilizer, generation of vacuum is important for proper sterilization of items. For testing the efficacy of the vacuum system in a pre-vacuum sterilizer, three consecutive empty cycles are run with a Bowie-Dick test, which is a class 2 chemical indicator. The test is also used each day the vacuum-type steam sterilizer is used, before the first processed load. Air that is not removed from the chamber will interfere with steam contact. The Bowie-Dick test detects air leaks and inadequate air removal, and consists of clean and preconditioned- folded 100% cotton surgical towels, in the centre of which is placed a sheet having chemical indicator. The sheet shows uniform color change with satisfactory steam contact as a result of proper vacuum generation **(Fig. 12.5)**. The test kit simulates the product to be sterilized and pockets of air act as a barrier that prevents steam from penetrating the load. Entrapped air thus causes a spotty or non-uniform change in the test sheet, due to the inability of the steam to reach the chemical indicator. Thus no or non-uniform color change indicates unsuccessful run. If the

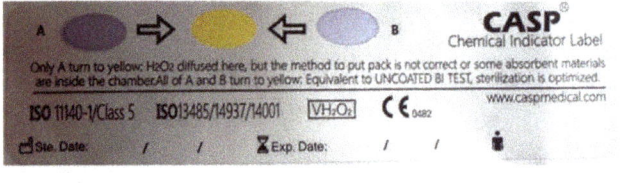

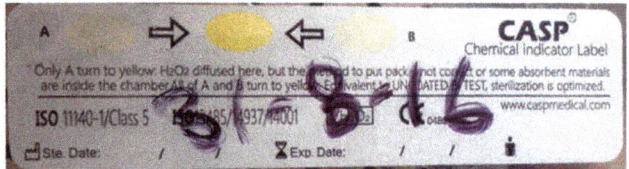

Figure 12.3 Chemical indicator strips for plasma sterilization with colour change to yellow from purple suggestive of adequate sterilization

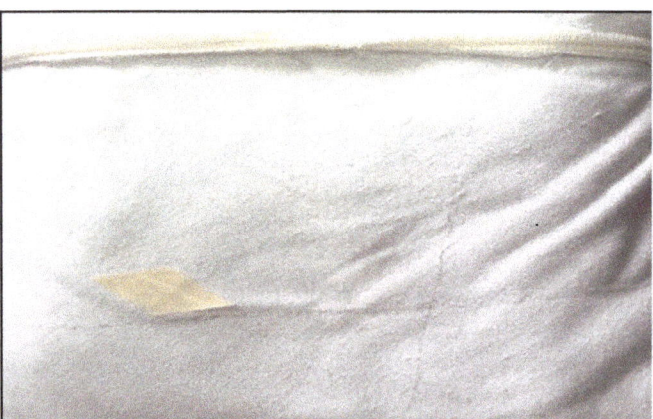
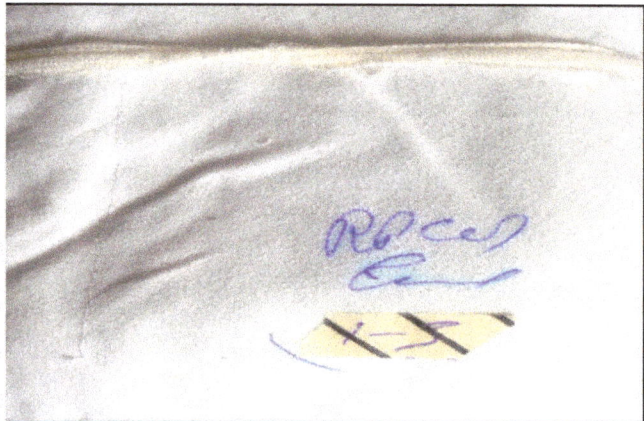

Figure 12.4 Chemical indicator strips pasted outside the linen packages with color change from white to black

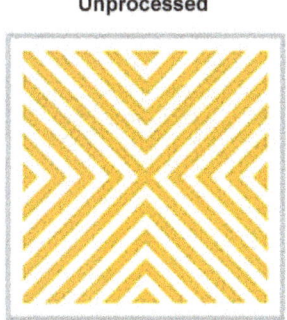 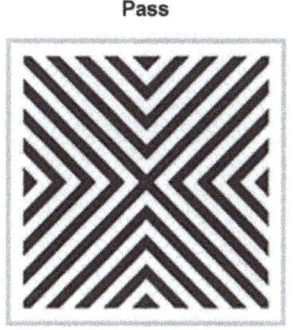 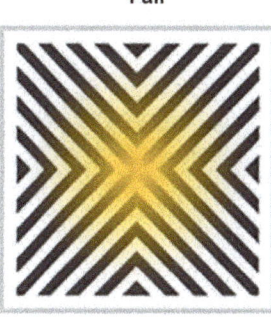

Figure 12.5 Bowie-Dick test sheet. Left one is unprocessed sheet, middle one is showing uniform change in color indicative of satisfactory steam contact as a result of proper vacuum generation, and the right one is showing nonuniform color change indicating an unsuccessful run

sterilizer fails the Bowie-Dick test, it is not to be used for patient care items, until it is inspected by the sterilizer maintenance personnel. After the cause of failure is rectified, three consecutive empty cycles of Bowie-Dick tests should be passed by the sterilizer before patient-care articles are sterilized.[2,4]

Chemical indicators monitor individual pack/package, whereas biological indicators monitor the whole load. Thus, it is extremely advantageous to use chemical indicator as it allows you to single out individual packs that weren't exposed to sufficient sterilization parameters. So if the load passes biological testing, but the chemical indicator on a pack fails, you only need to recall and reprocess that particular pack.

Biological Indicators

Biological indicators are closest to the ideal monitors of the sterilization process because they measure the sterilization process directly by using the spores of most resistant microorganisms and not merely by testing the physical and chemical conditions necessary for sterilization. Since the spores used in biological indicators are more resistant and present in greater numbers than are the common microbial contaminants found on patient-care equipment, the demonstration that the biological indicator has been inactivated strongly implies that other potential pathogens in the load have been killed.[1,9-11]

Ideal biological indicator: An ideal biological indicator of the sterilization process should be easy-to-use, be inexpensive, not be subject to exogenous contamination, provide positive results as soon as possible after the cycle so that corrective action may be accomplished, and provide positive results only when the sterilization parameters (e.g. steam-time, temperature, and/or saturated steam; EtO-time, temperature, relative humidity and/or EtO concentration) are inadequate to kill microbial contaminates.[1,8]

Biological indicators directly monitor the lethality of a given sterilization process. Spores used to monitor a sterilization process are more resistant than the bioburden found on medical devices.[10,11] *Bacillus atrophaeus* spores (10^6) are used to monitor EtO and dry heat, and *Geobacillus stearothermophilus* spores (10^5) are used to monitor steam sterilization, hydrogen peroxide gas plasma, and liquid peracetic acid sterilizers. Steam and low-temperature sterilizers (e.g. hydrogen peroxide gas plasma, peracetic acid) should be monitored at least weekly with the appropriate commercial preparation of spores. If a sterilizer is used frequently (e.g. several loads per day), daily use of biological indicators should be done, as it allows earlier discovery of equipment malfunctions or procedural errors.[1-4]

Biological indicators, though close to ideal, are time and procedure intense. The spores in the indicator strips need to be incubated in their ideal conditions to interpret the growth or absence of it, in order to call a sterilizing cycle unsuccessful or successful. Incubation temperature of *G. stearothermophilus* is 55–60°C, and that of *B. atrophaeus* is 35–37°C. Originally, spore-strip biological indicators were required up to 7 days of incubation to detect viable spores. The next generation of biological indicators was self-contained in plastic vials containing a spore-coated paper strip and a growth medium in a crushable glass ampoule **(Figs 12.6A to C)**. This indicator had a maximum incubation of 48 hours but significant failures could

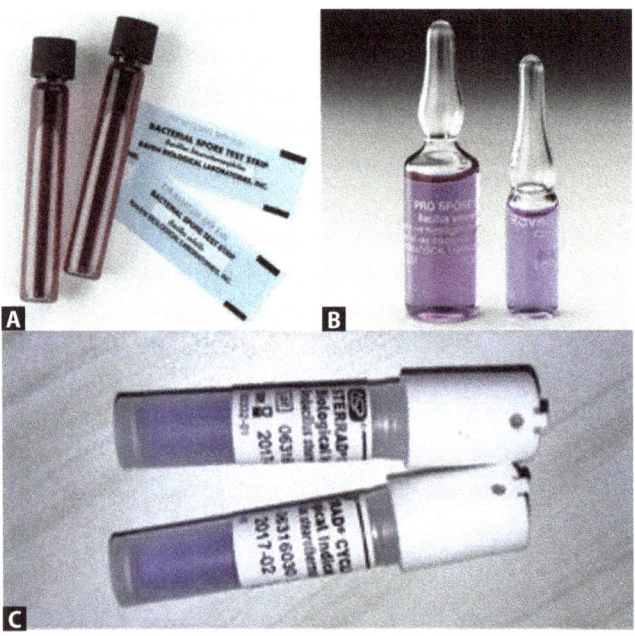

Figures 12.6A to C Biological indicators: Various formulations of biological indicators in the form of spore strips (A), spore suspensions (B) and sealed vials with self-contained indicators of growth (C)

be detected in ≤24 hours. Later rapid-readout biological indicators were introduced that detected the presence of enzymes of *G. stearothermophilus* by reading a fluorescent product produced by the enzymatic breakdown of a non-fluorescent substrate. The sensitivity of rapid-readout tests for steam sterilization (1 hour for 132°C gravity sterilizers, 3 hours for 121°C gravity and 132°C vacuum sterilizers) parallels that of the conventional sterilization-specific biological indicators.[1,8,12] The rapid-readout biological indicator is a dual indicator system as it also detects acid metabolites produced during growth of the *G. stearothermophilus* spores. Recently, rapid-readout EtO biological indicator has been designed for rapid and reliable monitoring of EtO sterilization processes. It detects the presence of *B. atrophaeus* by detecting a fluorescent signal indicating the activity of an enzyme present within the *B. atrophaeus* organism, beta-glucosidase. The fluorescence indicates the presence of an active spore-associated enzyme and a sterilization process failure. The standard biological indicator used for monitoring full-cycle steam sterilizers does not provide reliable monitoring of flash sterilizers. However, rapid-readout biological indicators can be used for monitoring of flash sterilization.[1,8,13]

Positive biological indicator test: For positive biological indicator test of steam sterilizer, the CDC recommendation is that 'objects, other than implantable objects, do not need to be recalled because of a single positive spore test unless the steam sterilizer or the sterilization procedure is defective.' The rationale for this recommendation is that single positive spore tests in sterilizers may occur for reasons such as slight variation in the resistance of the spores, improper use of the sterilizer, and laboratory contamination during culture (uncommon with self-contained spore tests). If the mechanical indicators, e.g. time, temperature, and pressure in the steam sterilizer suggest that the sterilizer was functioning properly, a single positive-spore test probably does not indicate sterilizer malfunction but the spore test should be repeated immediately. If the repeat spore test is positive, use of the sterilizer should be discontinued until it is serviced, and the biological indicators are satisfactory.[1,13,14]

A more conservative approach has been recommended for sterilization methods other than steam (e.g. EtO, hydrogen peroxide gas plasma). This approach requires that following a positive biological indicator test, all materials processed in that sterilizer, dating from the sterilization cycle having the last negative biologic indicator to the next cycle showing satisfactory biologic indicator challenge results, must be considered non-sterile and retrieved, if possible, and reprocessed. However, no action is necessary if there is strong evidence for the biological indicator being defective or the growth medium contained a *Bacillus* contaminant.[1,15,16]

Continuous Quality Improvement

Continuous quality improvement encompasses all the efforts to ensure that the guidelines for sterilization and disinfection are being followed, the cycles and all indicators are being properly documented, any failures are being notified within time, timely rectification methods are implemented and appropriate tracking of events is taking place to follow any infections occurring due to use of treated patient-care items and space. It also includes continuous training, education and motivation of personnel involved to keep the quality of procedures up to the mark.

MICROBIOLOGICAL SAMPLING

Operation theatres (OTs) can be considered the '*Sanctum Sanctorum*[17]' of a healthcare setting. In OTs, the sites and tissues which are normally not exposed to external milieu are ventured into; hence it is essential to ensure the 'purity' of the OT environment. Ideally, to endorse that the environment is free from pathogenic micro-organisms, microbiological processing of samples from air and inanimate objects and surfaces is done. Consequently, the two types of specimens which are collected from OT are environmental swabs and air samples. However, it is imperative to mention that of the various attributes which risk a patient for surgical infections, the role of environment contaminants is the least.

Collection of Specimens from Surfaces and Inanimate Objects

Historically, swabs from OT floor, walls and other inanimate objects were collected and processed to identify aerobic bacteria and anaerobes (*Clostridium tetani*) to ensure that post-sterilization the OT was aptly free of aerobic and anaerobic bacteria. However, this concept has now become obsolete; firstly because even when it was a routine practice, the results of environmental swabs from OTs had never correlated with the occurrence of surgical infections—as a positive result applies only to a particular moment and place; secondly, with the advent of clean and ultraclean OTs-the treatment of air and surfaces and equipment has become so much sophisticated and proficient, that if quality controls, standards and maintenance of sterilization and disinfection are kept up to the mark, barely will any case of surgical infection occur because of environment contaminant. Thus, in the current scenario, there are only two indications of collecting swabs from surfaces and inanimate objects in OTs:

1. To validate a particular method of surface cleaning and disinfection, i.e. to determine the efficiency of the procedure in removing contamination. Swabs may be collected post-treatment to check for presence of bacteria and bacterial spores.
2. If there is a clustering of surgical infections for which the source is suspected to be OT environment, swabs may be collected from surfaces and articles in the vicinity of place of patient intervention. However, the results have to be correlated with the moment and location of the specimen collection.

Method of collection of swabs: Conventionally, the swabs are collected from operation table at the head end, over head lamp, instrument trolley, drug rack, microscope handles (in ophthalmic OTs), floor below the head end of the table, wall near electrical switches, four walls and filters of air conditioning units.[18,19] Ordinary dry sterile swabs or those with a plastic shaft and a synthetic tip, can be used. Before taking the sample, it is necessary to ensure that the surface to be sampled is dry. The swab is removed from the receptacle, it is moistened with sterile normal saline, and is wiped over the sample area in close parallel streaks, using firm even pressure and rotating the swab between fingers to maximize sample pick-up. The swab should be held at a 30° angle to the contact surface. With the same swab, the process is repeated at right angles to the first streaks to ensure that the entire sample area is swabbed. The swab should be replaced in the receptacle and should be transported for immediate processing. If delay in processing is expected, the swab should be placed in a receptacle containing Amies' transport medium, which is capable of sustaining the viability of the microorganism until the swab can be plated.

Processing of swabs: The swabs collected are inoculated on blood agar for culture of aerobic bacteria, Robertson's cooked meat medium and subsequently taken for anaerobic culture for detecting anaerobes, and on Sabouraud's dextrose agar for fungal culture. From the culture, identification of organisms is done based on standard microbiological techniques. The results obtained should be carefully interpreted based on the indication for which environment sampling was done, and correlation of the result with the time and place of specimen collection and their relatedness with any surgical infections occurring in close proximity.

Collection of Swab Specimens from Instruments

A used instrument, for all practical purposes, has been exposed to external environment and has been tampered with; hence it is not appropriate for collecting specimen for microbiological processing. Any results generated with such sampling will be erroneous.

An unused instrument tray does not need to be sampled if it is run with proper mechanical, external and internal chemical, and biological controls; and the results of all quality controls are satisfactory. In special circumstances, if internal (inside the package) controls are not run and there is doubt about the performance of the sterilization process, one instrument tray of the processed load may be opened and sampled as stated in sampling of inanimate objects above. The results of microbiological processing of the tray/its instruments can be used as control for the whole load of the run. Such a tray which has been opened for sampling should not be used for surgery.

Air Sampling

Regarding routine bacteriological surveillance of air, there are mixed views. At one end, with the modern well-designed OTs—having conditioned ventilation and air filtration, and appropriate surface disinfection, it is not advocated;[20,21] at the other end, evaluation of microbial air contamination is considered to be an important criterion for determining the safety of OTs.[22,23] According to the latter view, regular microbial monitoring can represent a useful tool to assess environmental quality and to identify critical situations which require corrective intervention. Thus, air sampling should be conducted with a plan for interpreting and acting on the results obtained. While considering the use of air sampling, it should be kept in mind that the results represent indoor air quality at singular points in time, and these may be affected by a variety of factors, including (a) indoor traffic, (b) visitors entering the facility, (c) temperature, d) time of day or year, (e) relative humidity, (f) relative concentration of particles or organisms, and (g) the performance of the air-handling system components. Given the different kinds of operation theatres being used for various surgeries in different healthcare settings in India, it is important to know the different air sampling procedures and their interpretations. The knowledge can be used as a reference for formulating guidelines of checking air quality, depending on the type of healthcare facility. The microbiological content of the air can be monitored by two main methods—active and passive.

Active Air Sampling[20-25]

This involves active collection of a measured volume of air, which is brought in contact with a nutrient medium by various techniques. The medium is then incubated and observed for the growth of bacteria and/or fungi. Results are noted in colony-forming units (CFU)/m^3 of air. Since the sample volume can be calculated using the flow rate and sampling time, the result is quantitative. Interpretations are based on the standard guidelines for the type of operation theatre and the kind of technique used. Active air samplers are based on following principles:

1. *Impingement in liquids:* Impingers use a liquid medium for particle collection. The sampled air is drawn by a suction pump through a narrow inlet tube into a small flask containing the collection medium. This accelerates the air towards the surface of the collection medium with the flow rate being determined by the diameter of the inlet tube. When the air hits the surface of the liquid, it changes direction abruptly and any suspended particles are impinged into the collection liquid. Once the sampling is complete, the collection liquid can be cultured to count any viable microorganisms in the sample.

2. *Impaction on solid surfaces:* Impactors use a solid or adhesive medium, such as agar gel, rather than a liquid for particle collection. Typically, air is drawn into a sampling head by a pump or fan and accelerated, usually through a perforated plate (sieve samplers), or through a narrow slit (slit samplers, **Fig. 12.7**). This produces a laminar air flow onto the collection surface, often a standard agar plate filled with a suitable medium. The velocity of the air is determined by the diameter of the holes in sieve samplers and the width of the slit in slit samplers. When the air hits the collection surface, it makes a tangential change of direction and any suspended particles are thrown out by inertia, impacting onto the collection surface. When the correct volume of air has been passed through the sampling head, the agar plate can be removed

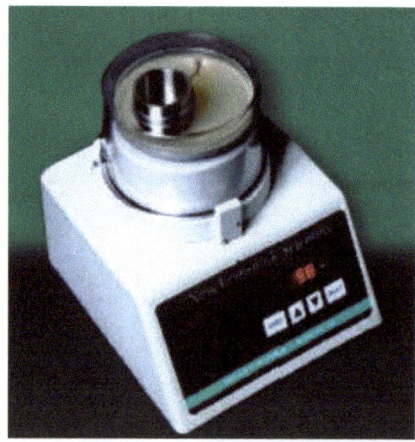

Figure 12.7 Slit sampler for air microbiological sampling (Active air sampling)

and incubated directly without further treatment. After incubation, counting the number of visible colonies gives a direct quantitative estimate of the number of colony-forming units in the volume of air sampled. Samplers based on impaction principle are convenient to use.

3. Other less popular principles used in active air sampling are filtration, centrifugation, electrostatic precipitation and thermal precipitation.

Interpretation: In volumetric air samplers, the microbial air contamination can be measured by counting the number of CFU/m^3 of air. Most official standards for air control are based primarily on the measurement of CFU/m^3, hence can be directly applied to the results obtained. The counts obtained are, however, not proportional to the risk of surgical infection as the forcible sampling leads to capture of suspended particles also. This is not representative of the infection which might occur due to settling of pathogens on surgical wound during patient intervention. **Table 12.2** shows the advantages and disadvantages of active air sampling, and **Table 12.3** shows example of a guideline used to interpret the active air sampling results.

Table 12.2 Advantages and disadvantages of active air sampling
Advantages
Sample collection is rapid and measured
Most official guidelines refer to CFU/m^3, hence interpretation is easy
Results obtained are quantitative
Disadvantages
Device is difficult to sterilize
Device is expensive
The process is noisy
Frequent calibrations of device are required
Correlation with surgical infection is usually out of proportion

Table 12.3 Interpretation of active air sampling results[21]	
Environment at risk	*Maximum acceptable level of CFU/m^3*
Ultraclean ventilated OTs	10–20
Conventionally ventilated OTs, at rest	50–150
Conventionally ventilated OTs, during activity	180

Passive Air Sampling[20-25]

This method employs settle plates—petri dishes containing appropriate culture media, which are opened and kept near the operating area, and exposed for a given time and then incubated to allow visible bacterial and fungal colonies to develop and be counted **(Fig. 12.8)**. Settle plates are only capable of monitoring those viable biological particles that sediment out of the air and settle onto a surface over the time of exposure. They will not detect smaller particles or droplets that remain suspended in the air and they cannot sample specific volumes of air, so the results can only be considered semi-quantitative. Settle plates are inexpensive and easy-to-use, they require no special equipment. When correctly used, they are a more realistic indicator of airborne bacterial contamination at the site of patient procedure, as only the particles which settle, pose a risk of surgical infection. **Table 12.4** shows the advantages and disadvantages of passive air sampling.

Interpretation: Traditionally, in sedimentation method, the interpretation of results was based on conversion of the colony counts obtained to CFU/m^3, as most official guidelines for interpretation of air quality referred to CFU/m^3. In the year 2000, Pasquerella *et al.* published the concept of index of microbial air contamination (IMA); in which standardization of the results obtained

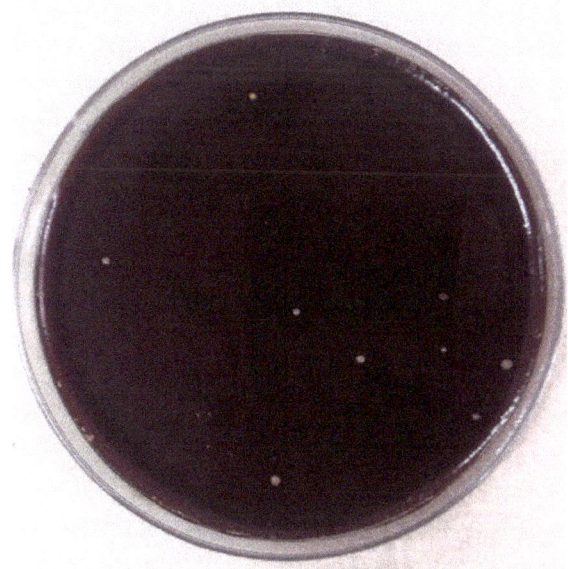

Figure 12.8 Settle plate method with bacterial colonies (Passive air sampling)

Table 12.4 Advantages and disadvantages of passive air sampling
Advantages
Easy to use
Inexpensive
Requires no special equipment
More realistic indicator of airborne bacterial contamination which might settle in surgical wound to cause infection
Disadvantages
Semi-quantitative results
Most official guidelines refer to CFU/m³, hence interpretation involves careful conversion of counts

Table 12.5 Interpretation of passive air sampling results[24]

Environment at risk	Maximum acceptable level of IMA*
Ultraclean OTs (Neurosurgery, cardiothoracic surgery, joint replacement surgery)	5
Other OTs	25
Other clean rooms of the healthcare facility (recovery rooms, OT corridors etc)	50
Other facilities	75

* IMA = Index of microbial air contamination, equals to the colony-forming units obtained in 90 mm petri plate.

The original standardization was based on 1/1/1 scheme (refer text); evidence-based modifications may be done depending on size of petri plate used, exposure time (in hours, and whether exposed to OT at rest or during activity), length of surgical procedure, and the correlation with the active air sampling results in CFU/m³.

Considering the high pathogenicity of *Staphylococcus aureus*, and invasiveness and difficult treatment of fungal infections; most facilities consider detection of even a single fungal colony, or that of *S. aureus* not to be acceptable.[18]

on passive air sampling was done based on literature review and performing a large number of tests in different environments. The standardization was based on 1/1/1 scheme, in which a standard petri dish of 9 cm in diameter containing nutrient medium is left open to air for one hour, one meter from the floor, and at least one meter away from walls or any relevant physical obstacle. After 48 hours of incubation at 37°C, the CFU are counted. The number of CFU obtained is the IMA **(Table 12.5)**. For ophthalmic OT, the acceptable levels are ≤ 5 CFU/9 cm diameter plate/h at rest and ≤ 25 CFU/9 cm diameter plate/h in operational time. Many facilities using sedimentation method for checking quality of air in OTs use IMA for interpreting their results.

HOSPITAL STERILIZATION AND DISINFECTION POLICY

Proper sterilization and disinfection are obligatory for prevention of procedural infections in OTs. Along with the articles which come in direct contact with the sterile sites of the patient's body, the OT environment also consists of a variety of items that do not come in direct contact with the patient. Although the chances of such items being related to post-operative infections are remote; every effort must be made to keep them also as germ free as possible.[25] Hence, there is a flexibility to choose from the previously described methods depending on the type of facility, patient load, the procedures being undertaken and the resources (monitory and manpower) available. It is imperative to lay down guidelines to be followed for all procedures in the form of hospital sterilization and disinfection policy. Along with the knowledge of all cleaning, disinfection and sterilization procedures and their applications and quality controls, certain things need to be followed while making hospital sterilization and disinfection policy.

Choosing a Method of Sterilization[1,26-30]

- Steam is the preferred method for sterilizing critical medical and surgical instruments that are not damaged by heat, steam, pressure or moisture.
- Dry-heat sterilization (e.g. 340°F for 60 minutes) can be used to sterilize items (e.g. powders, oils) that can sustain high temperatures.
- Steam- or heat-sterilized items should be cooled before they are handled or used in the operative setting.
- Low-temperature sterilization technologies (e.g. EtO, hydrogen peroxide gas plasma) are used for reprocessing critical patient-care equipment that are heat or moisture sensitive.
- Complete aeration is mandatory for surgical and medical items that have been sterilized in the EtO sterilizer (e.g. polyvinylchloride tubing requires 12 hours at 50°C, 8 hours at 60°C) before using these items in patient care.
- Sterilization using the peracetic acid immersion system can be used to sterilize heat-sensitive immersible medical and surgical items.

- Critical items that have been sterilized by the peracetic acid immersion process must be used immediately; long-term storage is unacceptable in sterilization by peracetic acid.
- As narrow-lumen devices provide a challenge to all low-temperature sterilization technologies and direct contact is necessary for the sterilant to be effective, it is important to ensure that the sterilant has direct contact with contaminated surfaces (e.g. scopes processed in peracetic acid must be connected to channel irrigators).
- Compliance with the sterilizer manufacturer's instructions regarding the sterilizer cycle parameters (e.g. time, temperature, concentration) and other recommended operating parameters is essential.

Packaging[1-4,31]

- Packaging materials should be compatible with the chosen sterilization process, and must be FDA approved.
- Packaging should be sufficiently strong to resist punctures and tears to provide a barrier to microorganisms and moisture.

Flash Sterilization[1,4,8,32,33]

- Flash sterilization should not be used for implantable surgical devices unless doing so is unavoidable.
- Flash sterilization should not be used for convenience, as an alternative to purchasing additional instrument sets, or to save time.
- While using flash sterilization, proper cleaning of the item, prevention of exogenous contamination of the item, and monitoring of the cycle using mechanical, chemical, and biological (if possible) indicators should be done.
- Flash sterilization should be used for patient-care items that will be used immediately (e.g., to reprocess an inadvertently dropped instrument).
- Flash sterilization should be used for processing patient-care items that cannot be packaged, sterilized, and stored before use.

Monitoring of Sterilizers[1-16]

- Mechanical, chemical, and biological monitors should be used to ensure the effectiveness of the sterilization process.
- Each load should be monitored with mechanical (e.g. time, temperature, pressure) and chemical (internal and external) indicators. If the internal chemical indicator is visible, an external indicator is not needed.
- Processed items should not be used if the mechanical (e.g. time, temperature, pressure) or chemical (internal and/or external) indicators suggest inadequate processing.
- Biological indicators should be used to monitor the effectiveness of sterilizers at least weekly with an FDA-cleared commercial preparation of spores intended specifically for the type and cycle parameters of the sterilizer (e.g. *Geobacillus stearothermophilus* for steam).
- After a single positive biological indicator used with a method other than steam sterilization, all items that have been processed in that sterilizer should be treated as non-sterile, dating from the sterilization cycle having the last negative biological indicator to the next cycle showing satisfactory biological indicator results. These nonsterile items should be retrieved if possible and reprocessed.
- After a positive biological indicator with steam sterilization, objects other than implantable objects do not need to be recalled because of a single positive spore test unless the sterilizer or the sterilization procedure is defective as determined by maintenance personnel or inappropriate cycle settings or results of mechanical or/and chemical indicators. If the sterilization procedure is proved to be defective or additional spore tests remain positive; the items should be considered nonsterile, and recall and reprocessing of the items from the implicated load(s) needs to be done.

Load Configuration[4,34]

The items should be placed correctly and loosely into the basket, shelf, or cart of the sterilizer so as not to impede the penetration of the sterilant.

Storage of Sterile Items[1,3,4,34-37]

- It should be ensured that the sterile storage area is a well-ventilated area that provides protection against dust, moisture, insects, and temperature and humidity extremes.
- Sterile items should be stored in a manner so that the packaging is not compromised (e.g. punctured, bent).

- Sterilized items should have a label that indicates the sterilizer used, the cycle or load number, the date of sterilization, and, if applicable, the expiration date.
- The shelf-life of a packaged sterile item depends on the quality of the wrapper, the storage conditions, conditions during transport, the amount of handling, and other events (e.g. moisture) that compromise the integrity of the package. If event-related storage of sterile item is used, then packaged sterile items can be used indefinitely unless the packaging is compromised.
- The packages should be evaluated before use for loss of integrity (e.g. torn, wet, or punctured). The pack can be used unless the integrity of the packaging is compromised.
- If the integrity of the packaging is compromised (e.g. torn, wet, or punctured), it should be repacked and reprocessed before use.
- If time-related storage of sterile items is used, the pack should be labeled at the time of sterilization with an expiration date. Once this date expires, the pack should be reprocessed.

Occupational Health and Exposure[1,38,39]

The healthcare workers involved in the procedures of cleaning, disinfection and sterilization are at risk of occupational hazard due to (a) exposure to contaminated spaces, articles and biomedical waste; and (b) exposure to the cleaning agents, disinfectants and sterilants. While making the hospital sterilization and disinfection policy, occupational health should be appropriately addressed. The key components to be borne in this subject matter are given below.
- Each worker should be informed of the possible health effects of his or her exposure to infectious agents (e.g. hepatitis B virus, hepatitis C virus, human immunodeficiency virus), and/or chemicals (e.g. EtO, formaldehyde). The information should be consistent with Occupational Safety and Health Administration (OSHA) requirements.
- Wherever indicated, vaccination should be provided to the workers, depending upon the potential infective agent the worker is exposed to.
- Areas and tasks in which potential exists for specific exposures should be identified.
- Healthcare workers should be educated for selection and proper use of personal protective equipment (PPE). The appropriate type of PPE depends on the infectious or chemical agent and the anticipated duration of exposure.
- Systems should be in place to ensure that workers wear appropriate PPE to preclude exposure to infectious agents or chemicals through the respiratory system, skin, or mucous membranes of the eyes, nose, or mouth.
- The PPE equipment and training should be available to the workers.
- A program should be in place for monitoring occupational exposure to regulated chemicals (e.g. formaldehyde, EtO).
- Healthcare workers with open wounds or dermatitis should be excluded from direct contact with patient-care equipment.

Quality Assurance[1-4,33]

Quality assurance does involve the use of quality control indicators in each sterilization cycle, which determine the success or failure of the procedure; and proper storage and transport of the processed articles. Equally importantly, it includes the events before and after the procedure, which if properly followed, give surety of the success of the whole process. Thus quality assurance is a promise of the excellence of the whole sphere of a hospital's sterilization and disinfection policy. By and large, careful inclusion of certain general things should be a part of sterilization and disinfection policy of all healthcare settings.
- Education of staff to make certain that they understand the importance of proper procedures.
- Comprehensive and intensive training of all staff assigned to reprocess semicritical and critical medical/surgical instruments.
- Supervision of the work done until competency is documented for each reprocessing task.
- Periodic competency testing.
- Review of the written reprocessing instructions regularly to ensure they comply with the scientific literature and updates.
- Conduction of infection control rounds periodically in high-risk reprocessing areas.
- Documentation of all deviations from policy, and identification and implementation of corrective actions.
- Retention of sterilization records (mechanical, chemical, and biological) for a time period that complies with standards of federal regulations.

- Periodic review of policies and procedures.
- Maintenance of sterilizers by qualified personnel who are guided by the manufacturer's instruction.

REFERENCES

1. Ruthala WA, Weber DJ. Healthcare Infection Control Practices Advisory Committee (HICPAC), Centre for Disease Control and Prevention, Atlanta, USA. Guideline for Disinfection and Sterilization in Healthcare Facilities, 2008.
2. Association for the Advancement of Medical Instrumentation. Steam sterilization and sterility assurance in healthcare facilities. ANSI/AAMI ST46. Arlington, VA, 2002:ANSI/AAMI ST46:2002.
3. Association for the Advancement of Medical Instrumentation. Ethylene oxide sterilization in healthcare facilities: Safety and effectiveness. AAMI. Arlington, VA, 1999.
4. Association for the Advancement of Medical Instrumentation. Comprehensive guide to steam sterilization and sterility assurance in health care facilities: ANSI/AAMI ST79. 2006.
5. Coulter WA, Chew-Graham CA, Cheung SW, Burke FJT. Autoclave performance and operator knowledge of autoclave use in primary care: a survey of UK practices. J. Hosp Infect. 2001;48:180-5.
6. Baird RM. Sterility assurance: Concepts, methods and problems. In: Russell AD, Hugo WB, Ayliffe GAJ (eds). Principles and practice of disinfection, preservation and sterilization. Oxford, England: Blackwell Scientific Publications; 1999. pp. 787-99.
7. Kurowski JA. Chemical Indicators 101: Applications for Use. Infection Control Today; 2004.
8. Rutala WA, Gergen MF, Weber DJ. Evaluation of a rapid readout biological indicator for flash sterilization with three biological indicators and three chemical indicators. Infect. Control Hosp. Epidemiol.1993;14:390-4.
9. Greene VW. Control of sterilization process. In: Russell AD, Hugo WB, Ayliffe GAJ (Eds). Principles and practice of disinfection, preservation and sterilization. Oxford, England: Blackwell Scientific Publications; 1992. pp. 605-24.
10. Nystrom B. Disinfection of surgical instruments. J. Hosp Infect. 1981;2:363-8.
11. Rutala WA, Gergen MF, Jones JF, Weber DJ. Levels of microbial contamination on surgical instruments. Am J Infect. Control. 1998;26:143-5.
12. Koncur P, Janes JE, Ortiz PA. 20 second sterilization indicator tests equivalent to BIs. Infect Control Steril Technol. 1998:26-8,30,32-4.
13. Perkins RE, Bodman HA, Kundsin RB, Walter CW. Monitoring steam sterilization of surgical instruments: a dilemma. Appl Environ Microbiol. 1981;42:383-7.
14. Mathur P. Cleaning, disinfection and sterilization. In. Hospital acquired infections-Prevention and Control, 1st edition. Published Wolters Kluver Health, India, 2010. pp. 143-220.
15. Centers for Disease Control. False-positive results of spore tests in ethylene oxide sterilizers - Wisconsin. MMWR. 1981;30:238-40.
16. Kleinegger CL, Yeager DL, Huling JK, Drake DR. The effects of contamination on biological monitoring. Infect. Control Hosp. Epidemiol. 2001;22:391-2.
17. *https://en.wikipedia.org/wiki/Sanctum_sanctorum.* Accessed. 16-09-2016.
18. Kelkar U, Kelkar S, Bal AM, Kulkarni S, Kulkarni S. Microbiological evaluation of various parameters in ophthalmic operating rooms. The need to establish guidelines. Indian J Ophthal. 2003;51(2):171-6.
19. Gupta C, Vanathi M, Tandon R. Current Concepts in Operative Room Sterilisation. Delhi J Ophthalmol. 2015;25(3):190-4.
20. Dharan S, Pittet D. Environmental controls in operating theatres. J Hosp Infect. 2002;51(2):79-84.
21. Mathur P. Operating Rooms. In: Hospital acquired infections-Prevention and Control, 1st edn. Published Wolters Kluver Health, India; 2010. pp. 249-74.
22. Sabharwal ER, Sharma R. Estimation of microbial air contamination by settle plate method: are we within acceptable limit. Sch Acad J Biosci. 2015;3(8):703-7.
23. Napoli C, Marcotrigiano V, Montagna MT. Air sampling procedures to evaluate microbial contamination: a comparison between active and passive methods in operating theatres. BMC Public Health. 2012;12:594.
24. Pasquarella C, Pitzurra O, Savino A. The index of microbial air contamination. J Hosp Infect. 2000;46:241-56.
25. Sharma S, Bansal AK, Gyanchand R. Asepsis in ophthalmic operating room. Indian J Ophthalmol. 1996;44(3):173-7.
26. Joslyn L. Sterilization by heat. In: Block SS, (ed). Disinfection, sterilization, and preservation. Philadelphia: Lippincott Williams & Wilkins; 2001. pp. 695-728.
27. Rutala WA, Gergen MF, Weber DJ. Evaluation of a rapid readout biological indicator for flash sterilization with three biological indicators and three chemical indicators. Infect. Control Hosp. Epidemiol. 1993;14:390-4.
28. Burgess DJ, Reich RR. Industrial ethylene oxide sterilization. In: Morrissey RF, Phillips GB (eds.) Sterilization technology: a practical guide for manufacturers and users of health care product. New York: Van Nostrand Reinhold; 1993. pp. 120-51.
29. Conviser CA. Ethylene oxide sterilization: sterilant alternatives. In: Reichert M, Young JH (eds). Sterilization technology for the healthcare facility. Gaithersburg, MD: Aspen Publication; 1997. pp. 189-99.

30. Rutala WA, Weber DJ. Clinical effectiveness of low-temperature sterilization technologies. Infect Control Hosp Epidemiol. 1998;19:798-804.
31. Rutala WA, Weber DJ. Choosing a sterilization wrap. Infect Control Today. 2000;4:64,70.
32. Barrett T. Flash sterilization: What are the risks? In: Rutala WA (ed). Disinfection, sterilization and antisepsis: principles and practices in healthcare facilities. Washington, DC: Association for Professional in Infection Control and Epidemiology; 2001. pp. 70-6.
33. Association for the Advancement of Medical Instrumentation. Flash sterilization: Steam sterilization of patientcare items for immediate use. AAMI. Arlington, VA, 1996.
34. American Society for Healthcare Central Service Professionals. Training Manual for Health Care Central Service Technicians. In: Association AH (Ed). Chicago: The Jossey Bass/American Hospital Association Press Series; 2001. pp. 1-271.
35. Mayworm D. Sterile shelf-life and expiration dating. J Hosp Supply, Process. Distri. 1984;2:32-5.
36. Cardo DM, Sehulster LM. Central sterile supply. In: Mayhall CG, (ed). Infect. Control and Hosp Epidemiol. Philadelphia: Lippincott Williams & Wilkins; 1999. pp. 1023-30.
37. Japp NF. Packaging: Shelf life. In: Reichert M, Young JH (eds). Sterilization Technology. Gaithersburg, Maryland: Aspen; 1997. pp. 99-102.
38. Occupational Health and Safety Administration. Hazard Communication Standard. 29 CFR 1910.1200,OSHA, Washington, DC.
39. Edens AL. Occupational Safety and Health Administration: Regulations affecting healthcare facilities. In:Rutala WA (Ed). Disinfection, Sterilization and Antisepsis: Principles and practices in healthcare facilities. Washington, DC: Association for Professionals in Infection Control and Epidemiology Inc. 2001. pp. 49-58.

CHAPTER 13

Post-Cataract Surgery Endophthalmitis

Anubha Rathi, Rohan Chawla, Atul Kumar

Endophthalmitis is a rare, but potentially devastating complication of any intraocular surgery. Such a complication becomes even more serious, both for the surgeon as well as the patient, in case of cataract surgery which, in the recent past, has become equivalent to any refractive surgery in terms of visual expectation and outcome. This chapter covers in detail the various risk factors, causes, clinical features, management and most importantly the prophylaxis of this sight threatening complication post-cataract surgery.

Post-cataract surgery endophthalmitis is defined as the inflammation of the internal layers of the eye presenting with exudation into the vitreous cavity occurring after cataract surgery in the perioperative period. Any intraocular surgery causes a breach in the ocular coats through which colonization of the microbes may occur and potentially lead to endophthalmitis. Although its reported incidence in the last decade has decreased from 1% to 0.05–0.1%, yet it still remains one of the most dreaded complications.[1,2]

MICROBIAL SPECTRUM OF POST-OPERATIVE ENDOPHTHALMITIS

The source of the infective micro-organisms in cases of post-operative endophthalmitis may be any of the following:
- Patient's own ocular surface microbial flora. This is the most common culprit. Patients with poor or delayed wound healing such as cases of diabetes mellitus are more at risk of microbial colonization from their own flora.
- Patients with blepharitis or active eyelid infection or inflammation at the time of surgery are at risk of the same micro-organism gaining entry into the eye and causing endophthalmitis post-operatively.
- Contaminated surgical instruments, irrigating fluids, machine tubing or OT environment may be the source of the infective organism.

The organisms isolated from cases of post-operative endophthalmitis may show regional variation. Overall coagulase negative staphylococci (CNS) are the most commonly (33–77%) isolated microorganisms in these cases.[2] *Staphylococcus aureus* is second on the list accounting for 10–21% cases.[2] Other causes in order of frequency include β-hemolytic streptococci, *Streptococcus pneumoniae* and gram-negative bacilli such as *Pseudomonas aeruginosa*. Fungi such as *Candida*, *Aspergillus* and *Fusarium* are known to cause up to 8% cases of post-operative endophthalmitis.[2] The incidence of gram negative bacilli and fungi causing endophthalmitis is reported to be higher in Indian and Chinese studies. *Propionibacterium acnes*, *Corynebacterium diphtheriae*, *Staphylococcus epidermidis* and fungi are reported in cases of chronic post-operative endophthalmitis.

MRSA AND MRSE: INCREASING RESISTANCE TO TOPICAL ANTIBIOTICS

In the recent past, reports of isolation of MRSA (Methicillin-resistant *Staphylococcus aureus*) and MRSE (Methicillin-resistant *Staphylococcus epidermidis*) have increased from the post-operative endophthalmitis samples. A retrospective study (1995–2008) from Bascom Palmer Eye Institute USA in 2010 reported 41% of the 32 cases caused by *Staphylococcus aureus* to be methicillin resistant. About 62% of these, MRSA showed resistance to fourth generation flouroquinolones as well. The incidence of MRSA/E varies with geographical region. It is reportedly higher in Asian countries including India. The current drug of choice for MRSA/E is vancomycin. The prophylactic use of vancomycin has been discouraged by most reports in view of the looming risk of VRSA/E (Vancomycin-resistant *Staphylococcus aureus/epidermidis*).

RISK FACTORS AND INCIDENCE OF POST-CATARACT SURGERY ENDOPHTHALMITIS

Various risk factors have been identified for post-operative endophthalmitis. Their frequency varies from region to region. The important ones are highlighted here under:

Type of Cataract Surgery

Historically, rate of endophthalmitis was much higher (10%) in the intracapsular cataract extraction (ICCE) era. The rates decreased with the advent of extracapsular cataract extraction (ECCE) with suture and intraocular lens (IOL) to 0.12%. This rate showed a mild increase though with clear corneal incision phacoemulsification.

Type and Location of Incision

Clear corneal incision (CCI) is reported to have a higher incidence of post-operative endophthalmitis as compared to scleral tunnel incision or corneo-scleral incision. CCI in phacoemulsification was first identified as a risk factor for endophthalmitis in 1992-2003 with reported 0.189% incidence as compared to 0.074% with scleral incision. The European Society of Cataract and Refractive Surgeons (ESCRS) study reported 5.88 times more risk of CCI cataract surgery developing endophthalmitis as compared to scleral tunnel incision.[2] Some reports have highlighted that suturing the CCI may reduce this rate considerably.

Nature of Intraocular Lens

Implantation of an intraocular lens is known to decrease the incidence of post-cataract surgery endophthalmitis as it introduces a barrier between the anterior and posterior chambers, hence avoiding spill over of infective material, if any into the vitreous cavity. Among various intra-ocular lenses available, several studies have shown silicone IOLs to have a higher rate of endophthalmitis post operatively. As per ESCRS study, patients with implanted silicone IOLs were 3.13 times more likely to contract post-operative endophthalmitis as compared to acrylic IOLs.[2] Also lesser endophthalmitis rates have been seen with foldable IOLs with injectors.

Surgical Complications

Intra-operative posterior capsular tear or vitreous loss has been associated with a higher risk of post-operative endophthalmitis than an uneventful cataract surgery. As per ESCRS study, this risk is almost 4.95 fold.[2]

Patient-related Factors

Older age, male gender, immunocompromised status, patients on immune modulators or anticancer drugs, history of diabetes mellitus, presence of active eye infection at the time of surgery and low socioeconomic conditions with poor eye hygiene post-operatively are some of the patient-related factors associated with higher incidence of postcataract surgery endophthalmitis.

PROPHYLAXIS OF POST-CATARACT SURGERY ENDOPHTHALMITIS

Several measures have been suggested in various studies for prophylaxis of the catastrophic complication of cataract surgery that is endophthalmitis. These may be subdivided into pre-operative, intra-operative and post-operative measures.

Pre-operative Period

In the pre-operative period, measures directed towards decreasing the load of colonizing micro-organisms are known to reduce the risk of postcataract surgery endophthalmitis.

Treating Pre-existing Ocular Conditions

Conditions such as blepharitis, meibomitis, conjunctivitis, canaliculitis and nasolacrimal duct obstruction should be addressed first and surgery deferred till the eye is completely quiet. Eyelid position abnormalities such as entropion and ectropion also increase the risk of post-surgery endophthalmitis, and hence should be tackled before undertaking cataract surgery.

Pre-operative Antisepsis: Preparing the Patient

- *Role of povidone-iodine in patient preparation:* There seems to be a generalized consensus on the prophylactic role of povidone-iodine for ocular surface preparation prior to cataract surgery. The very first reports on its role came in 1986, when it was shown to decrease the ocular surface flora load by up to 90%. Recent literature also shows similar trend and prophylactic povidone-iodine continues to remain the most important prophylactic measure in the pre-operative period. Applying 5–10% povidone-iodine in the conjunctival sac and periorbital skin for at least 3 minutes before the surgery is the recommended protocol. In cases of true iodine allergy or in cases of hyperthyroidism, povidone-iodine may be replaced with 2% chlorhexidine.
- *Role of topical antibiotics in the pre-operative period:* There are conflicting reports regarding the efficacy of pre-operative prophylactic use of topical antibiotics in case of cataract surgery. Despite that, they continue to be widely prescribed pre-operatively. Most studies reveal no definite benefit of using pre-operative topical antibiotics in preventing post-operative endophthalmitis. There seems to be no additional benefit of increasing the frequency of antibiotic administration as well. Few studies have compared a 3 day versus 1 day antibiotic regimen and have reported no significant difference between them.[3]
- *Careful and meticulous draping of the operating field:* The eyelids and eyelashes are home to several commensals and should be kept away from the operating field using a sterile eye drape and meticulously placed lid speculum. Trimming of eyelashes on the operating table is not recommended.
- *Preparation of the surgeon:* Proper scrubbing with meticulous handwash and use of sterile gowns and towels are required. Facemasks covering the nasal area of the surgeon and the assisting staff is a necessity. A recent case control study has shown that face masks when used properly by the surgeon and the assisting staff are associated with reduction in the rate of endophthalmitis significantly.[4]

Intra-operative Period

During the intra-operative period, measures that may reduce the rate of post-operative endophthalmitis include making a water tight incision or securing the incision with a suture in case of suspected wound leak. Placement of an intraocular lens and avoiding any posterior capsular tear or vitreous loss may also reduce endophthalmitis rate as mentioned earlier.

Role of intracameral antibiotics needs to be highlighted at this stage. Two antibiotics have been used majorly for this purpose, namely vancomycin and cefuroxime.

Intracameral use of vancomycin in the prevention of post-operative endophthalmitis has been controversial. There are reports in literature which reveal up to a nine-fold reduction in the rate of acute post-operative endophthalmitis with the use of intracameral vancomycin in cataract surgery.[5,6] In the recent past, there have been arguments regarding the intracameral use of vancomycin with Centers for Disease Control and Prevention in the US issuing caution against prophylactic vancomycin in cataract surgery.[7] Recent reports have suggested that the dosage and time for which the antibiotic is in the anterior chamber is not enough for its microbicidal activity to occur.[8] On the other hand rampant use of this drug may lead to increased microbial resistance. Cystoid macular edema and hemorrhagic retinopathy following the use of prophylactic intracameral vancomycin have also been reported.[9,10]

The use of intracameral cefuroxime has shown better results.[2,11,12] Its role in prophylaxis of post-cataract surgery endophthalmitis was studied in detail in the ESCRS study. Over 16000 patients undergoing cataract surgery were included in the study with almost a three-year recruitment period. The results were presented in 2007 and revealed that the use of 1 mg intracameral cefuroxime in 0.1 mL normal saline at the end of surgery significantly lowers the incidence of post-operative endophthalmitis. The study comprised four study groups:

- *Group A:* Control group, patients received placebo pre-operative drops but no injection
- *Group B:* Patients received placebo drops and intracameral cefuroxime injection
- *Group C:* Patients received topical levofloxacin drops but no injection
- *Group D:* Patients received both topical antibiotic drops and intracameral injection

Patients in all the groups also received povidone-iodine prophylaxis and topical antibiotics in the post-operative period. The results of ESCRS study are highlighted in **Table 13.1**.

Table 13.1 Summary of the ESCRS* study results showing the role of intracameral cefuroxime in preventing post-operative endophthalmitis				
Parameter	Result			
	Group A@	Group B#	Group C$	Group D&
No. of patients	4054	4056	4049	4052
Incidence rate of endophthalmitis				
Total	0.345%	0.074%	0.247%	0.049 %
Proven	0.247%	0.049%	0.173 %	0.025%

@Group A: Control group, patients received placebo pre-operative drops but no injection
#Group B: Patients received placebo drops and intracameral cefuroxime injection
$Group C: Patients received topical levofloxacin drops but no injection
&Group D: Patients received both topical antibiotic drops and intracameral injection
*Adapted from Barry P, Seal DV, Gettinby G, et al. ESCRS study of prophylaxis of post-operative endophthalmitis after cataract surgery: preliminary report of principal results from a European multicenter study. J Cataract Refract Surg. 2006;32:407-10.

After the ESCRS study, the use of intracameral cefuroxime during cataract surgery has become a routine in the European countries. In other parts of the world, it is still not widely accepted. A large scale study of more than 14000 patients conducted in India has shown marginal efficacy of intracameral cefuroxime in preventing post-operative endophthalmitis.[13] Some reports suggest that use of reconstituted cefuroxime intracamerally may increase the incidence of TASS,[14] though this is not widely believed. There are till date no reports of macular or retinal pathology associated with intracameral use of cefuroxime.

Intracameral moxifloxacin (50-500 μg/mL) has recently been tried with favorable results for prevention of post-operative endophthalmitis.[15-17] Its concentration dependent effect is considered better than the time dependent effect of cefuroxime.

Role of subconjunctival antibiotic injection at the end of surgery has been studied as well. Such an injection has shown promising results in reducing endophthalmitis rates post-operatively. The antibiotic concentration delivered to the anterior chamber is higher with a subconjunctival injection as compared to topical administration. However, various other studies fail to establish the usefulness of administering subconjunctival antibiotics at the end of the surgery for the prevention of endophthalmitis.

Post-operative Period

Topical antibiotics in the post-operative period are essential to reduce endophthalmitis developing in the immediate post-operative period. Clean surroundings and patient's eye hygiene practice also plays a role in the post-operative period.

Flow chart 13.1 summarizes the measures that may help in reducing the rates of post-operative endophthalmitis after cataract surgery.

DIAGNOSIS AND MANAGEMENT

Post-operative endophthalmitis may be acute or chronic depending on the time of presentation. Most of these cases are acute and present within six weeks post-cataract surgery. In two of the major endophthalmitis trials, namely Endophthalmitis Vitrectomy Study (EVS)[11] and ESCRS,[2] majority of the cases had presented in the first 1–2 weeks after cataract surgery. Diagnosis of post-operative endophthalmitis is based on clinical presentation and investigations. An important differential diagnosis of this condition is toxic anterior segment syndrome (TASS). High index of suspicion must be kept for endophthalmitis in any case presenting with pain, blurred vision, red eye, anterior chamber (AC) reaction, hypopyon or lid swelling in the post-operative period after a cataract surgery. TASS is a sterile inflammatory reaction that occurs usually due to noninfective toxic substances entering the eye. It can mimic endophthalmitis to a great extent.

Once the suspicion is in favor of endophthalmitis, it calls for an urgent management plan. The basic protocol in diagnosis of acute post-operative endophthalmitis is highlighted in **Flow chart 13.2**.

Post-Cataract Surgery Endophthalmitis

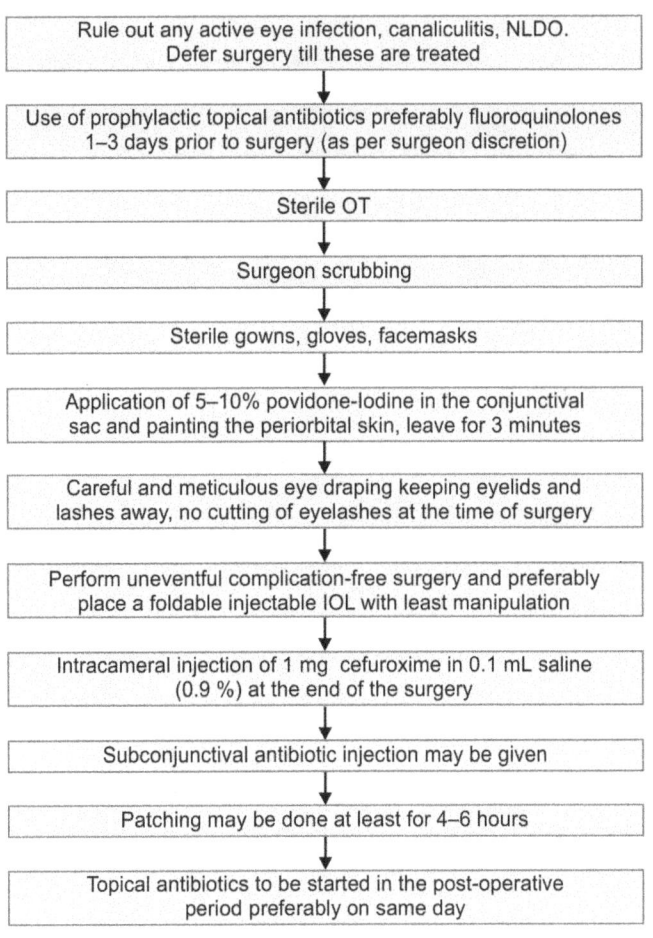

Flow chart 13.1 Guidelines for prophylaxis of postcataract surgery endophthalmitis

Adapted from: The ESCRS study. J Cataract Refract Surg. 2006;32:407-410

In a suspected case of endophthalmitis occurring in the post-operative period, a vitreous tap should be taken and sent for microbiological assessment as early as possible. An empirical dose of intravitreal antibiotics covering a broad-spectrum of micro-organisms may be given even before the microbiology reports become available. A timely administered intravitreal antibiotic injection aids in the resolution of acute post-operative endophthalmitis **(Figures 13.1A and B)**. Some reports have suggested the use of dexamethasone intravitreally at this stage along with the antibiotics in order to reduce the inflammation. It is not routinely practiced though and is purely based on surgeon's preferance. Once the microbiology reports are obtained, a second dose of intravitreal antibiotics according to the culture sensitivity may be administered 48 hours after the first. A repeat posterior segment analysis is done after each injection. If the endophthalmitis does not show any improvement, a complete three port pars plana vitrectomy is advisable. EVS study had suggested that vitrectomy may be done only in those cases where the presenting visual acuity was only perception of light. More recent studies such as ESCRS suggest an early and complete vitrectomy for post-operative endophthalmitis. With advances in vitrectomy surgery, it is now possible to achieve good visual outcomes with a timely performed vitrectomy. The management protocol is summarized in **Flow chart 13.3**.

Among intravitreal antibiotics ceftazidime (2.25 mg/0.1 mL) and vancomycin (1 mg/0.1 mL) are the most commonly used empirically. Specific antimicrobial agents may be administered intravitreally in cases of

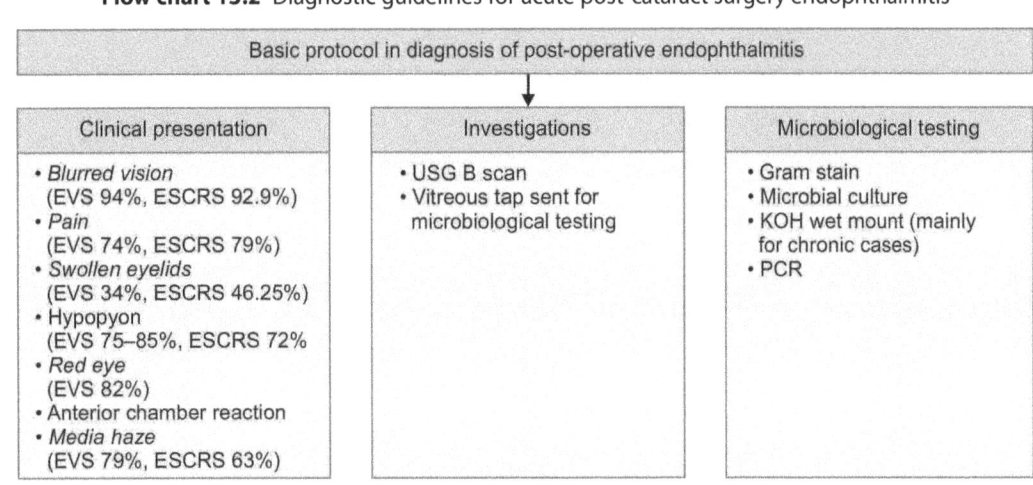

Flow chart 13.2 Diagnostic guidelines for acute post-cataract surgery endophthalmitis

Adapted from: EVS study and ESCRS study

Ocular Infections: Prophylaxis and Management

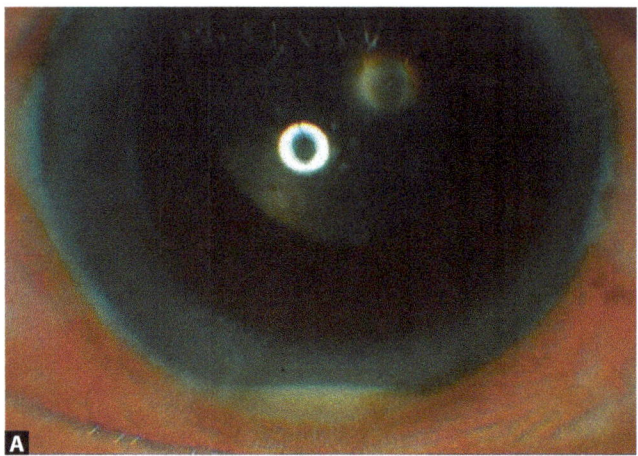
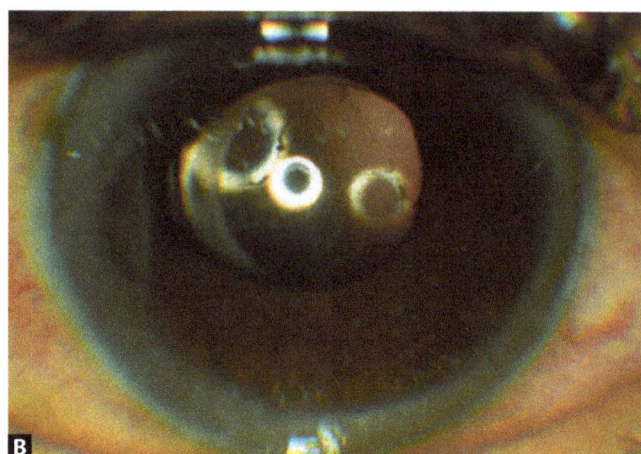

Figures 13.1A and B (A) Clinical photograph of acute post-operative endophthalmitis one week after phacoemulsification; (B) Clinical photograph at Day 4 after intravitreal antibiotics with resolution of hypopyon and exudates

Flow chart 13.3 Management protocol of a case of acute post-operative endophthalmitis

- Establish the diagnosis of endophthalmitis
- Earliest possible vitreous tap to be taken through pars plana route, sent for microbiological assessment
- Empirical intravitreal antibiotics (Ceftazidime 2.25 mg in 0.1 mL; Vancomycin 1 mg in 0.1 mL) administered through separate syringes
- Intravitreal injection dexamethasone (400 µg) may be given alongside but in separate syringe
- Repeat ultrasound B scan post-injection
- If there is severe non-resolving endophthalmitis, surgeon may go for PPV at this stage as well
- Repeat intravitreal injection 48 hours after first
- Repeat USG B scan to look for any improvement
- Three port complete pars plana vitrectomy: in case of no improvement
- Systemic antibiotics may be continued in the follow-up period

Adapted from: ESCRS study

Table 13.2 Dosage for intravitreal administration of antimicrobial agents

Ceftazidime	2.25 mg/0.1 mL
Vancomycin	1 mg/0.1 mL
Imipenem	50–100 µg/0.1 mL
Fluconazole	25 µg/0.1 mL
Amphotericin B	5 µg/0.1 mL
Piperacillin/Tazobactam	225 µg/0.1 mL
Voriconazole	50 µg/0.1 mL
Amikacin	125 µg/0.1 mL
Moxifloxacin	400 µg/0.1 mL
Gatifloxacin	400 µg/0.1mL
Clindamycin	250 µg/0.1 mL
Tobramycin	200 µg/0.1 mL
Ganciclovir	2 mg/0.1 mL

culture positivity of the vitreous tap. Antifungals such as fluconazole (25 µg/0.1 mL), voriconazole (50 µg/0.1 mL) and amphotericin B (5 µg/0.1 mL) are effective intravitreally in cases of fungal endophthalmitis. In case of pseudomonas endophthalmitis, combination of piperacillin-tazobactam (225 µg/0.1 mL) may be used intravitreally. The intravitreal dosage of various antimicrobial agents is summarized in **Table 13.2**.

Dilemmas in the Prevention of Post-cataract Surgery Endophthalmitis

There may be certain situations where a process by process algorithm may not work for the prevention of post-operative endophthalmitis. One such situation is patients with an allergy to cefuroxime or cephalosporins in general. In such cases, intracameral moxifloxacin or vancomycin may be used. In cases of penicillin allergy, intracameral cefuroxime may still be used. Administration of subconjunctival antibiotics at the end of surgery is left to the surgeon's discretion.

CONCLUSION

Post-cataract surgery endophthalmitis is a rare but potentially serious complication. Measures to prevent such a situation begin right from the pre-operative patient assessment. It requires a systematic approach including topical prophylactic antibiotics, pre-operative antisepsis, sterile OT techniques and post-operative antibiotic treatment. Timely diagnosis and management is the key in case such an event does occur.

REFERENCES

1. Lundström M. Endophthalmitis and incision construction. Curr Opin Ophthalmol. 2006;17:68-71.
2. Endophthalmitis Study Group, European Society of Cataract and Refractive Surgeons. Prophylaxis of postoperative endophthalmitis following cataract surgery: results of the ESCRS multicenter study and identification of risk factors. J Cataract Refract Surg. 2007;33:978-88 2.
3. He L, Ta CN, Hu N, et al. Prospective randomized comparison of 1-day and 3-day application of topical 0.5% moxifloxacin in eliminating preoperative conjunctival bacteria. J Ocul Pharmacol Ther. 2009;25:373-8.
4. Alwitry A, Jackson E, Chen H, Holden R. The use of surgical facemasks during cataract surgery: is it necessary? The British Journal of Ophthalmology. 2002;86(9):975-7.
5. Anijeet DR, Palimar P, Peckar CO. Intracameral vancomycin following cataract surgery: An eleven-year study. Clinical Ophthalmology (Auckland, NZ). 2010;4:321-6.
6. Au CP, White AJ, Healey PR. Efficacy and cost-effectiveness of intracameral vancomycin in reducing postoperative endophthalmitis incidence in Australia. Clin Exp Ophthalmol. 2016 Jun 17. doi: 10.1111/ceo.12789. [Epub ahead of print]
7. Hospital Infection Control Practices Advisory Committee (HICAC) Recommendations for preventing the spread of vancomycin resistance. Infect Control Hosp Epidemiol. 1995;16:105-13.
8. Montan PG, Wejde G, Setterquist H, Rylander M, Zetterstom C. Prophylactic intracameral cefuroxime: Evaluation of safety and kinetics in cataract surgery. J Cataract Refract Surg. 2002;28:982-7.
9. Axer-Seigel R, et al. Cystoid macular edema after cataract surgery with intraocular vancomycin. Ophthalmology. 1999;106(9):1660-4.
10. Witkin AJ, et al. Postoperative Hemorrhagic Occlusive Retinal Vasculitis: Expanding the Clinical Spectrum and Possible Association with Vancomycin. Ophthalmology. 2015;122(7):1438-51.
11. Endophthalmitis Vitrectomy Study Group. Results of the Endophthalmitis Vitrectomy Study. A randomized trial of immediate vitrectomy and of intravenous antibiotics for the treatment of postoperative bacterial endophthalmitis. Arch Ophthalmol. 1995;113:1479-96.
12. Barry P, Gardner S, Seal D, et al. ESCRS Endophthalmitis Study Group. Clinical observations associated with proven and unproven cases in the ESCRS study of prophylaxis of postoperative endophthalmitis after cataract surgery. J Cataract Refract Surg. 2009;35:1523-3.
13. Sharma S, Sahu SK, Dhillon V, Das S, Rath S. Reevaluating intracameral cefuroxime as a prophylaxis against endophthalmitis after cataract surgery in India. J Cataract Refract Surg. 2015;41:393-9.
14. Montan PG, Wejde G, Koranyi G, Rylander M. Prophylactic intracameral cefuroxime. Efficacy in preventing endophthalmitis after cataract surgery. J Cataract Refract Surg. 2002;28:977-81.
15. Lane SS, Osher RH, Masket S, Belani S. Evaluation of the safety of prophylactic intracameral moxifloxacin in cataract surgery. J Cataract Refract Surg. 2008;34:1451-9.
16. Arbisser LB. Safety of intracameral moxifloxacin for prophylaxis of endophthalmitis after cataract surgery. J Cataract Refract Surg. 2008;34:1114-20.
17. Shorstein NH, Winthrop KL, Herrinton LJ. Decreased postoperative endophthalmitis rate after institution of intracameral antibiotics in a Northern California eye department. J Cataract Refract Surg. 2013;39:8-14.

CHAPTER 14

Post-Intravitreal Injection Infections

Raghav Ravani, Rohan Chawla, Atul Kumar

INTRODUCTION

In recent times, with the advent and use of anti-VEGF (vascular endothelial growth factor) agents for intraocular use, there has been a paradigm shift in the management of various medical retinal pathologies including neovascular age-related macular degeneration (AMD), diabetic retinopathy and macular edema and retinal vein occlusion. It is now known that VEGF plays a pivotal role in the pathogenesis of these conditions and intravitreal anti-VEGF agents are the first agents which have shown to improve visual acuity, rather than just prevent vision loss.

Endophthalmitis is one of the most dreaded complications of any intraocular procedure including intravitreal injections, causing severe ocular morbidity and vision loss.

INCIDENCE AND RISK FACTORS

The incidence of post-intravitreal injection endophthalmitis (PIE) is low. The incidence of post-cataract surgery endophthalmitis ranges between 0.09% and 0.33% in various studies,[1] whereas that of suspected PIE has been reported to be around 0.038% and varies from 0.021 to 0.045%.[2,3] Although the incidence is low, there is a worldwide dramatic increase in the number of injections performed annually, including India. Intravitreal injections is the most commonly performed medical procedure in the United States with numbers about twice as that of cataract surgery.[4,5] Thus, PIE is a matter of grave concern, especially with confirmed reports of series of cluster endophthalmitis from our country following intravitreal injections. Cluster endophthalmitis has been defined as 5 or more cases occurring on a single surgical day and the same operating room at the center involved. Various risk factors predispose to the occurrence of PIE, including the condition for which the injection is given. The risk of infection seems to be lower in eyes with macular edema secondary to retinal vein occlusion as the indication of injection.[6] The risk is more in patients with diabetic eye disease and neovascular AMD, with impaired or waning immunity as the hypothesized mechanism in both.[6] Other risk factors (summarized in **Table 14.1**) include multiple patients undergoing the procedure in one sitting, improper storage of the drug or lapse in cold-chain (especially in drugs used as multidose vials, e.g. off-label use of bevacizumab), procurement of counterfeit drugs and multiple use of multi-dose vials, etc.

CLINICAL PRESENTATION

Clinical presentation, characteristics and suspected organisms causing infection in PIE is quite different from post-operative endophthalmitis (POE), with the former being more fulminant with a worse prognosis if not treated aggressively **(Fig. 14.1)**.

Post-operative endophthalmitis may present as fulminant (<4 days), acute (5–7 days) or chronic form (>4 weeks). The time period of occurrence of PIE from injection to presentation is early and ranges from within 24 hours to even up to 26 days as reported, with an average of 4 days.

Post-Intravitreal Injection Infections

Table 14.1 Risk factors for post-intravitreal injection infections

Associated with increased risk	Indication for injection (e.g. More risk in diabetes and AMD compared to vein occlusion)
	Improper storage/Lapse in cold chain
	Multiple use of multi-dose vials by repeated puncture of vials
	Counterfeit drugs
	Procedure performed in office-setting (risk if more when compared to operation theatre setting)
	Contaminated OT/irrigation fluids/failure of aseptic technique
Not associated with increased risk[8]	Type of intravitreal anti-VEGF agent use
	Hemisphere or quadrant of injection
	Conjunctival displacement during procedure

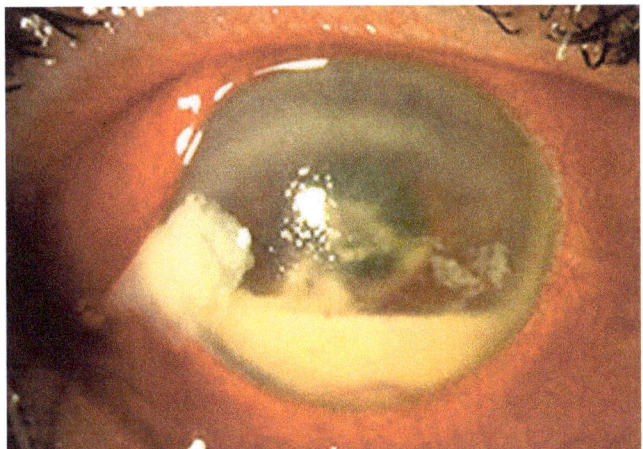

Figure 14.1 Post-intravitreal injection fulminant endophthalmitis

The most common symptom in both types of endophthalmitis is vision loss. The most frequent pathogens reported in PIE are gram positive bacteria (91.3%), especially coagulase-negative *Staphylococcus* (78.3%). *Streptococcus viridans*, a component of human oral flora has been reported to be present three times more often in PIE as compared to POE.[7] Postintravitreal injection endophthalmitis needs to be differentiated from culture-negative sterile endophthalmitis, resembling toxic anterior segment syndrome (TASS) seen after intraocular surgery.[9-11] A case series of such patients presenting with sterile endophthalmitis following intravitreal injection and their successful treatment with intravitreal antibiotics along with topical antibiotics and steroids has been reported from our center, highlighting the possibility of sterile endophthalmitis following intravitreal injection of bevacizumab.[12]

DIAGNOSIS AND MANAGEMENT

Diagnosis of endophthalmitis following intravitreal injection is primarily clinical. As mentioned earlier, patients receiving intravitreal injection of bevacizumab may present with sterile endophthalmitis.[9-12] In cases of doubt, it is important to consider all unexpected inflammatory response following injection or surgery to be endophthalmitis unless proven otherwise. The diagnosis can be confirmed by culture of causative organisms *in vitro* from intraocular samples. Samples that can be collected are aqueous tap or vitreous sample (higher yield) or both (preferred). A vitreous sample can be obtained by vitreous tap using 23-G needle through pars plana route before intravitreal antibiotic injections. However, due to the inadequacy of sample for analysis and theoretical risk of producing vitreous traction during aspiration, vitreous biopsy is preferred by many surgeons especially without infusion line to safely obtain adequate volume of sample that provides higher yield of organisms (**Fig. 14.2**). This may be performed as a sole procedure or just before pars plana vitrectomy for endophthalmitis. The sample is then sent for staining for microscopic evaluation and culture and sensitivity. Apart from confirmation of diagnosis in patients presenting with intraocular inflammation, it is also important to maintain and check records of the batch number of the drug used, and patients receiving injection on same day or injection from the same batch number. A drug vial from that particular batch number may also be sent for smear and culture which can help to trace the source of infection and early detection of other cases of endophthalmitis in the cluster if any.

Treatment in POE can be initiated following Endophthalmitis Vitrectomy Study (EVS) guidelines.[13]

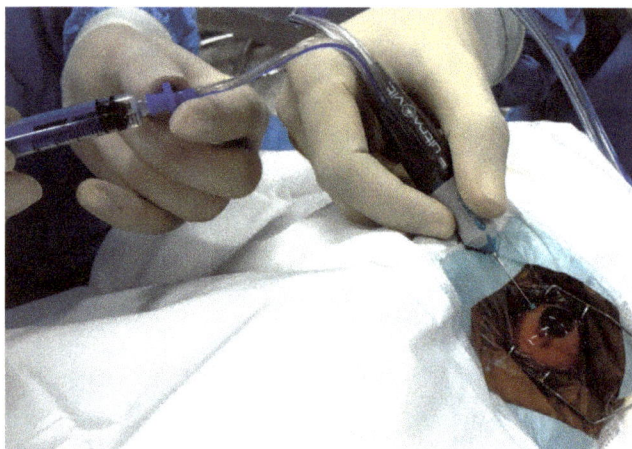

Figure 14.2 The technique of intravitreal biopsy (single port) under strict aseptic precautions

This includes anti-bacterial therapy in the form of intravitreal antibiotics, anti-inflammatory therapy, supportive therapy or surgery. Concentrated topical antibiotics should be considered empirically till the culture results are awaited, especially if the route of infection spread seems to be from the anterior segment. Concentrated topical antibiotics may include cefazolin 5% and tobramycin 1.3%. Commonly used empirical intravitreal antibiotics include vancomycin 1 mg/0.1 mL and ceftazidime 2.25 mg/0.1 mL.

However, the treatment of PIE needs be tailored depending upon individual cases. The treatment in PIE should be more aggressive as the infection tends to have a worse prognosis.

Though EVS concluded that there is no additional benefit of parenteral antibiotics in post-cataract surgery endophthalmitis, parenteral antibiotics help in augmenting and sustaining an adequate concentration of antibiotics in the vitreous cavity for a more prolonged period. Also, with the use of newer generations of antibiotics adequate MIC levels of the antimicrobial drugs in vitreous may be achieved when given parenterally, especially in cases of endophthalmitis, due to associated inflammation and resultant breakdown of the blood-retinal barrier. Thus parenteral antibiotics may be used, especially in post-intravitreal injection endophthalmitis which are usually fulminant and aggressive.

Like post-cataract surgery endophthalmitis, intravitreal antibiotics is the most common first line treatment in post-intravitreal injection endophthalmitis, however vitrectomy may be required for persistent vitritis, especially with atypical organisms. Early surgical intervention may be preferred in fulminant PIE. With the advancement in surgical techniques and equipment, the aim of surgery is to achieve complete vitrectomy with PVD induction, thereby removing the nidus of infection and significantly decreasing toxic and inflammatory load.

Undiluted specimen should be sent for culture studies and antibiotics should be injected in the vitreous cavity at the end of the surgery thereby achieving increased intraocular antibiotic concentration. A prospective randomized controlled trial at our center for post-traumatic endophthalmitis compared outcomes in patients that underwent core vitrectomy alone, to patients that underwent complete vitrectomy with silicone oil endotamponade.[15] The study showed that complete vitrectomy with primary silicone oil endotamponade improved anatomical and functional results in post-traumatic endophthalmitis. Apart from being used as an internal tamponade after vitrectomy, silicone oil has been suggested to possess antimicrobial activity and could be preferred in post-intravitreal injection endophthalmitis.

PROPHYLAXIS

Pre-operative Patient Screening and Precautions

- The need and choice of intravitreal injection should be tailored to the individual patient as required in the best clinical judgment of the attending/injecting physician.
- Patients with uncontrolled systemic conditions like uncontrolled diabetes should first be treated for it.
- All patients should be screened to ensure patency of the nasolacrimal duct by a negative regurgitation test.
- Patients with active infection of the ocular adnexa (blepharitis, meibomitis), or a blocked nasolacrimal duct/positive regurgitation test are at high risk for endophthalmitis and should be treated for the active infection first. Injection should be postponed until the active infection is cleared.
- Surgical/Procedural time-out to verify patient's name, intravitreal agent and laterality should be practiced before injection in each patient.
- Bilateral injections are *not* recommended and injection in the other eye should be spaced at least one to two weeks apart.

Post-Intravitreal Injection Infections

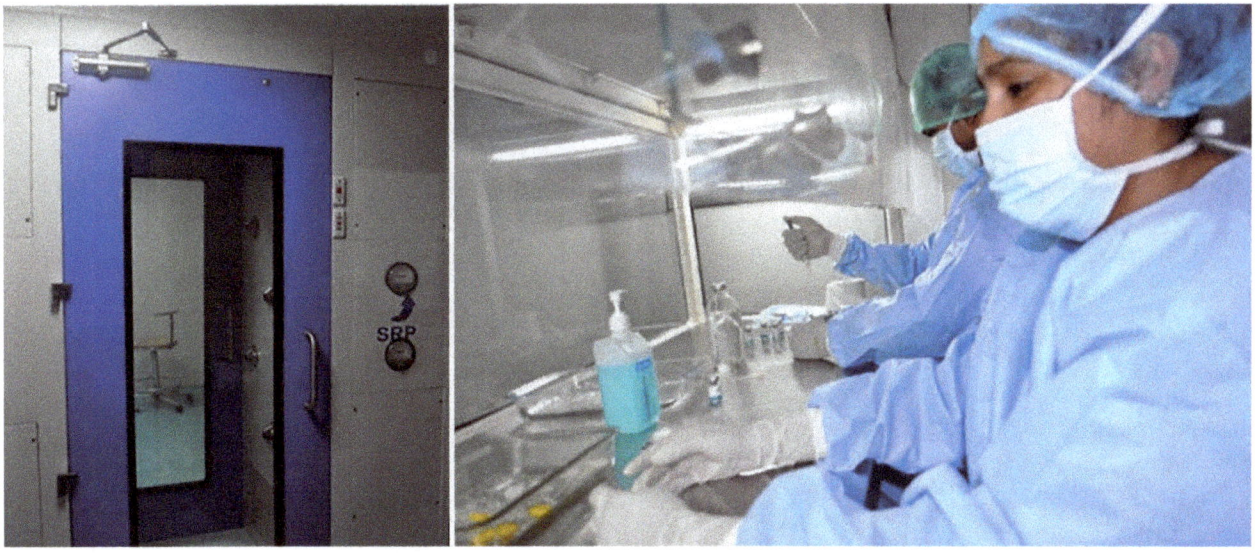

Figure 14.3 Dispensing of drug from multidose vials to single dose ampoules by a trained pharmacist under sterile GMP dispensing facility (class 10000 and class 10)

Drug Procurement or Preparation—Precautions for use of Drugs with Multi-Dose Vials

- Drug should be purchased from recognized dealers with proper receipt.
- Cold chain is to be maintained at each stage with proper temperature log maintenance.
- Note the batch number of each vial before opening.

Options for multiple injections from one vial (especially bevacizumab)

- *Ideally*: *Compounding pharmacy* to provide *single dose ampoules*. This constitutes dispensing of drug from vial (100 mg/4 mL) to sterile ampoules containing 0.2 mL for single use of 0.05 mL injection. This includes various tests including test of drug formulation for counterfeits (before dispensing), quality control tests and dispensing in sterile dispensing Good Manufacturing Practice (GMP) facility (class 10 and class 10,000 environment) under laminar flow hood as is done at our center **(Figs 14.3 and 14.4)**.
- Prepare multiple syringes by single puncture of vial under laminar hood. Store the syringes in a sterile container. Send 2 such syringes for culture. If culture negative, use the syringes for injection. The stored syringes are to be discarded after 2 weeks as there is minimal degradation of anti-VEGF activity of bevacizumab over first 2–3 weeks.[16]

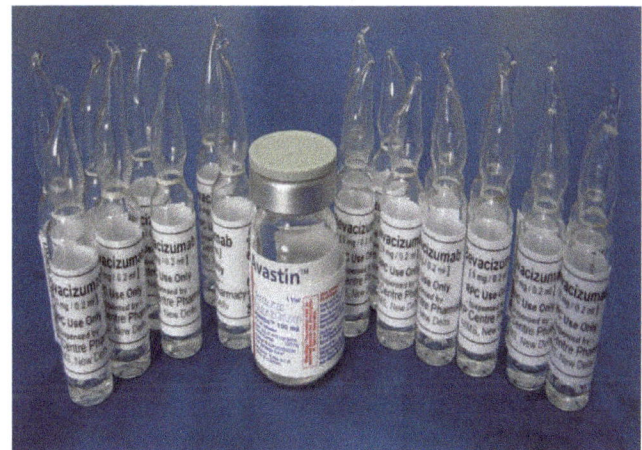

Figure 14.4 Single use ampoules prepared from a multi-dose vial

- In case the facility for above two is not available (least preferred):
  - Pool up to 7 patients on the day of injection (the number has been empirically decided keeping in mind the financial viability of the procedure on one hand and prevention of loss of vision in many eyes in case of a cluster endophthalmitis)
  - Prepare 7 aliquots of around 0.2 mL per syringe (one syringe for one patient) inside the OT by single puncture of the vial after proper scrubbing and using aseptic technique
  - Re-cap the syringes with fresh sterile needles
  - Keep these syringes on a sterile surface

- Only use these for the patients in the same session
- Discard the vial—It is *not* to be re-used or re-punctured

Prophylactic Topical Antibiotics

The studies on the role of topical antibiotics in the prevention of PIE concluded lack of evidence to support the administration of peri or post-injection topical antibiotics.[3,17,18] Thus pre-injection and post-injection topical antibiotics do not reduce the risk, in fact some studies showed a trend towards higher incidence.[3,18] However, short course of post-procedure prophylactic antibiotics is used on surgeon's personal experience and discretion.

Patient Preparation

- A written-informed consent should be taken from all patients, explaining the procedure and the risks involved. Off label use of bevacizumab is to be included in consent and explained to the patient.
- Each patient is to be given clean OT gown, protective cap and shoe-cover before entering the pre-operative holding area/operating room **(Fig. 14.5)**.
- In the pre-operative holding area/or on table, the periocular skin should be cleaned with povidone-iodine 10% solution.
- 10% povidone iodine should be used to clean the skin and ocular adnexa, 5% povidone iodine for instillation into the cul de sac with contact time of atleast 3 minutes **(Figs 14.6A and B)**.
- Surgical area should be draped using sterile linen and a separate plastic eye-drape for each patient to isolate the field. A sterile speculum is placed to isolate the eyelashes away from the field **(Figs 14.6C and D)**.

Sterilization of Operating Room and Operating Room Milieu

- *Location*: Intravitreal injection should be administered in the operating-room setting, and *not* in office-setting.
- *Sterilization and quality control*: should be done prior to intravitreal injections as discussed in detail in relevant chapters of the book.

Intra-operative Precautions

Surgeon Factors

- Surgeon should wear washed OT clothes, OT slippers, cap and mask.
- Surgeon should perform 3 scrubs with a solution equivalent to 2% w/v of chlorhexidine gluconate for at least 5–7 minutes under running water as per WHO recommendation. Details of scrubbing, gowning and gloving have been discussed in detail in the relevant chapters of the book.
- The surgeon/staff/patient should minimize speaking on table during preparation or during the injection procedure to minimize spread of aerosolized droplets containing oral contaminants.[6]

Peri-injection Precautions

- Topical anesthetic drops should be preferred over anesthetic gel as the latter may interfere with povidone iodine contact with the conjunctiva/injection site.
- Reapply povidone-iodine after anesthetic drop use. Before injection, povidone-iodine (5%) should be the last agent applied to the intended injection site.
- Routine anterior chamber paracentesis is not recommended.

Post-operative Precautions

- Proper lid hygiene should be maintained in the post-operative period
- Post-injection topical antibiotics do *not* reduce the risk of infection/endophthalmitis.

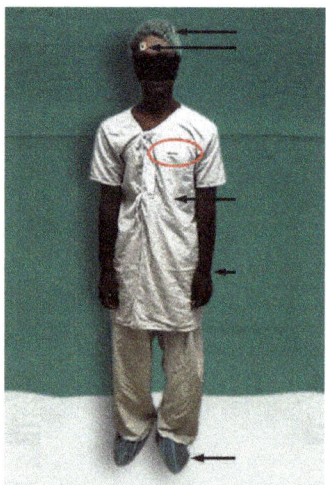

Figure 14.5 Pre-operative preparation of patient wearing protective cap and shoe-cover, clean operation theatre dress, eye marked for laterality check during surgical time-out, label on chest with name and unique ID no./registration number, removal of any bands or ornaments

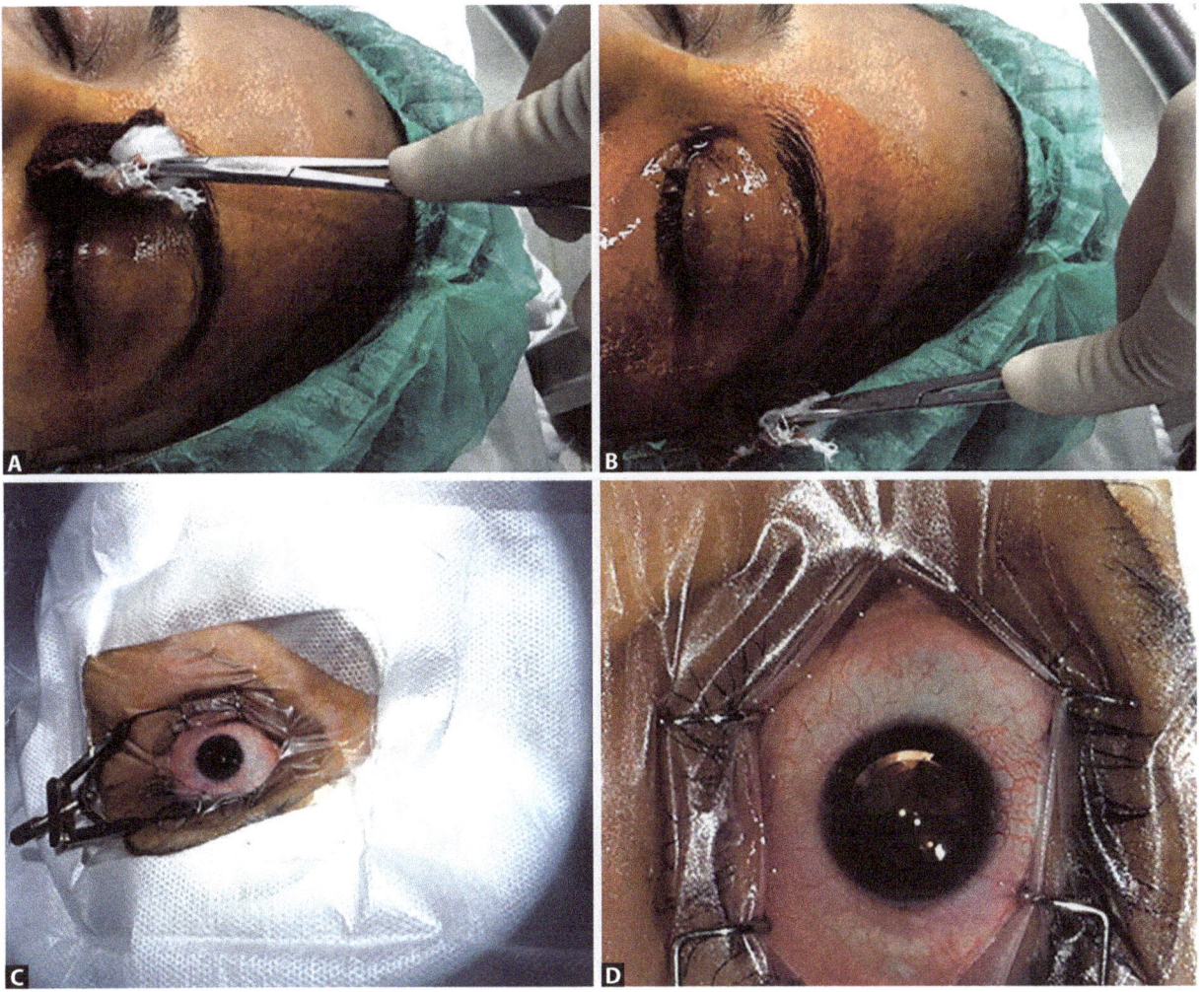

Figures 14.6A to D Pre-operative cleaning (A and B), use of sterile plastic drape (C) and use of sterile speculum (D) to isolate the eyelashes away from the field before intravitreal injection

- Post-injection IOP should be monitored and topical antiglaucoma drugs may be prescribed for post-injection IOP spike as and when warranted.
- All patients should be given a discharge card mentioning the injection details, post-operative instructions, symptoms of infection (pain, redness, dimness of vision, swelling, discharge etc.) and 24-hour emergency contact information.
- Follow-up of each patients should be tailored as per the indication for the intravitreal injections.

Intravitreal injection of bevacizumab (Avastin©) for ophthalmic disorders may be considered at treating physician's discretion, under strict aseptic precautions and following the recommended guidelines after informed consent of the patient. Intravitreal injection of medications for various posterior segment disorders has become one of the most common procedure performed worldwide. With extensive ongoing trials worldwide for various disorders involving intravitreal injection of different pharmacological agents, intravitreal injections have become a standard protocol and mainstay treatment for various pharmacological disorders. Endophthalmitis following intravitreal injection, though rare, is a dreaded complication causing significant ocular morbidity and vision loss. Following standard surgical procedures, precautions and maintaining asepsis can go a long way in preventing this complication and provide better outcomes.

REFERENCES

1. Taban M, Behrens A, Newcomb RL, et al. Acute endophthalmitis following cataract surgery: A systematic review of the literature. Arch Ophthalmol. 2005;123: 613-20.
2. Dossarps D, et al. Endophthalmitis After Intravitreal Injections: Incidence, Presentation, Management, and Visual Outcome. Am J Ophthalmol. 2015;160:17-25.
3. Storey P, et al. The role of topical antibiotic prophylaxis to prevent endophthalmitis after intravitreal injection. Ophthalmology. 2014;121:283-9.
4. Ramulu PY, Do DV, Corcoran KJ, Corcoran SL, Robin AL. Use of retinal procedures in medicare beneficiaries from 1997 to 2007. Arch Ophthalmol. 2010;128:1335.
5. Colin A. McCannel, et al. Updated Guidelines for Intravitreal Injection. Review of Ophthalmology, 7/6/2015.
6. Rayess N, et al. Incidence and clinical features of post-injection endophthalmitis according to diagnosis. Br J Ophthalmol. 2015 Nov 19. pii: bjophthalmol-2015-307707.
7. Chen E, et al. Endophthalmitis after intravitreal injection: the importance of viridans streptococci. Retina. 2011;31:1525-33.
8. Shah CP, et al. Outcomes and risk factors associated with endophthalmitis after intravitreal injection of anti-vascular endothelial growth factor agents. Ophthalmology. 2011;118:2028-34.
9. Sato T, Emi K, Ikeda T, Bando H, Sato S, Morita S, et al. Severe intraocular inflammation after intravitreal Injection of Bevacizumab. Ophthalmology. 2010;117:512-6.
10. Yamashiro K, Tsujikawa A, Miyamoto K, Oh H, Otani A, Tamuara H, et al. Sterile endophthalmitis after intravitreal injection of bevacizumab obtained from a single batch. Retina. 2010;30:485-90.
11. Wickremasinghe SS, Michalova K, Gilhotra J, Guymer RH, Harper CA, Wong TY, et al. Acute intraocular inflammation after intravitreous injections of bevacizumab for treatment of neovascular age related macular degeneration. Ophthalmology. 2008;115:1911-5.
12. Sinha S, Vashisht N, Venkatesh P, Garg SP. Managing bevacizumab-induced intraocular inflammation. Indian J Ophthalmol. 2012;60:311-3.
13. Endophthalmitis Vitrectomy Study Group. Results of the Endophthalmitis Vitrectomy Study. A randomized trial of immediate vitrectomy and of intravenous antibiotics for the treatment of post-operative bacterial endophthalmitis. Arch Ophthalmol. 1995;113:1479-96.
14. Sachdeva MM, Moshiri A, Leder HA, Scott AW. Endophthalmitis following intravitreal injection of anti VEGF agents: Long-term outcomes and the identification of unusual micro-organisms. Journal of Ophthalmic Inflammation and Infection. 2016;6(1):2.
15. Azad R, Ravi K, Talwar D, Rajpal, Kumar N. Pars plana vitrectomy with or without silicone oil endotamponade in post-traumatic endophthalmitis. Graefes Arch Clin Exp Ophthalmol. 2003;241:478-83.
16. Bakri SJ, et al. Six-month stability of bevacizumab (Avastin) binding to vascular endothelial growth factor after withdrawal into a syringe and refrigeration or freezing. Retina. 2006;26:519-22.
17. Li AL, Wykoff C, Wang R. et al. Endophthalmitis after intravitreal injection: Role of Prophylactic Topical Ophthalmic Antibiotics. Retina. 2016;36(7):1349-56.
18. Cheung CS, Wong AW, Lui A, et al. Incidence of endophthalmitis and use of antibiotic prophylaxis after intravitreal injections. Ophthalmology. 2012;119(8): 1609-14.

CHAPTER 15

Endophthalmitis after Pars Plana Vitrectomy

Karthikeya R, Rohan Chawla, Atul Kumar

INTRODUCTION

Endophthalmitis after pars plana vitrectomy (PPV) is a rare entity.[1-5] Unlike the aqueous, vitreous is stationary, without a turn over and in a gel form which impedes migration of bacteria as well as cells and mediators from the blood. This makes it an ideal culture medium for pathogens inoculated into the cavity to proliferate. With the removal of the vitreous gel, as a consequence, the risk of endophthalmitis drastically falls and, therefore, vitrectomy has the least incidence of endophthalmitis among the intraocular surgeries. However, it does occur and with an incidence of 0.03–0.14% for 20-G PPV and 0.058–1.55% for small gauge transconjunctival sutureless vitrectomy (TSV).[6] Over the last few years, the incidence has been found to be decreasing possibly owing to better surgical techniques and wound construction.[7] Most studies exclude vitrectomies for lens matter drop, recent ocular trauma, retained intraocular foreign body and endophthalmitis from the case definition of post PPV endophthalmitis.

CLINICAL FEATURES

Endophthalmitis after PPV is usually diagnosed in the first post-operative week, usually on the third day of surgery with disproportionately high intraocular inflammation.[2,3,8] Symptoms are similar to those of other causes of post-operative endophthalmitis like pain, redness and diminution of vision. Signs include circumciliary congestion, anterior chamber and/or posterior segment cells, hypopyon, fibrinous exudates and in severe cases exudation from the ports **(Fig. 15.1)**. Increasing media haze is an important sign early in the course. Chronic forms of endophthalmitis after vitrectomy have not been described in literature.

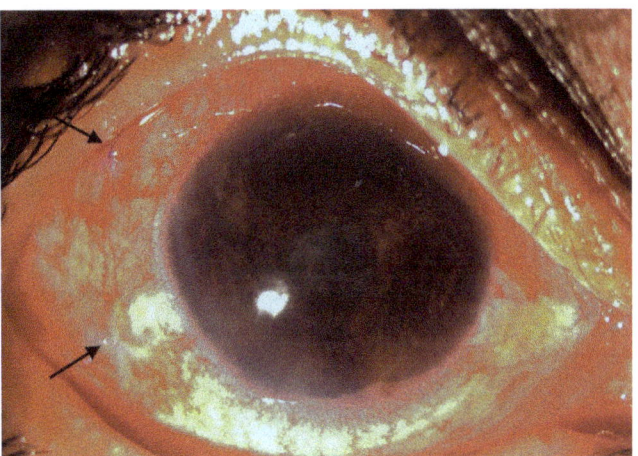

Figure 15.1 Post pars plana vitrectomy endophthalmitis with vitreous exudates and anterior chamber inflammation one week after pars plana vitrectomy. Note the vicryl sutures which are still present at the port sites (arrows)

The most common organism isolated in many studies is coagulase-negative staphylococci. Other organisms reported are *Pseudomonas* species, *Propionibacterium*, *Enterococci*, and *Bacillus* species.[6] Culture of the vitreous aspirate is positive in about 70% of the cases.[6]

RISK FACTORS

The debate over whether or not sutureless minimally invasive TSV was a risk factor for endophthalmitis raged for over a decade after the introduction of 25-G and 23-G systems. It now appears largely settled owing to numerous prospective studies and a few systematic reviews. Initially, sutureless nature and wound construction techniques of TSV were blamed for the post-operative contamination of vitreous cavity and subsequent development of endophthalmitis. Early retrospectives studies showed ambiguous results for the incidence of post PPV endophthalmitis with TSV as compared to the 20G surgeries—some studies showing higher rates of endophthalmitis after PPV and some showing similar rates.[3,6,9] But many prospective studies since then have shown unequivocally that there is no difference in the rates of endophthalmitis between the 20G and TSV systems.[7,10] Govetto et al. have analyzed the same in a systematic review and found no increased risk of endophthalmitis with Micro Incision Vitrectomy Surgery (MIVS) as compared to standard 20G vitrectomy.[5] Currently MIVS remains the most widely used system for vitrectomy in India and world over.

Post-operative wound leak and hypotony are important risk factors.[11] Wound leak and hypotony promotes exchange of conjunctival fluid with the vitreous fluid thereby causing intraocular contamination. Sutured ports have been shown to reduce post-operative hypotony, wound leak and flux of extraocular fluid into the intraocular space.[12] A straight incision, as opposed to a beveled incision,[5,8,11] fluid filled cavity as compared to air or gas filled cavity,[3,13] and mechanical disturbance of the wound by the patient[3,8] have all been found to be a risk factor for the development of endophthalmitis. All these factors increase the risk of endophthalmitis by increasing the risk of post-operative hypotony and wound leak due to inefficient port closure. Fluid as opposed to air/gas or silicone oil has a lower surface tension which prevents the efficient sealing of ports.

Vitreous wick syndrome is the condition of persisting herniation of a 'bead' or strand of vitreous within the sclerotomy after closure, at the end of pars plana vitreous surgery.[14] This herniation of vitreous occurs due to multiple factors: higher intraocular pressure due to infusion fluid or gas in relation to the atmospheric pressure, repeated instrumentation, difficulty in removing the sub-sclerotomy vitreous, need for multiple ports and difficulty in visualizing the prolapsed vitreous. This 'wick' of vitreous can act as a conduit to carry extraocular fluids and commensal bacteria into the vitreous cavity and set up endophthalmitis.

Diabetes mellitus and elderly age can also predispose to endophthalmitis post PPV due to the poor immune status in these individuals. In most studies describing endophthalmitis, a substantial proportion of the patients were diabetic.[1-4,6,7] A prospective study from UK also found pre-operative immunosuppression in the form of topical steroid use as an independent risk factors for the development of endophthalmitis post PPV.[7] In this study, pre-operative topical steroid use had an odds ratio (confidence interval) of 131.4 (21.8 to 792.7). The same study also showed that surgery for retinal detachment was associated with a reduced risk of endophthalmitis, perhaps because of a more complete vitrectomy in these cases.

Surgeon's learning curve has also been implicated as a risk factor for endophthalmitis after PPV. It was noted that surgeons transitioning from 20-G to TSV had a higher incidence of post-operative hypotony and endophthalmitis.[6]

PROPHYLAXIS

General pre-operative screening and prophylactic measures employed in other ocular surgeries need to be also observed for vitrectomy. Active ocular or adnexal infection should be considered a contraindication for an elective vitreous surgery. Diabetes needs to be well controlled before an elective intraocular surgery is contemplated. The use of perioperative topical antibiotics is suggested as well, acknowledging a lack of evidence to justify this practice.[15] Povidone-iodine preparation of the periocular skin and ocular surface remains the central measure to achieve presurgical asepsis.[16,17] In cases of suspected povidone-iodine allergy, a pre-operative skin test can be performed to confirm the reaction. In proven cases of allergy, chlorhexidine gluconate can be used instead to prepare the periocular skin. Lid speculum and an adhesive surgical drape are to be used to keep the lashes out of the surgical field.

Special attention needs to be paid while constructing wounds. As discussed earlier, straight incisions increase the risk of endophthalmitis as opposed to beveled entries. Conjunctival displacement while making trocar entry can reduce the flux of ocular fluids into the vitreous cavity in case of unsealed ports and hypotony. This may also reduce the chances of vitreous wick prolapsing out on to the ocular surface. Good port site vitrectomy ensures less residual vitreous at the sclerotomy site and reduces the risk of vitreous wick syndrome. During the surgery, slow removal of instruments from the ports minimizes any vacuum effects which would promote vitreous incarceration. Suturing leaky ports at the end of the surgery is prudent. In this regard, it is best to consider 23-G, 25-G and 27-G systems as "minimally invasive" or "microincision" rather than strictly sutureless. Subconjunctival antibiotics injected over the sclerotomy sites at the end of the surgery may have a protective effect against endophthalmitis by delivering the drug into the subconjunctival space as a depot which is often the source of the infecting flora and repositioning any vitreous that may have prolapsed out of the conjunctival incision[5,18] Post-operative topical and systemic antibiotics are widely used for prophylaxis of endophthalmitis, but the scientific basis for the same is poor.[17]

MANAGEMENT

Early detection of the condition improves the outcomes. Pain and blurring of vision are important symptoms that require immediate attention. Management includes vitreous tap to identify the infecting organism followed by intravitreal antibiotics. If the vitreous cavity is filled with gas or silicone oil, anterior chamber tap can be an alternative. Broad spectrum oral and topical antibiotics can be started after the tap. The choice of antibiotic for intravitreal and oral therapy can be similar to post cataract surgery endophthalmitis since the profile of infecting organisms is similar. Ceftazidime (2.25 mg/0.1 mL) and Vancomycin (1 mg/0.1 mL) are currently the authors choice of intravitreal antibiotics. An alternative to ceftazidime is Piperacillin + Tazobactam (225 μg/0.1 mL). Ciprofloxacin is the empirical oral antibiotic of choice with a dose of 750 mg BD. Topical broad spectrum antibiotics like a fourth generation fluoroquinolone can also be started. If there is co-existing keratitis, fortified antibiotics such as Cefazolin 50 mg/mL and Tobramycin 14 mg/mL are administered. Antibiotic therapy can be changed according to sensitivity reports as and when they become available. Intravitreal injection can be repeated if there is a response. In cases of lack of a response or worsening, a repeat vitrectomy/vitreous lavage with intravitreal antibiotics and silicone oil injection can be considered. Repeat vitrectomy may help by washing out the exudates and the infecting inoculum, clearing the residual vitreous and by providing opportunity to inject antibiotics and silicone oil. Silicone oil also has bacteriostatic properties.[19]

OUTCOMES

Most patients have a poor final visual acuity. The outcomes also depend on the nature of infecting organism—*Streptococci* usually have poor prognosis.[1] Prognosis also importantly depends on the underlying condition that required vitrectomy and time since onset of symptoms to initiation of therapy. Although good visual recovery has been reported in some patients with endophthalmitis after PPV, in general the prognosis remains poor.[2,6,8,9]

REFERENCES

1. Cohen SM, Flynn HW, Murray TG, Smiddy WE. Endophthalmitis after pars plana vitrectomy. The Postvitrectomy Endophthalmitis Study Group. Ophthalmology. 1995;102(5):705-12.
2. Eifrig CWG, Scott IU, Flynn HW, Smiddy WE, Newton J. Endophthalmitis after pars plana vitrectomy: Incidence, causative organisms, and visual acuity outcomes. Am J Ophthalmol. 2004;138(5):799-802.
3. Kunimoto DY, Kaiser RS, Wills Eye Retina Service. Incidence of endophthalmitis after 20- and 25-gauge vitrectomy. Ophthalmology. 2007;114(12):2133-7.
4. Mollan SP, Mollan AJ, Konstantinos C, Durrani OM, Butler L. Incidence of endophthalmitis following vitreoretinal surgery. Int Ophthalmol. 2009;29(3):203-5.
5. Govetto A, Virgili G, Menchini F, Lanzetta P, Menchini U. A systematic review of endophthalmitis after microincisional versus 20-gauge vitrectomy. Ophthalmology. 2013;120(11):2286-91.
6. Dave VP, Pathengay A, Schwartz SG, Flynn HW. Endophthalmitis following pars plana vitrectomy: a literature review of incidence, causative organisms, and treatment outcomes. Clin Ophthalmol Auckl NZ. 2014;8:2183-8.
7. Park JC, Ramasamy B, Shaw S, Prasad S, Ling RHL. A prospective and nationwide study investigating endophthalmitis following pars plana vitrectomy: incidence and risk factors. Br J Ophthalmol. 2014;98(4):529-33.
8. Scott IU, Flynn HW, Dev S, Shaikh S, Mittra RA, Arevalo JF, et al. Endophthalmitis after 25-gauge and 20-gauge pars plana vitrectomy: incidence and outcomes. Retina Phila Pa. 2008;28(1):138-42.
9. Scott IU, Flynn HW, Acar N, Dev S, Shaikh S, Mittra RA, et al. Incidence of endophthalmitis after 20-gauge vs 23-gauge vs 25-gauge pars plana vitrectomy. Graefes Arch Clin Exp Ophthalmol Albrecht Von Graefes Arch Für Klin Exp Ophthalmol. 2011;249(3):377-80.
10. Oshima Y, Kadonosono K, Yamaji H, Inoue M, Yoshida M, Kimura H, et al. Multicenter survey with a systematic

overview of acute-onset endophthalmitis after transconjunctival microincision vitrectomy surgery. Am J Ophthalmol. 2010;150(5):716-725.e1.
11. Acar N, Kapran Z, Unver YB, Altan T, Ozdogan S. Early postoperative hypotony after 25-gauge sutureless vitrectomy with straight incisions. Retina Phila Pa. 2008;28(4):545-52.
12. Chen D, Lian Y, Cui L, Lu F, Ke Z, Song Z. Sutureless vitrectomy incision architecture in the immediate postoperative period evaluated in vivo using optical coherence tomography. Ophthalmology. 2010;117(10):2003-9.
13. Chiang A, Kaiser RS, Avery RL, Dugel PU, Eliott D, Shah SP, et al. Endophthalmitis in microincision vitrectomy: outcomes of gas-filled eyes. Retina Phila Pa. 2011; 31(8):1513-7.
14. Venkatesh P, Verma L, Tewari H. Posterior vitreous wick syndrome: a potential cause of endophthalmitis following vitreo-retinal surgery. Med Hypotheses. 2002;58(6):513-5.
15. Miño de Kaspar H, Kreutzer TC, Aguirre-Romo I, Ta CN, Dudichum J, Bayrhof M, et al. A prospective randomized study to determine the efficacy of pre-operative topical levofloxacin in reducing conjunctival bacterial flora. Am J Ophthalmol. 2008;145(1):136-42.
16. Speaker MG, Menikoff JA. Prophylaxis of endophthalmitis with topical povidone-iodine. Ophthalmology. 1991; 98(12):1769-75.
17. Shah RE, Gupta O. The microsurgical safety task force: guidelines for minimizing endophthalmitis with vitrectomy surgery. Curr Opin Ophthalmol. 2012;23(3): 189-94.
18. Hu AYH, Bourges JL, Shah SP, Gupta A, Gonzales CR, Oliver SCN, et al. Endophthalmitis after pars plana vitrectomy a 20- and 25-gauge comparison. Ophthalmology. 2009;116(7):1360-5.
19. Chrapek O, Vecerova R, Koukalova D, Maresova K, Jirkova B, Sin M, Rehak J. The in vitro anti microbial activity of silicone oils used in ophthalmic surgery. Biomed Pap Med Fac Univ Palacky Olomouc Czech Repub. 2012;156(1):7-13.

CHAPTER 16

Post-LASIK Infections

Divya Singh, Neelima Aron, Prafulla K Maharana, Namrata Sharma

INTRODUCTION

Laser *in situ* keratomileusis (LASIK) is a very commonly performed refractive procedure. This is because it offers several advantages over other refractive procedures which include rapid visual rehabilitation and minimal amount of pain. However, this procedure requires the disruption of corneal integrity thereby exposing the stroma to the risk of invasion by the various infectious organisms. Infectious keratitis after LASIK is becoming an increasingly recognized and a potentially sight threatening complication of the surgery.

The incidence of infectious keratitis after LASIK ranges from 1 in 1000 to 1 in 5000 procedures.[1-5] The various risk factors include dry ocular surface, blepharitis and breaks in the epithelial barrier,[6] intra-operative contamination,[7] history of previous corneal surgery,[8] excessive surgical manipulation,[9] temporary use of contact lens post-operatively, use of topical steroids, and delayed post-operative re-epithelialization of the cornea.[10-13]

MICROBIAL SPECTRUM

Infectious keratitis is becoming an increasingly profound and devastating complication of LASIK surgery. It is indeed important to differentiate this from diffuse lamellar keratitis, another common complication after LASIK. The microbial organisms frequently isolated from infectious keratitis after LASIK are *Staphylococcus aureus*,[6,14-18] *Streptococcus viridans*,[17,19] coagulase negative *Staphylococcus*,[6,20] *Streptococcus pneumoniae*,[9,21] *Mycobacterium* species,[8,10,22,23] *Nocardia*[5,24,25] and *Pseudomonas aeruginosa*[26] (**Figs 16.1A to C**). The time of onset of symptoms could provide an important clue in arriving at the etiology of infection. Infections occurring within 10 days are usually classified as *early onset* whereas those occurring after 10 days are classified as *delayed onset*. *Early onset infectious keratitis* is usually caused by bacteria with a preponderance of the gram-positive organisms. On the other hand, the organisms most commonly causing the *delayed onset* symptoms are atypical mycobacteria, fungi, and *Nocardia*. The mycobacteria species most frequently belong to nontuberculous mycobacteria group, which are widely present in the environment, including distilled water, body fluid and surfaces, soil, and in healthy individuals. These are resistant to the chemical disinfectants which accounts for their likelihood of occurrence after any surgical procedure. The diagnosis is often delayed because the acid fast stains and the Lowenstein-Jensen media are not routinely used for cultures, and also because of the location of the organisms in the lamellar interface from where it is very difficult to take the scrapings and hence such infections often go unnoticed.

RISK FACTORS

The various risk factors which have been associated with infectious keratitis in the post-LASIK period are listed in **Table 16.1**.

Ocular Infections: Prophylaxis and Management

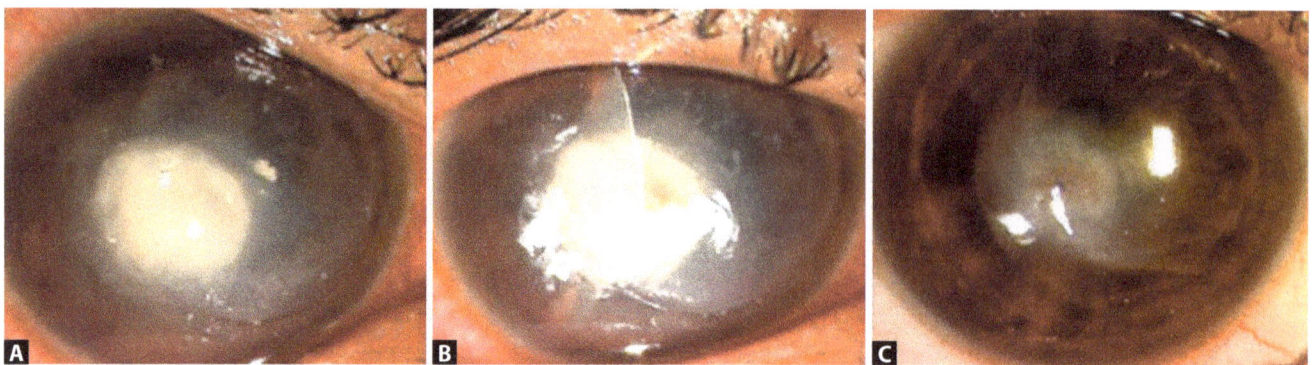

Figures 16.1A to C Infective keratitis 2 weeks post-LASIK with *Pseudomonas aeruginosa* (A) Worsening of infection with corneal perforation (B) Resolution of infection after a change of topical antibiotic therapy according to the culture sensitivity report (C)

Table 16.1 Risk factors for post-LASIK keratitis
Pre-operative
Blepharitis and dry eye
Previous refractive surgery like radial keratotomy and photorefractive keratectomy (PRK)
Immunocompromised status as in HIV-positive patients
Intra-operative
Breach in aseptic technique
Intra-operative epithelial defects
Intra-operative interface debris
Post-operative
Use of bandage contact lens
Use of tap water to wash the eye
Post-traumatic flap dehiscence or dislocation

CLINICAL DIAGNOSIS

Patients usually present with redness, photophobia, diminution of vision and pain. However, it is difficult to differentiate it from post-operative eye pain. Moreover, the subjective sensation of pain may be reduced post-operatively due to severing of the corneal nerves during flap creation. Post-LASIK infectious keratitis usually starts 2–3 days after the surgery and occurs as an inflammatory reaction which is not confined to the lamellar interface and can extend up to the flap, even beyond the flap, and also deeper into the stroma. It is often associated with anterior chamber reaction. This can even lead to flap melts, corneal scarring and resulting irregular astigmatism. The gram-positive infections are usually seen at the flap edge and have distinct and sharp margins. The fungal and mycobacterial infections are usually seen in the interface, with indistinct or feathery margins. A high degree of suspicion is required for rapid diagnosis and quick visual recovery. In cases of suspected post-LASIK infectious keratitis, it may be required to lift the flap, scrape the infiltrate and culture it on appropriate media including the blood agar, chocolate agar, thioglycolate broth, Sabouraud's dextrose agar, non nutrient agar with *E. coli* overlay, and Lowenstein-Jensen medium. The staining should also be performed with Gram's stain, Gomori methenamine silver stain, and Ziehl-Neelsen stain to rule out atypical causative agents. Viral swabs can also be sent for polymerase chain reaction (PCR) for *Herpes simplex*, *Herpes zoster*, and adenovirus infections. **Figures 16.2A to C** depicts post-LASIK keratitis caused by *Staphylococcus aureus* 3 days post-surgery.

Confocal Microscopy: Role in *Acanthamoeba* and Fungal Keratitis

This is an instrument used for non-invasive imaging of the cornea. This modality can provide high magnification images of the corneal layers. One of the main advantages of the confoscan is to assist in the rapid detection of fungal hyphae, *Acanthamoeba* trophozoites and cysts such that appropriate treatment can be started while the culture is still awaited. This can have a significant effect on the visual outcomes of the patient. However, bacterial and viral keratitis cannot be reliably diagnosed with confocal microscopy.

Polymerase Chain Reaction: Role in Viral, Fungal and *Acanthamoeba* Keratitis

This technique has been successfully used in the diagnosis of fungal, *Acanthamoeba* and viral keratitis and the high sensitivity, specificity, and the rapidity of this test make it an important modality of investigation in microbial keratitis.

PROPHYLAXIS

Over the years, it has been realized that the most important factor which is truly within our control is the prevention of infection. This commences right from the pre-operative period and continues till the post-operative period.

Pre-operatively, meibomian gland disease should be duly taken care of, as it poses the most significant risk factor for early onset infections. Subjects with meibomian gland dysfunction should be given instructions on lid hygiene at least 2 weeks before the surgical procedure and therapy with oral doxycycline should be started. Proper sterilization of instruments is equally important.

Intra-operatively, all aseptic and sterile precautions should be followed by the surgeon and the assisting staff. Adequate scrubbing is mandatory and the use of sterile gloves and drapes is warranted. The subjects should be prepared with 10% povidone iodine and draped to remove the lashes from the surgical field. The instruments should be sterile and care should be taken so as to avoid irrigating the meibomian secretions into the interface. Suction lid speculum may be of use in keeping away the debris.

Post-operatively, the patients should be instructed to use eyeshields and avoid eye rubbing. Swimming, gardening, and contact with pets should be preferably avoided in the post-operative period. In subjects with dry eye, the role of frequent lubrication with artificial tears is imperative. Prophylactic antibiotics should be prescribed for the initial few days post-operatively. These antibiotics should have a broad spectrum coverage. Fourth generation fluoroquinolones remain the prophylactic agent of choice amidst the bewildering array of drugs. However, these prophylactic agents are not effective against atypical mycobacteria.

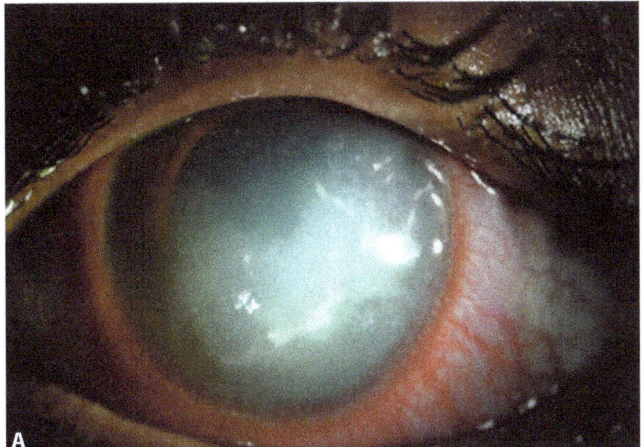
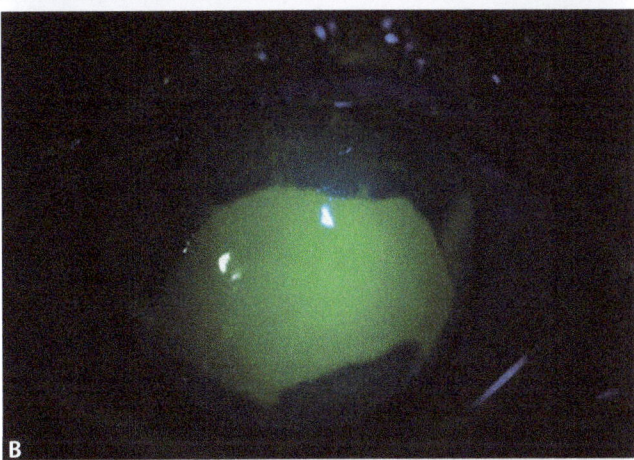
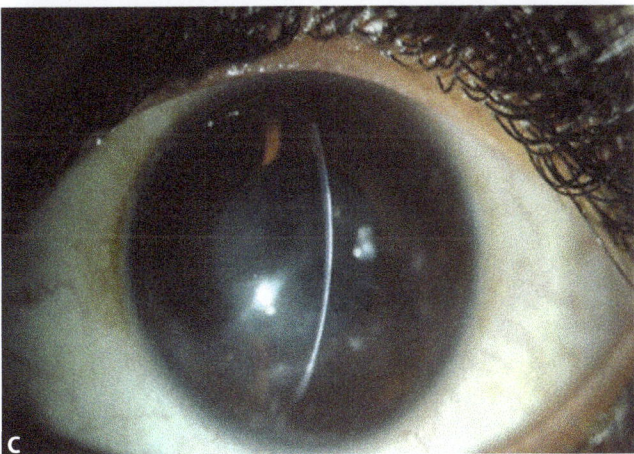

Figures 16.2A to C Post-LASIK keratitis with *Staphylococcus aureus*. (A and B) Clinical photograph and fluorescein staining of corneal ulcer involving the flap and interface 3 days after the surgery. The visual acuity of the patient dropped to 3/60 on Snellen's chart; (C) The patient was treated with topical fortified antibiotics with resolution of the ulcer. The uncorrected distance visual acuity improved to 6/18

TREATMENT: MEDICAL AND SURGICAL THERAPY

As previously discussed, even a very small infiltrate should be treated as an infection unless proved otherwise. Cases of suspected post-LASIK infectious keratitis should be managed by lifting the flap, scraping, and irrigating the stromal bed with a broad spectrum antibiotic such as fortified vancomycin 50 mg/mL for early onset and fortified amikacin 35 mg/mL for delayed onset keratitis. The choice of empirical therapy may vary depending upon the time of onset of symptoms. This empirical therapy may later be modified in light of the culture sensitivity reports.

For early onset keratitis, usually caused by gram-positive organisms, the treatment regimen includes fortified tobramycin (14 mg/mL) and vancomycin (25–50 mg/mL) or a fourth-generation fluoroquinolone and cefazolin (50 mg/mL) every 30 minutes. The steroid therapy should be tapered off immediately.

Delayed onset keratitis is usually due to atypical mycobacteria, *Nocardia*, or fungus infection. Topical clarithromycin (10 mg/mL), oral clarithromycin (500 mg bid), and topical amikacin (35 mg/mL) every 30 minutes are recommended for the treatment of mycobacterial infections. Natamycin (50 mg/mL) is used for filamentous fungi, amphotericin (1.5 mg/mL) for yeast infections, and topical voriconazole (10 mg/mL) with oral voriconazole (400 mg bid) is useful for treating both filamentous fungi and yeast infections. The corticosteroid therapy should be stopped.

If the infection fails to respond to any of these therapies, it might become necessary to amputate the corneal flap to allow better penetration of the antibiotic drugs. A partial flap amputation in the area of infiltrate might suffice. However, in cases of extensive involvement, a complete flap amputation may be needed. The resolution of infection leads to corneal scar formation the depth of which depends upon the extent of infiltrates. Corneal scar leads to vision loss due to the opacity as well as irregular astigmatism. A lamellar/penetrating keratoplasty may be performed at a later date for restoration of vision.

If the patient deteriorates further or there is no improvement with the above mentioned therapies, an emergency penetrating therapeutic keratoplasty should be performed to reduce the infectious load of the disease and prevent any devastating complications like endophthalmitis or panophthalmitis.

To conclude, infections after LASIK is disturbing both to the patient as well as the surgeon who performed the procedure. An early diagnosis, prompt institution of treatment and timely surgical intervention may help to maximize visual and functional outcomes.

REFERENCES

1. Machat JJ. LASIK complications. In: Machat JJ, Slade SG, Probst LE (Eds). The Art of LASIK, 2nd edn. Thorofare, NJ: Slack Inc. 1999. pp. 371-416.
2. Gimbel HV, Anderson-Penno EE. Laser Complications: Prevention and Management. Thorofare, NJ: Slack Inc. 1999. pp. 81-91.
3. Lin RT, Maloney RK. Flap complications associated with lamellar refractive surgery. Am J Ophthalmol. 1999;127:129-36.
4. Stulting RD, Carr JD, Thompson KP, et al. Complications of laser in situ keratomileusis for the correction of myopia. Ophthalmology. 1999;106:13-20.
5. Pe´rez-Santonja JJ, Sakla HF, Abad JL, et al. Nocardial keratitis after laser in situ keratomileusis [case report]. J Refract Surg. 1997;13:314-7.
6. Levartovsky S, Rosenwasser GOD, Goodman DF. Bacterial keratitis after laser in situ keratomileusis. Ophthalmology. 2001;108:321-25; errata, 1012.
7. Sridhar MS, Garg P, Bansal AK, Sharma S. Fungal keratitis after laser in situ keratomileusis. J Cataract Refract Surg. 2000;26:613-5.
8. Gelender H, Carter HL, Bowman B, et al. *Mycobacterium* keratitis after laser in situ keratomileusis. J Refract Surg. 2000;16:191-5.
9. Dada T, Sharma N, Dada VK, Vajpayee RB. Pneumococcal keratitis after laser in situ keratomileusis. J Cataract Refract Surg. 2000;26:460-1.
10. Garg P, Bansal AK, Sharma S, Vemuganti GK. Bilateral infectious keratitis after laser in situ keratomileusis; a case report and review of the literature. Ophthalmology. 2001;108:121-5.
11. Chung MS, Goldstein MH, Driebe WT Jr, Schwartz B. Fungal keratitis after laser in situ keratomileusis: a case report. Cornea. 2000;19:236-7.
12. Sridhar MS, Garg P, Bansal AK, Gopinathan U. *Aspergillus flavus* keratitis after laser in situ keratomileusis. Am J Ophthalmol. 2000;129:802-4.
13. Gupta V, Dada T, Vajpayee RB, et al. Polymicrobial keratitis after laser in situ keratomileusis. J Refract Surg. 2001;17:147-8.
14. Hovanesian JA, Faktrorovich EG, Hoffbauer JD, et al. Bilateral bacterial keratitis after laser in situ kerato-

mileusis in a subject with human immunodeficiency virus infection. Arch Ophthalmol. 1999;117:968-70.
15. Watanabe H, Sato S, Maeda N, et al. Bilateral corneal infection as a complication of laser in situ keratomileusis [letter]. Arch Ophthalmol. 1997;115:1593-4.
16. Webber SK, Lawless MA, Sutton GL, Rogers CM. Staphylococcal infection under a LASIK flap. Cornea 1999;18:361-5.
17. Quiros PA, Chuck RS, Smith RE, et al. Infectious ulcerative keratitis after laser in situ keratomileusis. Arch Ophthalmol. 1999;117:1423-7.
18. Al-Reefy M. Bacterial keratitis following laser in situ keratomileusis for hyperopia. J Refract Surg 1999;15:S216-7.
19. Kim HM, Song JS, Han HS, Jung HR. Streptococcal keratitis after myopic laser in situ keratomileusis. Korean J Ophthalmol. 1998;12:108-11.
20. Karp KO, Hersh PS, Epstein RJ. Delayed keratitis after laser in situ keratomileusis. J Cataract Refract Surg. 2000;26:925-8.
21. Mulhern MG, Condon PI, O'Keefe M. Endophthalmitis after astigmatic myopic laser in situ keratomileusis [case report]. J Cataract Refract Surg. 1997;23:948-50.
22. Reviglio V, Rodriguez ML, Picotti GS, et al. *Mycobacterium chelonae* keratitis following laser in situ keratomileusis. J Refract Surg. 1998;14:357-60.
23. Chung MS, Goldstein MH, Driebe WT Jr, Schwartz BH. *Mycobacterium chelonae* keratitis after laser in situ keratomileusis successfully treated with medical therapy and flap removal. Am J Ophthalmol. 2000;129:382-4.
24. Nascimento EG, Carvalho MJ, de Freitas D, Campos M. Nocardial keratitis following myopic keratomileusis. J Refract Surg. 1995;11:210-1.
25. Kim EK, Lee DH, Lee K, et al. *Nocardia* keratitis after traumatic detachment of a laser in situ keratomileusis flap. J Refract Surg. 2000;16:467-9.
26. Sharma N, Sinha R, Singhvi A, Tandon R. *Pseudomonas keratitis* after laser in situ keratomileusis. J Cataract Refract Surg. 2006;32(3):519-21.

CHAPTER 17

Infections after Intrastromal Corneal Ring Segments

Deepali Singhal, Neelima Aron, Prasad Gupta, Rajesh Sinha

Intrastromal corneal rings segments (ICRS) implantation constitutes a promising and reversible refractive technique.[1] It consists of two clear polymethyl methacrylate segments, which are placed in semicircular channels between the stromal lamellae at a depth of two-thirds of the corneal stroma. These semicircular channels can be created either manually or by using femtosecond laser. The 2 main intrastromal corneal rings available are Intacs (Addition Technology Inc, Fremont, CA) and the Ferrara ring (Ferrara Ophthalmics, Belo Horizonte, Brazil). They are designed to achieve a refractive correction by regularization of the central cornea, flattening the meridian near the tip of the rings, and steepening the flattest meridian in relation with the ring body.[2] They lead to sparing of the central cornea and thus, preserve the corneal tissue, unlike excimer laser refractive surgery which has a high-risk of triggering or worsening ectasia in already weaker corneas.[3-5] This technique follows the Barraquer thickness law, which states that central corneal flattening is achieved by adding tissue to the corneal periphery,[6] and displacing the corneal apex closer to its physiologic position in front of the pupillary area.[7] Thus, they can be used in low to moderate myopia and keratoconus.

The ICRS have been associated with intra-operative complications like anterior chamber perforation as well as post-operative complications like extrusion, displacement of the segments[8] and infrequently infection also. Post ICRS infection is a grave and sight threatening complication if it occurs.[9,10]

RISK FACTORS

Microbial keratitis occurs as a complication in approximately 1.4–6.8% of cases post ICRS.[11-13] The various predisposing factors described can be either pre-operative, intra-operative and implant related or post-operative factors. Pre-operative factors include history of contact lens use, dry eye, ocular surface disease, lagophthalmos, recurrent infection, chronic topical steroid use and systemic factors such as diabetes mellitus.[2,9,14] Intra-operative factors include surgical or implant contamination and use of manual technique with low tension level at the suture incision.[15] A higher incidence of infection has been reported in patients who had undergone Ferrara ring implantation in a keratoconic cornea which can be explained by the triangular shape and depth of the Ferrara ring segments leading to superficialization of the ring, particularly in thin keratoconic corneas.[16] Also, multiple incisions are required in Ferrara rings, which further contribute as a risk factor. Post-operative factors include epithelial defect, loose sutures, wound gape and ocular trauma.[9,15,17] Bourcier et al reported that the risk factors for anaerobic infection include prior corneal surgery and anaerobic condition in the stromal channels.[10]

ETIOLOGICAL ORGANISMS

Major etiological organisms identified vary according to the time of onset of keratitis. *Staphylococcus aureus, Streptococcus viridans,* and *Pseudomonas species* were identified in early (<2 weeks) infections. *Nocardia species* and *Streptococcus pneumoniae* were identified in patients presenting with corneal infections between 2 and 4 weeks after the surgery. *Staphylococcus aureus*, *Klebsiella* species, and *Paecilomyces* species were isolated from eyes presenting with infection 2 months or more after implantation.[9] *Staphylococcus epidermidis* and *Clostridium perfringes* were identified in late bacterial keratitis (>3 months) post ICRS implantation.[10] Acanthamoeba keratitis has also been reported 1 month after Intacs insertion along with a history of contact lens use.[14]

Recently, *Candida parapsilosis* has also been identified to be the etiologic cause of infectious keratitis following insertion of corneal ring segments in the treatment of keratoconus.[17]

PATHOGENESIS

Several mechanisms can explain the presentation of channel infection after Intacs. The incisional keratotomy used to create the channel serves as a port of entry for microorganisms. The incision also puts the wound perpendicular to the corneal plane which tends to heal slowly. The presence of an intrastromal foreign body and post-operative use of topical steroids carry an additional risk for infections.[10] This procedure also causes disruption of the corneal integrity[18] and potentially exposes the stroma to infectious agents from the eyelids, eyelashes and conjunctiva.[10]

Late onset infective keratitis most probably results from the nidus of microorganisms, which are sequestered in the extremity of the stromal channels and are introduced at the time of surgery. Presentation can also be delayed because of the antibiotics given in the post-operative period.[10]

DIFFERENTIAL DIAGNOSIS

Infectious keratitis post ICRS should be differentiated from extracellular intrastromal deposits and channel haze.[10,15] Extracellular intrastromal deposits accumulate in the lamellar channel and consist of disorganized convolution of collagen lamellae and proteoglycan macromolecules. Lipid accumulation may also be seen on the external side of intrastromal ring segments.[17] Channel haze may be caused by the physical separation of stromal lamellae and should be differentiated from infectious keratitis.

CLINICAL FEATURES

Though the time between surgery and onset of symptoms is variable, early onset infections have been reported to develop within 2 weeks.[9] Late onset bacterial keratitis is seen to develop at 3 months after surgery.

General Symptoms

The general symptoms of infectious keratitis include pain, photophobia, redness, discharge and diminution of vision,[2,9,10] which have been reported in bacterial keratitis. Milder symptoms were noted in case of *Candida* keratitis, which was recognized as a small epithelial defect and infiltrates on the edge of the ring segment.[17]

General Signs

The precorneal tear film and meniscus are seen to contain debris and numerous cells. Corneal epithelial defect over the location of ring segments is seen in most of the cases with stromal infiltrates commonly at the extremity of the stromal channel (**Fig. 17.1**). Few cases have been reported with corneal melt and perforation.[14,18] Anterior chamber shows an inflammatory reaction and hypopyon in some cases.[15,18] Inflammatory membrane can also be seen over the pupil.

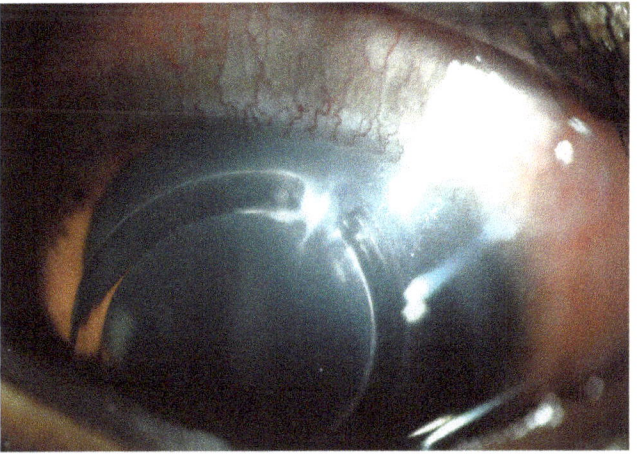

Figure 17.1 Tunnel infection associated with intrastromal ring implantation seen 2 weeks after the surgery. Note the presence of infiltrates at the site of Intacs insertion

MICROBIOLOGICAL WORK-UP

Corneal scraping should be sent in every case of an epithelial defect and the smear should be sent for staining which includes Gram's stain, Giemsa stain, potassium hydroxide (KOH) wet mount and Grocott-Gomori methenamine silver staining, especially if fungal infection is suspected. The scraping material should also be sent for culture sensitivity including Blood agar, Chocolate agar and Sabouraud's dextrose agar for fungal organisms. Conjunctival swab should be sent in case of purulent discharge.[18] Corneal biopsy may be required in case of stromal infiltrates. Removed intrastromal ring segment should be sent for culture sensitivity and also contact lens in cases with history of use of the same.

Newer diagnostic modalities include polymerase chain reaction of the scrapings, which can generate results in around four hours. In vivo confocal microscopy (IVCM) of the cornea can be of great help in suspicion of fungal or Acanthamoeba keratitis. Host corneal button should be sent for culture sensitivity as well as histopathological examination in cases where therapeutic keratoplasty is performed. Acanthamoeba keratitis post ICRS implantation was diagnosed with microscopic analysis of the host cornea showing basophilic cysts with eosinophillic rim and fungal elements found adjacent to the cysts.[14]

TREATMENT

Early diagnosis and management is of paramount importance because a delay in detection can often lead to increased complications like vision loss and corneal damage.[14] All patients post ICRS implantation should be explained about the symptoms of pain, redness, vision loss and photophobia and the importance of regular follow-up.

Medical Therapy

The empirical treatment with the broad-spectrum antibiotics should be started while waiting for the culture reports. A combination therapy consisting of a cephalosporin which acts against gram-positive cocci and some of the gram-negative rods and an aminoglycoside which acts against the gram-negative organisms is started. Combined fortified 5% cefazolin sodium and 1.3% tobramycin sulfate are given in hourly dosage for the initial 48 hours. Following an initial response to this therapy, frequency is tapered to two hourly and subsequently four hourly after 72 hours. Bourcier et al reported the use of fortified ticarcillin (6 mg/mL) combined with fortified gentamicin (15 mg/mL) and vancomycin (50 mg/mL) hourly which was gradually tapered.[10] These patients should be hospitalized and daily follow-up should be done with detailed drawings.

Adjunctive Therapy

Topical cycloplegic agents should be administered along with the antimicrobials which help to relieve the ciliary spasm and pain, and also help to prevent the formation of synechiae. Homatropine bromide eyedrops 2% is preferably used three to four times daily. Antiglaucoma medication should be started in cases of secondary glaucoma.

Low dose topical and subconjunctival steroids have been used after 3 days of antimicrobial therapy in order to decrease the inflammation and scarring.[10,17] They should be avoided in cases of fungal keratitis.

Further, the treatment should be modified according to the culture sensitivity reports. Systemic antimicrobial therapy should be started in case of severe keratitis with scleral melting, impending or frank perforation, one eyed patients or in children.

Surgical Therapy

Removal of the stromal ring segment should be performed in all the cases.[9,10,14,15] Following removal, stromal channel irrigation should be done with balanced salt solution and antimicrobial agent such as vancomycin.[2] In cases of corneal perforation or treatment failure therapeutic keratoplasty may need to be performed.[14,17] Smaller areas of perforation can also be managed with cyanoacrylate glue (up to 3 mm perforation) or patch graft (up to 5 mm perforation).

COMPLICATIONS AND SEQUELAE

Major sequelae of infectious keratitis post ICRS implantation include corneal scarring, thinning and vascularization. In severe cases it often leads to descemetocele, perforation or ectatic cicatrix.

PROPHYLAXIS

Various prophylactic measures should be taken to prevent such infections. Pre-operatively, eyelid hygeine of the patient should be improved. Intra-operatively, all aseptic precautions to maintain sterility should be maintained by the surgeon and the assistant. The implant should be handled with sterile instruments following aseptic precautions during insertion. Antibiotic irrigation within the stromal channels may be performed. A close follow-up of the patient should be done post-operatively to look for any signs of epithelial defect, loosening of suture, infiltrates and wound gape. These simple precautions at each level of patient care can prevent the occurrence of infections after ICRS implantation.

REFERENCES

1. Clinch TE, Lemp MA, Foulks GN, et al. Removal of intacs for myopia. Ophthalmology. 2002;109:1441-6.
2. Galvis V, Tello A, Delgado J, et al. Late bacterial keratitis after intracorneal ring segments (Ferrara ring) insertion for keratoconus. Cornea. 2007;26:1282-4.
3. Randleman JB. Post-laser in-situ keratomileusis ectasia: current understanding and future directions. Curr Opin Ophthalmol. 2006;17:406-12.
4. Schmitt-Bernard CF, Lesage C, Arnaud B. Keratectasia induced by laser in situ keratomileusis in keratoconus. J Refract Surg. 2000;16:368-70.
5. Kohnen T. Iatrogenic Keratectasia: current knowledge, current measurements. J Cataract Refract Surg. 2002;28:2065-6.
6. Barraquer J. Cirugia Refractiva de la Cornea, 1st edition. Bogota, Colombia: Instituto Barraquer de America-Bogota;1989.
7. Siganos D, Ferrara P, Chatzinikolas K, et al. Ferrara intrastromal corneal rings for the correction of keratoconus. J Cataract Refract Surg. 2002;28:1947-51.
8. Kwitko S, Severo NS. Ferrara intracorneal ring segments for keratoconus. J Cataract Refract Surg. 2004;30:812-20.
9. Hofling-Lima AL, Castelo B, Romano A, et al. Corneal infections after implantation of intraestromal corneal ring segments. Cornea. 2004;23:547-9.
10. Bourcier T, Bordiere V, Laroche L. Late bacterial keratitis after implantation of intraestromal corneal ring segments. J Cataract Refract Surg. 2003;29:407-9.
11. Mulet ME, Pérez-Santonja JJ, Ferrer C, et al. Microbial keratitis after intrastromal corneal ring segment implantation. J Refract Surg. 2010;26:364-9.
12. Ferrer C, Alio JL, Montanes AU, et al. Causes of intrastromal corneal ring segment explantation: clinicopathologic correlation analysis. J Cataract Refract Surg. 2010;36:970-7.
13. Miranda D, Sartori M, Francesconi C, et al. Ferrara intrastromal corneal ring segments for severe keratoconus. J Refract Surg. 2003;19:645-53.
14. Slade DS, Johnson JT, Tabin G. Acanthamoeba and fungal keratitis in a woman with a history of Intacs corneal implants. Eye Contact Lens. 2008;34:185-7.
15. Ibáñez-Alperte J, Pérez-García D, Cristóbal JA, Mateo AJ, Río BJ, Mínguez E. Keratitis after Implantation of Intrastromal Corneal Rings with Spontaneous Extrusion of the Segment. Case Rep Ophthalmol. 2010;1(2):42-6.
16. Silva FBD, Alves EAF, Cunha PFA. Utilização do Anel de Ferrara na estabilização e correção da ectasia corneana pós PRK. Arq Bras Oftalmol. 2000;63:215-8.
17. Zare MA, Hashemi H, Salari MR. Delayed Onset Bacterial keratitis after implantation of intrastromal corneal ring segments. Iranian Journal of Ophthalmology. 2008;20:1.
18. Mitchell BM, Kanellopoulos AJ, Font RL. Post intrastromal corneal ring segments insertion complicated by Candida parapsilosis keratitis. Clin Ophthalmol. 2013;7:443-8.

CHAPTER 18

Post-Collagen Cross-linking Infections

Jayanand Urkude, Neelima Aron, Anubha Rathi, Prafulla K Maharana, Namrata Sharma

Corneal collagen cross-linking (CXL/C3R) has emerged as a promising treatment option for keratoconus. Corneal CXL uses riboflavin and ultraviolet-A (UV-A) rays to increase the mechanical rigidity of corneal stroma which helps to halt/delay the progression of keratoconus.[1] As such, CXL is a very safe procedure as many studies have shown long-term stabilization of keratoconus after C3R without any sight threatening complications.[2,3] Alio et al[4] have showed that CXL can cause inhibition of bacterial replication because it causes oxidative damage to DNA and RNA processes and has been tried for managing resistant microbial keratitis, however infective keratitis after CXL has been seen and can be attributed to a variety of factors. This chapter will cover the incidence, risk factors, prophylaxis and management of microbial keratitis post-CXL.

INCIDENCE

Occurrence of microbial keratitis post-CXL in keratoconus patient is a rare complication with incidence varying from one region to another. In Asian countries, the frequency noted is 0.0017%.

RISK FACTORS

Various factors may be causative in the occurrence of post-CXL keratitis. They can be divided into pre-operative, intra-operative and post-operative factors and are mentioned further.

Pre-operative Factors

Lid hygiene and ocular surface health are two most very important factors that predict the occurrence of post-operative infection after any intraocular and extraocular surgery. CXL in the presence of blepharitis, lid margin abnormalities, trichiasis and meibomian gland dysfunction which is not fully controlled can lead to infection of the cornea after the procedure especially in the presence of near total epithelial defect. It is of utmost importance to treat these disorders with topical and oral antibiotics such as tetracycline and azithromycin, surgical correction of entropion and trichiasis and warm compresses before performing CXL.

Intra-operative Factors

Unsterile technique of scrubbing, gowning, gloving and draping are the most important intra-operative risk factors for contamination. Apart from these, specific factors such as creation of an epithelial defect, prolonged exposure by ultraviolet-A (UV-A) light and contaminated riboflavin solution may lead to post-CXL keratitis.

Epithelial Defect

CXL requires epithelial removal before corneal stromal irradiation by UV-A is done. The resultant epithelial defect takes 2–5 days to heal completely. An intact corneal epithelium is an important defence barrier as majority of bacteria cannot penetrate it, except

Neisseria gonorrhoeae, *Corynebacterium diphtheriae* and *Listeria monocytogenes*.[5] An epithelial defect increases the risk of superinfection by pathogenic microorganisms multifold leading to a full blown infection.

Prolonged Exposure to UV-A Radiation

Kymionis et al reported a patient with herpetic epithelial keratitis and iritis post-CXL treatment thus hypothesizing that UV-A light could lead to reactivation of latent herpes simplex virus even in those patients who have no history of previous clinical herpes virus infections.[6] Hence, prolonged exposure of cornea to UV-A rays like in conventional CXL may lead to increased risk of infection.

Contaminated Solution

Contaminated riboflavin solution can be another reason for post-collagen cross-linking infection. Thus, it is very important to check the expiry date of the solution, check if the package is sealed properly and rule out the presence of turbidity in the solution.

Post-operative Factors

Unhygienic practices followed by the patient in the post-operative period can lead to environmental contamination of the operated eye leading to infection. Apart from this, factors such as use of bandage contact lenses and steroids post-operatively facilitate superinfection.

Bandage Contact Lens

Bandage contact lens (BCL) is applied in post-operative period to aid in the healing of epithelial defect and for patient's comfort. However, improper handling of BCL, repeated application of same BCL or washing it with tap water which may be contaminated can lead to introduction of microorganisms in the cornea.

There have been cases of polymicrobial keratitis caused by *Streptococcus salivarius*, *Streptococcus oralis*, and coagulase negative *Staphylococcus* species because of poor contact lens hygiene.[7]

Use of Steroids

Use of steroids in the post-operative period is a potential risk factor for nonhealing epithelial defect leading to easy access of microorganisms in deeper corneal layer.

MICROBIAL PROFILE OF POST-COLLAGEN CROSS-LINKING INFECTION

The source of infective microorganisms in cases of post-C3R keratitis may be one of the following:
- Microbial flora from patient's own ocular surface may get entry into corneal stroma through debrided epithelium.
- Trivial trauma can introduce micro-organisms into the eye easily from the environment.
- Contaminated OT instruments and OT environment may be the source of infection.

Post-C3R keratitis can be caused by various microbial agents like bacteria (*Staphylococcus* species, *Streptococcus* species, *Pseudomonas aeruginosa*, *Escherichia coli*), Herpes virus, *Acanthamoeba* species, *Mycobacterium* species and fungi. *Staphylococcus aureus* is most frequently linked with post-C3R keratitis.[8]

Various cases have been reported in literature with infectious keratitis post-CXL. *Acanthamoeba* keratitis has been reported due to eye washing under tap water since the patient was unaware of a bandage contact lens being inserted in the eye.[9] Sharma et al reported a case of severe keratitis with patient's contact lens caused by *Pseudomonas aeruginosa*.[10]

PROPHYLAXIS

Various measures can be taken pre-operatively, intra-operatively and post-operatively to prevent post-collagen cross-linking infection.

Pre-operative Period

- *Treating pre-existing diseases:* Patients of atopic keratoconjunctivitis have been shown to be at a greater risk of infection due to the presence of pro-inflammatory factors. So, tackling pre-existing ocular diseases could lead to prevention of post-CXL keratitis.[1]

  Diseases like vernal keratoconjunctivitis (VKC), blepharitis, meibomitis, conjunctivitis, canaliculitis, nasolacrimal duct obstruction, entropion and ectropion should be treated before taking up the patient for collagen cross-linking.

- *Pre-operative medications:* Patients should be started on topical antibiotics in the pre-operative period to decrease the ocular flora. Patients who are on topical steroids should be advised to stop them or taper them as steroids create a local immunocompromised state and increase the risk of post-operative infections. Moxifloxacin is the preferred choice by most surgeons for surgical prophylaxis.[11] It has a broader spectrum of action, increased penetration into the eye and delivers a concentration greater than the minimum inhibitory concentration in the ocular system.[12,13]

- The ocular flora is altered in cases of VKC because of chronic use of steroids, which could be a cause of increased risk of post-operative keratitis.[14] Hence, the dose and frequency of steroids in VKC patients should be monitored and the patients should be informed about the increased risks associated with it. As it is hypothesized that a longer exposure to UV-A and duration of the conventional CXL might be a potential precipitating factor for infection, there could be a potential role for transepithelial and accelerated CXL as an alternative to conventional CXL, as the total procedure time is significantly reduced in these procedures.[6]

Intra-operative Period

- Aseptic precautions should be followed in the operation theatre:
  - *Surgeon preparation:* Proper scrubbing and use of sterile towel and gowns is recommended. Surgeon should use face mask during the complete procedure of CXL.
  - *Preparation of surgical field:* Use of povidone iodine 10% for cleaning the eye should be done before starting the procedure. Povidone iodine in 5% concentration should be applied to the conjunctival sac for a minimum of 3 minutes duration. Drape should be tightly adhered to the underlying skin and speculum should be properly applied taking care not to let eyelashes in the operating field. Use of sterile instruments for epithelial debridement during CXL procedure is of utmost importance.
- Twenty percent ethyl alcohol should be used for epithelial debridement which makes the procedure very easy and reduces trauma to the underlying corneal stroma, corneal nerves and Bowman's membrane. Application of bandage contact lens at the end of CXL procedure helps in faster healing of epithelial defect and reduces discomfort to the patient. Application of antibiotic drops at the completion of collagen cross-linking procedure should be done.

Post-operative Period

Wollensak et al have proposed the role of antibiotic eye drops and ointments in the post-operative period after CXL.[2] Various other studies have described the use of post-operative steroids and/or nonsteroidal anti-inflammatory drugs (NSAIDs) along with an antibiotic agent.[15,16] However, the use of topical corticosteroids and/or NSAIDs has the potential to exacerbate an infection and hence should be withheld until complete epithelial healing takes place.[17,18]

The patients should be followed up closely till the complete healing of epithelial defect and steroids should be started judiciously thereafter in tapering doses.

DIAGNOSIS AND MANAGEMENT

The patient presents with sudden onset pain, redness and discharge in the follow-up period after CXL in case of infection. The patient can present very early in the post-operative period like in case of *Pseudomonas* infection with aggressive involvement. There might be associated history of trauma or something falling into eye which could give a clue towards the diagnosis of causative microorganism.

On examination, an epithelial defect may be present which could be the one created during CXL but with associated infiltrates. The infiltrates can be superficial or deep, focal or diffuse like in corneal abscess. In cases of severe involvement, the sclera or anterior chamber can also be involved. Thus, it can be classified as a small ulcer or large ulcer and superficial or deep depending upon the extent of involvement **(Figs 18.1A to D)**.

In case of infection, the bandage contact lens should be immediately removed, cut into two halves and sent for bacterial and fungal culture and sensitivity examination. Corneal scraping should be done and the sample should be examined with Gram's stain and patassium hydroxide (KOH) stain under the microscope. The scraping material should be sent for bacterial and fungal culture and sensitivity. Corneal confocal microscopy may be performed for diagnosing infections caused by fungus and *Acanthamoeba*.

The treatment can be started according to the standard protocol followed during infective keratitis. Single drug antibiotic (fourth generation

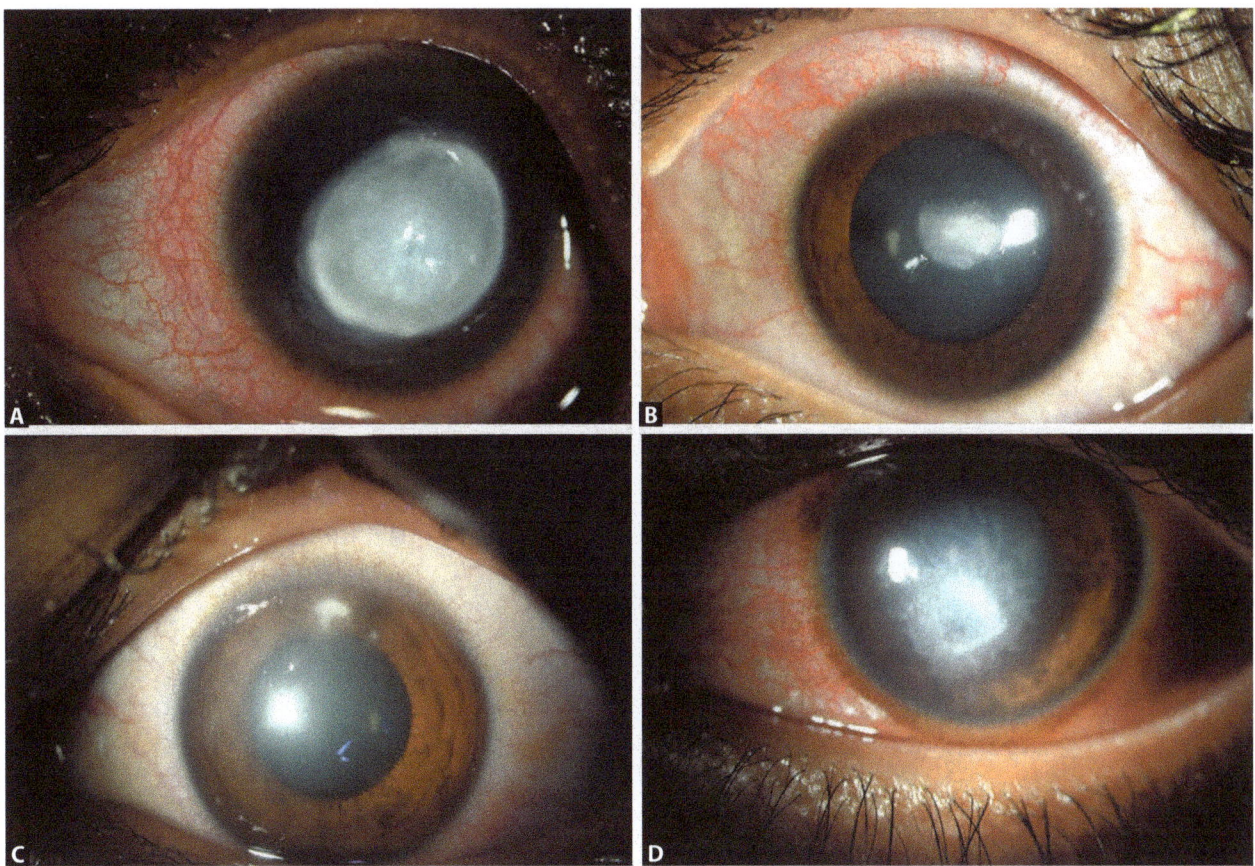

Figures 18.1A to D Varied presentations of post-CXL keratitis. (A) A large corneal ulcer in a 13-year-old child 3 days following hypo-osmolar CXL procedure. The causative organism was *Staphylococcus aureus*; (B) Central corneal ulcer 1 week after CXL caused by *Staphylococcus epidermidis*; (C) Small corneal ulcer near the superior limbus along with a satellite lesion 2 days after CXL. The cultures were sterile; (D) Post-CXL keratitis with *Streptococcus* species referred to our center in the healing phase

fluoroquinolone) for small paracentral ulcers and fortified drops for larger, deeper and central corneal ulcers is preferred. Drugs can later be changed according to the corneal scraping report. Various drugs show a decreased penetration through a cross-linked cornea such as ofloxacin[19] and voriconazole[19] but penetration of moxifloxacin into the anterior chamber remains unaltered by CXL.[20] Also, moxifloxacin is more potent than ciprofloxacin against *S. aureus* and also has higher bactericidal activity against highly resistant strains.[21] In cases of non resolution of symptoms, the corneal scrapings should be repeated and in addition sent for acid fast bacilli staining and culture on Lowenstein-Jensen media to rule out infection by *Mycobacterium* species.

Hence, though there is a risk of microbial keratitis post-CXL, given the revolutionary change CXL has brought about in the management of keratoconus, we cannot overlook the much greater benefit-risk ratio associated with it. CXL can continue to remain a safe procedure if the above mentioned safety protocols are followed both by the surgeon and the patient.

REFERENCES

1. Rana M, Lau A, Aralikatti A, Shah S. Severe microbial keratitis and associated perforation after corneal crosslinking for keratoconus. Cont Lens Anterior Eye. 2015;38(2):134-7.
2. Wollensak G, Spoerl E, Seiler T. Riboflavin/ultraviolet-a-induced collagen crosslinking for the treatment of keratoconus. Am J Ophthalmol. 2003;135:620-7.
3. Raiskup-Wolf F, Hoyer A, Spoerl E, Pillunat LE. Collagen crosslinking with riboflavin and ultraviolet—A light in keratoconus: Long-term results. J Cataract Refract Surg. 2008;34:796-801.
4. Alio JL, Abbouda A, Valle DD, Del Castillo JM, Fernandez JA. Corneal cross linking and infectious keratitis: a systematic review with a meta-analysis of reported cases. J Ophthalmic Inflamm Infect. 2013;3(1):47.

5. Kodavoor S, Sarwate N, Ramamurhy D. Microbial keratitis following accelerated corneal collagen cross-linking. Oman J Ophthalmol. 2015;8(2):111.
6. Kymionis GD, Portaliou DM, Bouzoukis DI, Suh LH, Pallikaris AI, Markomanolakis M, et al. Herpetic keratitis with iritis after corneal crosslinking with riboflavin and ultraviolet A for keratoconus. J Cataract Refract Surg. 2007;33(11):1982-4.
7. Zamora KV, Males JJ. Polymicrobial keratitis after a collagen cross-linking procedure with postoperative use of a contact lens: A case report. Cornea. 2009;28:474-6.
8. Shetty R, Kaweri L, Nuijts RMMA, Nagaraja H, Arora V, Kumar RS. Profile of microbial keratitis after corneal collagen cross-linking. Bio Med Res Int. 2014;2014:e340509.
9. Rama P, Di Matteo F, Matuska S, Paganoni G, Spinelli. *Acanthamoeba keratitis* with perforation after corneal crosslinking and bandage contact lens use. J Cataract Refract Surg. 2009;35(4):788-91.
10. Sharma N, Maharana P, Singh G, Titiyal JS. *Pseudomonas keratitis* after collagen crosslinking for keratoconus: case report and review of literature. J Cataract Refract Surg. 2010;36(3):517-20.
11. Chang DF, Braga-Mele R, Mamalis N, et al. Prophylaxis of postoperative endophthalmitis after cataract surgery. J Cataract Refract Surg. 2007;33(10):1801-5.
12. Stroman DW, Dajcs JJ, Cupp GA, Schlech BA. In vitro and in vivo potency of moxifloxacin and moxifloxacin ophthalmic solution 0.5%, a new topical fluoroquinolone. Surv Ophthalmol. 2005;50(Suppl 1):S16-31.
13. Mather R, Karenchak LM, Romanowski EG, Kowalski RP. Fourth generation fluoroquinolones: new weapons in the arsenal of ophthalmic antibiotics. Am J Ophthalmol. 2002;133(4):463-6.
14. Ermis SS, Aktepe OC, Inan UU, Ozturk F, Altindis M. Effect of topical dexamethasone and ciprofloxacin on bacterial flora of healthy conjunctiva. Eye. 2004;18(3):249-52.
15. Pollhammer M, Cursiefen C. Bacterial keratitis early after corneal crosslinking with riboflavin and ultraviolet-A. J Cataract Refract Surg. 2009;35(3):588-9.
16. Pérez-Santonja JJ, Artola A, Javaloy J, Alió JL, Abad JL. Microbial keratitis after corneal collagen crosslinking. J Cataract Refract Surg. 2009;35(6):1138-40.
17. Mian SI, Gupta A, Pineda R. Corneal ulceration and perforation with ketorolac tromethamine (Acular) use after PRK. Cornea. 2006;25(2):232-4.
18. Chen D, Lian Y, Li J, Ma Y, Shen M, Lu F. Monitor corneal epithelial healing under bandage contact lens using ultra high-resolution optical coherence tomography after pterygium surgery. Eye & Contact Lens. 2014;40(3):175-80.
19. Tschopp M, Stary J, Frueh BE, et al. Impact of corneal cross-linking on drug penetration in an ex vivo porcine eye model. Cornea. 2012;31(3):222-6.
20. Litvin G, Ben Eliahu S, Rotenberg M, Marcovich AL, Zadok D, Kleinmann G. Penetration of moxifloxacin through crosslinked corneas. J Cataract Refract Surg. 2014;40(7):1177-81.
21. Ince D, Zhang X, Hooper DC. Activity of and resistance to moxifloxacin in *Staphylococcus aureus*. Antimicrob Agents Chemother. 2003;47(4):1410-5.

CHAPTER 19

Post-Keratoplasty Infections

Neelima Aron, Prafulla K Maharana, Namrata Sharma

Infective keratitis post-keratoplasty is one of the most common causes of graft failure apart from graft rejection. The incidence of graft infection after full thickness penetrating keratoplasty has been reported to vary from 1.76% to 12.1%[1,2] with a higher incidence in the developing countries as compared to the developed world. With the rise in the number of lamellar corneal transplants being performed in view of their faster recovery and better visual outcomes, previously unseen interface infections are being increasingly reported due to the sequestration of microorganisms between the layers of the graft and the host. Data on the incidence of infectious keratitis following lamellar keratoplasties is limited. Studies in literature till date suggest an incidence of 0.5–11.11% in endothelial and anterior lamellar keratoplasty procedures.[3,4] This change in the spectrum of post-keratoplasty infections has been associated with novel methods of diagnosis and management protocols for the treatment of infections. Further, infection may not be limited to the graft and can spread easily into the vitreous cavity especially in aphakic patients leading to endophthalmitis with poor final visual outcomes despite adequate treatment. Thus, all measures should be taken to address the risk factors leading to infections in the first place in order to reduce the incidence of graft infection. Further, if the graft infection occurs, timely and appropriate intervention should be done to reduce further ocular morbidity.

RISK FACTORS FOR GRAFT INFECTION AND PREVENTION

One of the most important factors associated with infection in a corneal graft is the indication for which the keratoplasty was performed. Therapeutic penetrating keratoplasty which is performed in infected corneas carries the highest risk of re-infection, the most important factor being the inability to attain a clear margin of cornea free of infection while trephination.

In optical keratoplasties performed for healed viral keratitis, the chances of recurrence increases multifold if the eye is not quiet at the time of transplantation.[5] Further, herpes virus is notorious for reactivation which can occur anytime throughout life and hence the patient needs to be on lifelong follow-up. Thus, corneal transplantation in a case of herpetic keratitis should be performed only after the disease is in remission for a minimum period of 6 months. The patient should be administered oral acyclovir in a prophylactic dose of 400 mg bd started pre-operatively and continued for a minimum period of 1 year post-operatively (Herpetic Eye Disease Study-II).[6] The other indications of transplantation which are reported to have high chances of infection include bullous keratopathy[7] due to a compromised ocular surface and corneoiridic scars.[8]

Various risk factors have been implicated in the occurrence of graft infection. They can be divided into donor related problems, host related problems and graft related problems.

Donor-related Problems

Contamination of donor corneal tissue is one of the most important risk factor leading to graft infection. Various factors implicated in the causation include contamination of the cornea during retrieval or transportation to the eye bank, contaminated corneal preservation media and infection of the corneal button while grafting on to the recipient. Contamination of donor tissue can be easily prevented by following a sterile procedure of harvesting the cornea, maintenance of cold chain (4 degree Celsius) for the preservation media and regular microbiological surveillance of the same. A culture from the preservation media with the corneal button in-situ should preferably be sent when the death to preservation time is more than 12 hours and the cornea should be transplanted once the culture report is negative. An increased resistance to the antibiotics used in the preservation media may lead to higher chances of infection and thus use of alternative antibiotics must be considered.

Host-related Problems

Ocular Surface Disorders

Ocular surface disease (OSD) refers to poor tear film stability leading to ocular surface destabilization causing dry eye and epithelial breakdown. This has been implicated as a causative risk factor for graft infection in 60% of the eyes by Vajpayee et al.[8] It was found that OSD increases the risk of acquiring graft infection by more than 2 fold. Furthermore, a penetrating keratoplasty can further aggravate the pre-existing ocular surface disease by creating a graft host junction. This highlights the importance of pre-operative stabilization of ocular surface with preservative free lubricating eye drops, punctal plugs and eyelid surgery to correct ectropion and entropion. A keratoplasty should be deferred until then unless it is an emergency.

Recurrence of Previous Infection

An optical penetrating keratoplasty performed for healed herpetic keratitis may lead to reactivation of the disease in the transplanted cornea. This is especially true if the interval between disease remission and corneal transplant is less such that still some disease activity is present. It is recommended to perform the transplant procedure in an uninflamed eye and when the disease is under remission for at least 3-6 months otherwise the surgery should be deferred. Furthermore, the importance of prophylaxis with oral acyclovir following keratoplasty in healed herpetic keratitis cannot be undermined. In a randomized control trial, it was seen that the incidence of graft failure was 14% in acyclovir treated eyes compared with 56% without acyclovir due to reactivation of herpes virus in the full thickness graft.[9] Thus, oral acyclovir prophylaxis in a dose of 400 mg twice a day for at least 1 year is mandatory after all grafts performed for herpetic keratitis.

The other scenario where the graft can have recurrence of infection is in cases of therapeutic keratoplasty wherein an incomplete removal of the infectious foci has been performed. Hence, it should be ensured that maximum debulking is performed while performing keratoplasty along with administration of full dose antibiotic treatment post-operatively.

Topical Steroids

Although prolonged topical steroid therapy after keratoplasty has been suggested as a risk factor for the development of infection in the corneal graft, it is difficult to implicate its use in the pathogenesis of post-keratoplasty keratitis since a large number of patients receiving steroids on an extended basis do not develop any infection.[10,11] Nonetheless, steroids do lead to ocular surface compromise and cannot be overlooked as an important risk factor.

Use of Contact Lenses

Bandage contact lenses (BCL) have been used commonly to treat large epithelial defects in the corneal graft in the initial days after keratoplasty. Contact lenses have been known to induce corneal hypoxia which leads to a reduction in local immunity causing increased microbial adherence and a subsequent infection of the graft.[12] Thus, the patient should maintain proper hygiene when the BCL is *in situ*. Further, BCL should be used judiciously and should be reserved for grafts that develop persistent epithelial defects. They should be discontinued once complete epithelial healing takes place. It may be advisable to increase the frequency of topical prophylactic antibiotics when the BCL is *in situ*.

Systemic Diseases

Systemic diseases such as diabetes mellitus have been known to increase the risk of development of graft infection especially in those with uncontrolled and fluctuating blood sugar levels.[12] The random blood sugar should be at least less than 200 mg/dL when the patient is being taken up for surgery. These patients should be kept on close follow up especially till the time epithelial healing is complete.

Socioeconomic Status

Poor socioeconomic status has been associated with a higher risk of graft infection due to failure of maintenance of proper hygienic practices by the patient in view of poor living conditions leading to environmental contamination.[8,13,14] It has been seen that a lower socioeconomic status had a 28% higher risk of corneal graft failure and 2.5 times higher chance of infection being the causative factor of graft failure.[13,15]

Graft-related Problems

One of the most important risk factors for infection are the graft related factors and are enumerated below.

Suture-related Problems

Suture related problems are one of the most common causative risk factors for infection. Loose sutures, broken end of sutures and erosion of sutures cause a localized compromise of the surrounding epithelium leading to direct invasion of microorganisms at the site of suture. Further, the accumulation of mucus and debris at the site of suture acts as a nidus for colonization of microbes leading to keratitis.[2] In a study by Vajpayee et al,[8] continuous sutures have been proposed as having a higher risk of infection than interrupted sutures since interrupted sutures can be removed selectively thereby controlling the infection unlike continuous sutures.

It is, therefore, recommended to remove the loose and broken sutures and replace them as early as possible to prevent microbial colonization. Further, once complete wound healing takes place, all sutures should be removed starting at 1–1.5 years post-operatively.[16]

Persistent Epithelial Defect

Persistent epithelial defect has been found to be the most common predisposing factor for graft infection.[8,17,18] It was found that patients having persistent epithelial defects had a threefold higher risk of developing graft infection compared to patients who did not have persistent epithelial defects. Hence, all factors such as lid abnormalities, poor ocular surface, indiscriminate use of topical medications containing preservatives and use of steroids should be taken care of to enable faster healing of the epithelial defect.

Decompensated Graft

It has been reported that failed and decompensated grafts are predisposed to graft infection due to stromal and epithelial edema leading to a compromised ocular environment.[2]

Wound Leak/Graft Dehiscence

A positive Seidel's test post-keratoplasty should never be overlooked. A continuous aqueous leak can lead to invasion of microorganisms from the graft surface into the anterior chamber and further into the vitreous cavity leading to endophthalmitis. Graft dehiscence has been reported to be present in 4% of the cases of graft infection.[8]

History of Graft Rejection

Herpetic keratitis is known for recurrences in the corneal grafts performed for healed viral keratitis. An immune graft rejection can lead not only to a viral recurrence but also reactivation of the herpes virus in the trigeminal ganglion leading to a new herpetic infection after keratoplasty that never occurred in the eye before.[19]

Venting Incisions

Corneal venting incisions in cases of endothelial keratoplasty have been proposed to lead to the entry of organisms in the interface through these sites.[20]

CLINICAL FEATURES

Any history of sudden onset pain, redness and blurring of vision in a patient who has undergone keratoplasty should be looked upon with suspicion of having graft infection. The very close differential diagnosis is graft rejection. It is very important to differentiate between the two since the treatment of both the entities is poles apart.

Infections caused due to intra-operative contamination, donor infection, or previous host disease tend to present earlier in the post-operative course within 6–8 weeks post-operatively.[21] Environmental pathogens cause late post-operative infections generally considered to occur after 2 months post-operatively.[21]

The usual presentation is an epithelial defect with surrounding infiltrates that may be present either in the centre (**Figs 19.1A and B**) or in the periphery (**Figs 19.2A and B**). Central ulcers are usually caused due to persistent epithelial defects[8] whereas peripheral ulcers are generally due to suture related problems.[2] Peripheral ulcers are generally smaller (<4 mm) whereas central ulcers tend to be larger (>4 mm). The ulcer readily involves the graft host junction leading to loosening of sutures and vascularization (**Figs 19.3A and B**). In severe cases, it can cause a rapid corneal perforation with the spread of infection into the vitreous cavity.

Graft infection in cases of herpetic keratitis presents with an epithelial dendrite. In case of herpetic

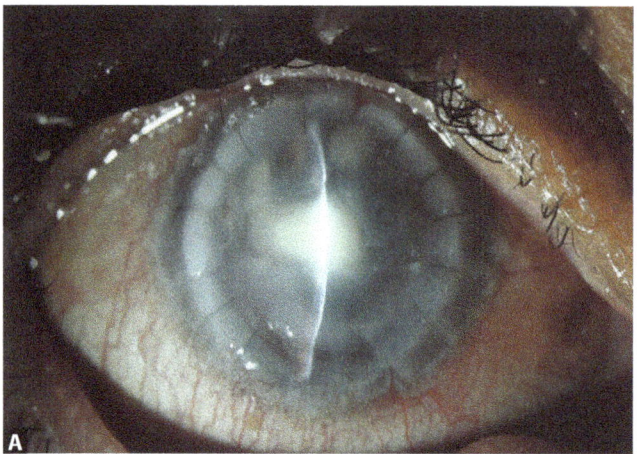 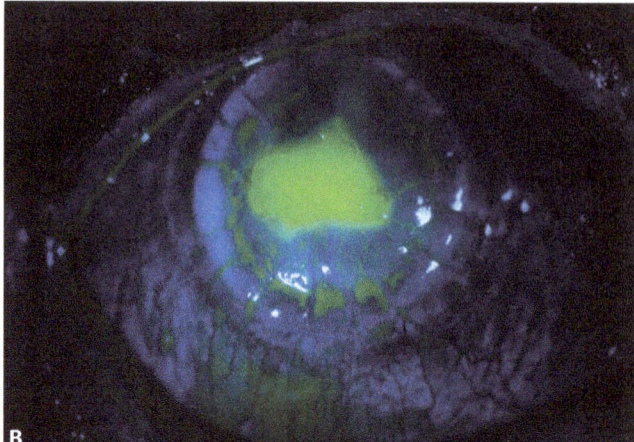

Figures 19.1A and B Infective keratitis 3 months post optical penetrating keratoplasty. The corneal ulcer is associated with deep seated infiltrates (A) and overlying epithelial defect (B)

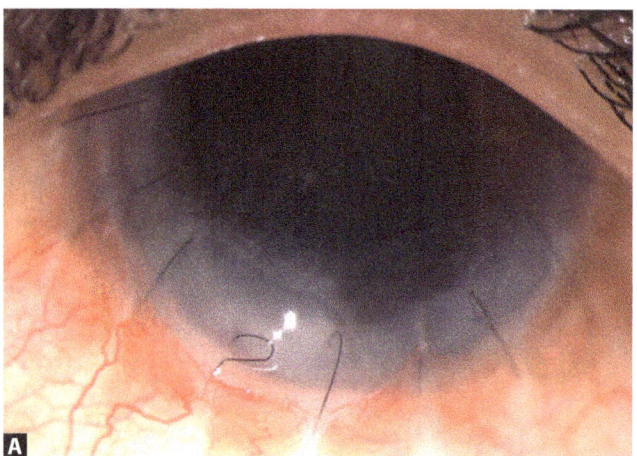 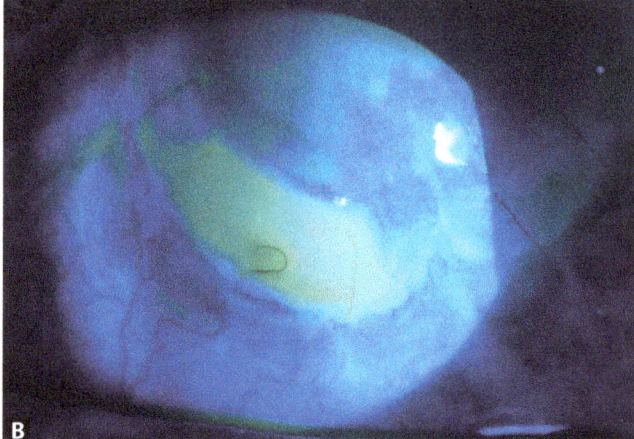

Figures 19.2A and B Corneal ulcer at the graft-host junction post penetrating keratoplasty associated with loose suture and graft edema one week post-operatively. The loose suture was removed and sent for culture and sensitivity examination

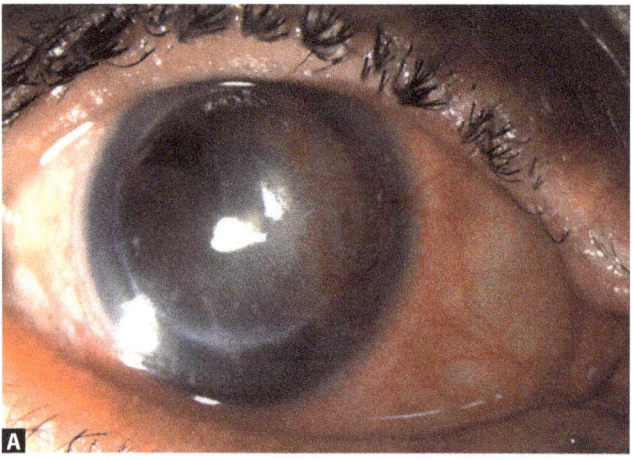 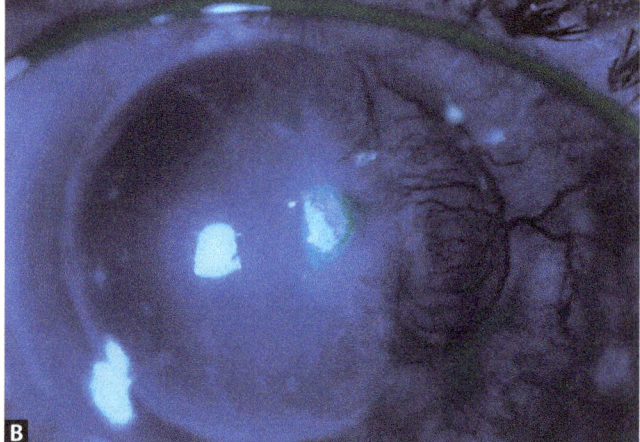

Figures 19.3A and B Resolving graft infection with a small corneal ulcer associated with vascularization from the limbus towards the donor cornea

keratouveitis, keratic precipitates along with anterior chamber reaction and stromal edema may be present. In such cases it becomes difficult to differentiate it from graft rejection. A differential graft edema and presence of khodadoust line may be helpful signs in favor of graft rejection.

Infectious crystalline keratopathy presents as a chronic, intralamellar infiltrate and is characterized by crystal-shaped opacities that are very slow to heal. It is usually caused by *Streptococcus* species though other micro-organisms have also been implicated for the same.[22]

Interface keratitis is the newer presentation of graft infections that has come into being due to the presence of an interface or the interlamellar space in lamellar keratoplasty. It is an infection of the host–donor interface either following endothelial keratoplasty (Figs 19.4A to D) or anterior lamellar keratoplasty. It presents as white or creamy deposits at the centre or periphery of the donor lenticule involving the interface and is most commonly caused by candidal infection.[23,24]

Untreated infections can lead to the spread of infection into the limbus, sclera, anterior chamber and finally the vitreous cavity leading to endophthalmitis and panophthalmitis after which the eye may go into pthisis bulbi.

INVESTIGATIONS

The most important and essential investigation in a case of post-keratoplasty infection is to find out the micro-organism causing it. Corneal scraping is done from the margin and base of the ulcer and the samples are sent for Gram's stain, potassium hydroxide 10% wet mount,

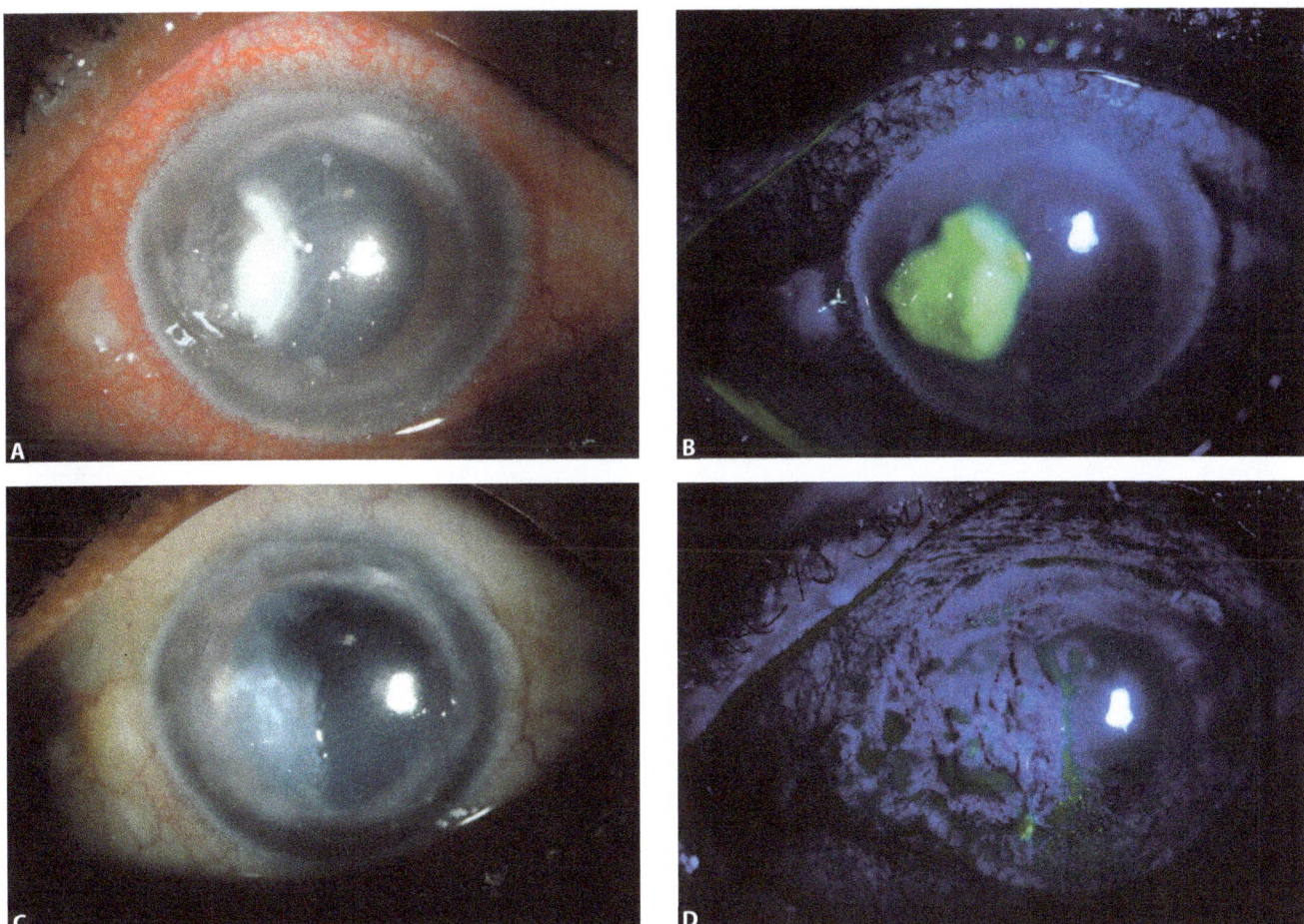

Figures 19.4A to D Graft infection post Descemet's stripping automated endothelial keratoplasty. (A and B) Infiltrates involving the epithelium and graft-host interface; (C and D) The infection resolved with medical therapy with concentrated fortified antibiotics leading to scarring. The patient had a final best corrected visual acuity of 6/24 on Snellen's chart

bacterial and fungal culture and sensitivity. The culture media commonly used are blood agar, chocolate agar, Sabouraud dextrose agar, and thioglycolate broth. Any loose suture is removed and sent for bacterial and fungal cultures. It was found that the culture positivity rate of post-keratoplasty infective keratitis may be higher than for non post-keratoplasty microbial ulcers (93% vs 54%), the reason being attributed to the more severe nature of infectious keratitis in cases following keratoplasty.[10] Ultrasound B scan is done to rule out coexisting endophthalmitis.

One of the newer modalities of diagnosis is the confocal microscopy. This is especially helpful in cases where the smears and culture reports are negative. Further, it gives the report within few minutes as opposed to cultures which take 3 days to 2 weeks for the organisms to grow. Confocal microscopy is most useful in visualization of fungal hyphae and cysts and trophozoites of *Acanthamoeba*. Bacteria appear as highly refractile bodies in the epithelium and the involved stroma.

MICROBIOLOGICAL SPECTRUM

Different patterns of microbial growth are seen in cases of graft infection in various parts of the world. The most common bacteria isolated are the gram positive cocci and the most common fungus reported is *Aspergillus* species. However, in lamellar keratoplasty, the organisms reported are predominantly fungal with only five reported cases caused by bacteria.

Bacteria

Of the gram-positive cocci, coagulase negative *Staphylococcus* species is the most frequently isolated.[2,25,26] This is closely followed by *Staphylococcus aureus*. The most commonly identified gram-negative bacteria is *Pseudomonas aeruginosa*. In regard to lamellar keratoplasty, two cases of *Pseudomonas aeruginosa* and two cases of *Streptococcus pneumoniae* have been reported following endothelial keratoplasty.[3,27] Infection by *Klebsiella pneumoniae*, coagulase-negative *Staphylococcus*, *Pseudomonas aeruginosa* and *Rhodotorula* have been reported following anterior lamellar keratoplasty.[4,28-30]

In cases of pediatric post-keratoplasty infections, *Staphylococcus* species followed by *Streptococcus pneumoniae* have been found to be the most common isolates.[31]

Fungi

Fungal keratitis is the second most common cause of post-keratoplasty infective keratitis following bacterial infections. As mentioned, *Aspergillus* accounts for most of the cases of infection caused by fungus. Although the number of cases reported after penetrating keratoplasty is small, fungal keratitis predominates among reports of infection after anterior lamellar and endothelial keratoplasty.[3,32-36] *Aspergillus flavus* tends to present early within few days with a rapidly progressive course which may require urgent intervention. *Candida* infections tend to present weeks to months after surgery and have a slow indolent course.

Viruses

Herpes simplex virus is the most commonly reported infection after keratoplasty. It generally occurs in grafts that were performed for healed viral keratitis in which reactivation of infection takes place.[37]

MANAGEMENT

The management of infective keratitis post-keratoplasty includes prompt diagnosis and institution of early and aggressive treatment to save the graft from failure. The initial management includes medical therapy with antibiotics. Cases of non resolution or worsening of symptoms require surgical intervention in various forms.

Medical Management

The first and foremost step after diagnosis of graft infection is a meticulous scraping from the base and margin of the ulcer. The patient is then put on topical concentrated fortified antibiotics such as cefazolin 5% and tobramycin 1.3% every hourly alternating half hourly round the clock for 48 hours after which the frequency is gradually reduced and the eye drops are instilled only during the waking hours. Newer antibiotics such as fourth generation fluoroquinolones (gatifloxacin and moxifloxacin) may be prescribed for peripheral small ulcers. Vancomycin 5% is reserved for cases nonresponsive to therapy. Cycloplegics such as homatropine 2% or atropine 1% is administered 3–4 times a day for relieving ciliary spasm. The treatment may then be modified based on smear and culture-sensitivity report. The practice of using prophylactic antibiotics for long-term has not been proven to be very beneficial because of the high incidence of infections by antibiotic resistant strains.[10,11,17] In a study performed by Vajpayee et al,[8] medical therapy was successful in 74% of the eyes that developed graft infection (n= 50).

In cases of fungal keratitis, topical natamycin 5% is the treatment of choice. In cases of deep seated infections, oral antifungals such as ketoconazole and voriconazole are started in twice daily dosing. Infection by *Candida* species is often treated with topical amphotericin B 0.15% and oral fluconazole.[33]

Viral keratitis is treated with topical and therapeutic dose of oral acyclovir. In cases of keratoplasty done for healed herpetic keratitis, oral acyclovir should be administered twice a day for prophylaxis for at least one year.[38]

Acanthamoeba infection is rare after keratoplasty. If it occurs, it is treated with propamidine isethionate or hexamidine, and biguanides, such as polyhexamethylene biguanide or chlorhexidine.[39]

Post-keratoplasty infections are generally severe and should preferably be treated in an inpatient setting. Only those patients who are compliant to therapy and are willing to follow-up every three days can be treated on an outpatient basis.[11,17]

Surgical Management

Surgical management is indicated in cases unresponsive to medical therapy or showing worsening of symptoms. Cases with <2 mm corneal perforations are treated with cyanoacrylate glue and bandage contact lens. Perforations less than 5 mm are managed with a full thickness patch graft. Larger perforations are treated with an emergency therapeutic keratoplasty. Cases associated with vitreous exudates are administered intravitreal antibiotics at the end of the procedure.

In cases of fungal keratitis, a trial of intracameral and intrastromal voriconazole (50–100 µg/0.1 mL) or amphotericin B (5–10 µg/0.1 mL) can be given before proceeding for therapeutic keratoplasty since the chances of reinfection in graft in such cases is very high.

Treatment of Post-lamellar Keratoplasty Infections

Aggressive medical therapy is required in cases of lamellar keratoplasty due to the sequestrated infectious foci in the interface. However, most of these cases ultimately require surgical intervention in some or the other form such as irrigation of the host-graft interface with antibiotics,[40] anterior lamellar graft removal[41] or exchange[35] and finally a therapeutic keratoplasty due to poor ocular penetration of the drugs.

PREVENTION

The importance of prevention of graft infection cannot be overemphasized. The risk factors for graft infection related to donor, host and graft should always be kept in mind. Thus, these three sources of infection should be addressed rigorously pre-operatively, intra-operatively and post-operatively.

Surveillance of obtaining the donor tissue, storage and its final use is of utmost importance. Donor corneas with a prolonged death to preservation time >12 hours should be screened for contamination by sending samples for bacterial and culture sensitivity. Pre-operatively, the ocular surface should be improved with copious lubrication, punctal plugs and anti-inflammatory drugs. Further, it should be emphasized that no optical graft should be performed in eyes with disease activity which has not fully resolved. This holds special importance in cases of viral keratitis which are highly prone for recurrence. Systemic diseases such as diabetes mellitus should be well controlled. Intra-operatively, all measures should be taken to maintain sterile precautions by the surgeon, assistant and the nursing staff. Post-operatively, steroids should be used judiciously and tapered slowly to bring them on a maintenance dose. Bandage contact lenses should be used only in cases of persistent epithelial defect to avoid contamination. On follow-up, any loose or broken suture should be immediately removed and replaced. Presence of any aqueous leak should be promptly addressed in the early post-operative period to avoid the microbes from entering the anterior chamber of the eye. Persistent epithelial defects should be treated with copious lubrication, bandage contact lens and amniotic membrane grafting if necessary.

Studies have shown that there is no role of long-term prophylactic antibiotics in preventing graft infection in view of emergence of antibiotic resistant strains.

OUTCOMES

Visual outcomes for patients with infectious keratitis after keratoplasty are not very encouraging. The rates of retained graft clarity range from only 30 to 50%.[1,8,17] This has been attributed to post infection corneal scar as well as endothelial decompensation due to severe inflammation and the infection eroding through the endothelium. Around 46% of cases have been reported to present with a visual acuity drop.[42] In another report, 63% cases have a final visual acuity of less than 20/200.[43] It has been seen that ulcers with size >4 mm resolve with medical therapy in only 11% of cases and hence such cases require a therapeutic keratoplasty.[2] Overall the rate of regraft in post penetrating keratoplasty infection cases is high ranging from 13% to 53%.[1,2,11,17]

Infectious keratitis is a serious vision threatening complication of keratoplasty that is distressing both to the patient as well as the surgeon especially after a well-performed keratoplasty. It is one of the most common cause of regrafts whose survival rate is much lower than the initial graft procedure. Measures aimed at reducing the rate of tissue contamination, improving surgical skills, and optimizing the host ocular mileu can play a very important role in bringing down the rates of post-keratoplasty infection to a minimum.

REFERENCES

1. Bates AK, Kirkness CM, Ficker LA, Steele AD, Rice NS. Microbial keratitis after penetrating keratoplasty. Eye 1990;4(Pt 1):74-8.
2. Akova YA, Onat M, Koc F, Nurozler A, Duman S. Microbial keratitis following penetrating keratoplasty. Ophthalmic Surg Lasers. 1999;30(6):449-55.
3. Basak SK, Basak S. Complications and management in Descemet's stripping endothelial keratoplasty: analysis of consecutive 430 cases. Indian J Ophthalmol. 2014; 62:209-18.
4. Sharma N, Gupta V, Vanathi M, et al. Microbial keratitis following lamellar keratoplasty. Cornea. 2004;23:472-8.
5. Panda A, Kumar TS: Prognosis of keratoplasty in viral keratitis. Ann Ophthalmol. 1991;23:410-3.
6. Dawson CR, Beck R, Wilhelmus KR, Cohen EJ: Herpetic Eye Disease Study. You can help. Arch Ophthalmol. 1996; 114:89-90.
7. Saini JS, Rao GN, Aquavella JV. Post-keratoplasty corneal ulcers and bandage lenses. Acta Ophthalmol (Copenh). 1988;66:99-103.
8. Vajpayee RB, Boral SK, Dada T, et al. Risk factors for graft infection in India: a case-control study. Br J Ophthalmol 2002;86:261-5.
9. Barney NP, Foster CS. A prospective randomized trial of oral acyclovir after penetrating keratoplasty for herpes simplex keratitis. Cornea. 1994;13(3):232-6.
10. Driebe WT, Stern GA. Microbial keratitis following corneal transplantation. Cornea. 1983;2:41.
11. Fong LP, Ormerod LD, Kenyon KR, et al. Microbial keratitis complicating penetrating keratoplasty. Ophthalmology. 1988;95:1269-75.
12. Saini JS, Rao GN, Aquavella JV. Post-keratoplasty corneal ulcers and bandage lenses. Acta Ophthalmologica. 1988;66:99-103.
13. Dandona L, Naduvilath TJ, Janarthanan M, et al. Causes of corneal graft failure in India. Indian J Ophthalmol. 1998;46:149-52.
14. Sinha R, Vanathi M, Sharma N, et al. Outcome of penetrating keratoplasty in patients with bilateral corneal blindness. Eye. 2004;20:451-4.
15. Dandona L, Naduvilath TJ, Janarthanan M, et al. Survival analysis and visual outcome in a large series of corneal transplants in India. Br J Ophthalmol. 1997;81: 726-31.
16. Christo CG, van Rooij J, Geerards AJ, et al. Suture-related complications following keratoplasty: a 5-year retrospective study. Cornea. 2001;20:816-9.
17. Harris DJ, Stulting RD, Waring GO, et al. Late bacterial and fungal keratitis after corneal transplantation. Spectrum of pathogens, graft survival, and visual prognosis. Ophthalmology. 1988;95:1450-7.
18. Tavakkoli H, Sugar J. Microbial keratitis following keratoplasty. Ophthalmic Surg. 1994;25:350-60.
19. Mannis MJ, Plotnik RD, Schwab IR, et al. Herpes simplex dendritic keratitis after keratoplasty. Am J Ophthalmol 1991;111:480-4.
20. Chew AC, Mehta JS, Li L, Busmanis I, Tan DT. Fungal endophthalmitis after descemet stripping automated endothelial keratoplasty–a case report. Cornea. 2010; 29:346-9.
21. Dubord PJ, Evans GD, Macsai MS, et al. Eye banking and corneal transplantation communicable adverse incidents: current status and project NOTIFY. Cornea 2013;32:1155-66.
22. Salabert D, Robinet A, Colin J. Infectious crystalline keratopathy occurring after penetrating keratoplasty. J Fr Ophtalmol. 1994;17:355-7.
23. Fontana L, Parente G, Di Pede B, Tassinari G. *Candida albicans* interface infection after deep anterior lamellar keratoplasty. Cornea. 2007;26:883-5.
24. Kanavi MR, Foroutan AR, Kamel MR, et al. *Candida* interface keratitis after deep anterior lamellar keratoplasty: clinical, microbiologic, histopathologic, and confocal microscopic reports. Cornea. 2007;26:913-16.
25. Al-Hazzaa SA, Tabbara KF. Bacterial keratitis after penetrating keratoplasty. Ophthalmology. 1988;95:1504-8.
26. Tseng SH, Ling KC. Late microbial keratitis after corneal transplantation. Cornea. 1995;14:591-4.
27. Sengupta J, Khetan A, Saha S, et al. Bacterial keratitis after manual Descemet stripping endothelial keratoplasty–a

different pathophysiology? Eye Contact Lens. 2010;36: 62-5.
28. Zarei-Ghanavati S, Sedaghat MR, Ghavami-Shahri A. Acute *Klebsiella* pneumoniae interface keratitis after deep anterior lamellar keratoplasty. Jpn J Ophthalmol. 2011;55:74-6.
29. Egrilmez S, Palamar M, Sipahi OR, Yagci A. Extended spectrum betalactamase producing *Klebsiella pneumoniae*-related keratitis. J Chemother. 2013;25:123-5.
30. Bajracharya L, Sharma B, Gurung R. A case of acute postoperative keratitis after deep anterior lamellar keratoplasty by multidrug resistant *Klebsiella*. Indian J Ophthalmol. 2015;63:344.
31. Kunimoto DY, Sharma S, Reddy MK, et al. Microbial keratitis in children. Ophthalmology. 1998;105:252-7.
32. Kitzmann AS, Wagoner MD, Syed NA, Goins KM. Donor-related *Candida* keratitis after descemet stripping automated endothelial keratoplasty. Cornea. 2009; 28:825-8.
33. Koenig SB, Wirostko WJ, Fish RI, Covert DJ. *Candida* keratitis after Descemet stripping and automated endothelial keratoplasty. Cornea. 2009;28:471-3.
34. Lee WB, Foster JB, Kozarsky AM, et al. Interface fungal keratitis after endothelial keratoplasty: a clinicopathological report. Ophthalmic Surg Lasers Imaging. 2011;42:e44-e48.
35. Jafarinasab MR, Feizi S, Yazdizadeh F, et al. *Aspergillus flavus* keratitis after deep anterior lamellar keratoplasty. J Ophthalmic Vis Res. 2012;7:167-71.
36. Le Q, Wu D, Li Y, et al. Early-onset *Candida glabrata* interface keratitis after deep anterior lamellar keratoplasty. Optom Vis Sci. 2015;92:e93-e96.
37. Jhanji V, Ferdinands M, Sheorey H, et al. Unusual clinical presentations of new-onset herpetic eye disease after ocular surgery. Acta Ophthalmol. 2012;90:514-8.
38. Tambasco FP, Cohen EJ, Nguyen LH, et al. Oral acyclovir after penetrating keratoplasty for herpes simplex keratitis. Arch Ophthalmol. 1999;117:445-9.
39. Oldenburg CE, Acharya NR, Tu EY, et al. Practice patterns and opinions in the treatment of *Acanthamoeba* keratitis. Cornea. 2011;30:1363-8.
40. Sedaghat MR, Hosseinpoor SS. *Candida albicans* interface infection after deep anterior lamellar keratoplasty. Indian J Ophthalmol. 2012;60:328-30.
41. Lyall DA, Srinivasan S, Roberts F. A case of interface keratitis following anterior lamellar keratoplasty. Surv Ophthalmol. 2012;57:551-7.
42. Tuberville AW, Wood TO. Corneal ulcers in corneal transplants. Curr Eye Res. 1981;1:479-85.
43. Tixier J, Bourcier T, Borderie V, Laroche L. Microbial keratitis after penetrating keratoplasty. J Fr Ophthalmol. 2001;24:597.

CHAPTER 20

Bleb-Related Infections

Neha Midha, Talvir Sidhu, Tanuj Dada

Bleb-related infections are a sight threatening complication of glaucoma filtering surgery that require immediate attention and treatment, as there can be a rapid spread of infection from the conjunctiva to the vitreous cavity due to the presence of limbal fistula created during the surgery. It is important for all eye care physicians to be aware of this complication, so that appropriate patient counseling can be done for all patients undergoing trabeculectomy surgery and early treatment can be initiated to salvage vision. Although bleb-related inflammation may be sterile, especially seen in patients with ocular surface disorders such as dry eyes and ocular allergies, a high degree of suspicion should be maintained for an infective pathology and topical antibiotics initiated along with anti-inflammatory therapy. This chapter highlights the risk factors, clinical signs and management protocol for bleb-related infections postfiltering surgery.

INCIDENCE

Bleb-related infection (BRI) is a potentially blinding complication which can develop in an eye that has remained quiet for months or years after glaucoma filtration surgery. Bleb-associated endophthalmitis (BAE) is the second most frequent (16.7%) cause of post-operative endophthalmitis after acute and chronic post-cataract surgery endophthalmitis.[1] The incidence of BAE after trabeculectomy has been reported from 0.5% to 1.3% and about 0.3–10% for patients undergoing trabeculectomy with mitomycin-C (superior bleb).[2-6] The incidence is highest (9.4%) in eyes with an inferior bleb due to the close proximity of the bleb to the tear meniscus and frequent rubbing against the inferior eyelid.[4] The Collaborative Bleb-Related Infection Incidence and Treatment Study (CBIITS) reported that the incidence of bleb-related infection was about 2.2% at the 5-year follow-up for all cases, whereas it was 7.9% for cases with a history of bleb leakage.[7]

The incidence of BRI also varies according to the conjunctival approach used in surgery. Many studies have shown BRI incidence between 5.7% and 20% with limbal-based flaps as compared to 0–2.2% with fornix-based flaps.[8-10] It is postulated that limbal-based flaps were associated with increased rate of thin cystic bleb and bleb leaks due to a localized large area of antimetabolite application, which could be the reason for increased rate of BRI with this technique.

CLASSIFICATION

Bleb-related infections (BRI) can be broadly classified into "Blebitis" and "Bleb-associated endophthalmitis" **(Table 20.1)**. Blebitis is the early form of bleb-related infection where mucopurulent infiltration is limited

Table 20.1 Classification of BRI

Stage I	Bleb is involved with milky white appearance of bleb with erythema around the bleb
Stage II	Bleb involvement with anterior chamber cells and flare present/hypopyon
Stage III	Vitreous involvement with exudates 1. IIIa: Mild involvement of vitreous, fundus is visible 2. IIIb: Extensive involvement of vitreous

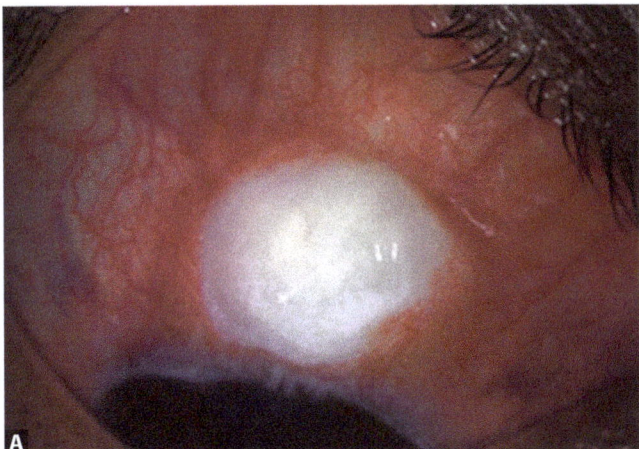
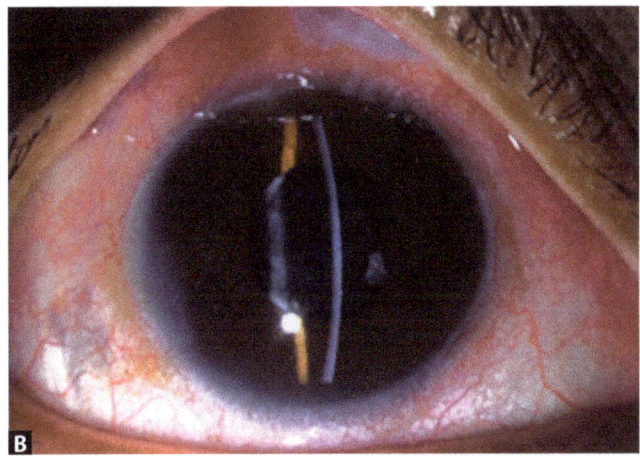

Figures 20.1A and B Bleb-related infection (Stage I). (A) Milky white appearance of bleb with erythema around the bleb-white on red appearance; (B) Anterior chamber is clear without hypopyon

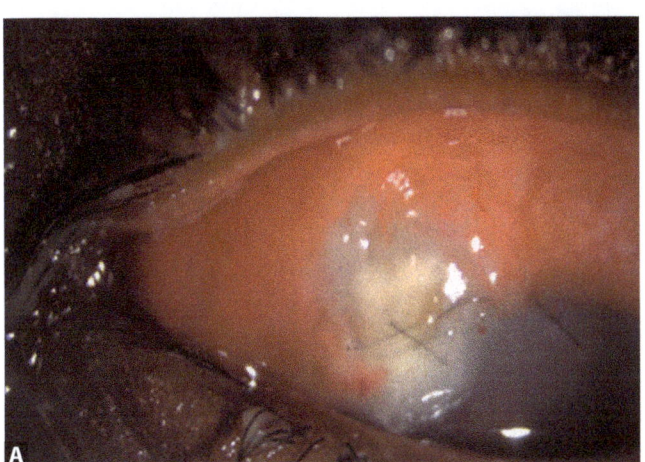
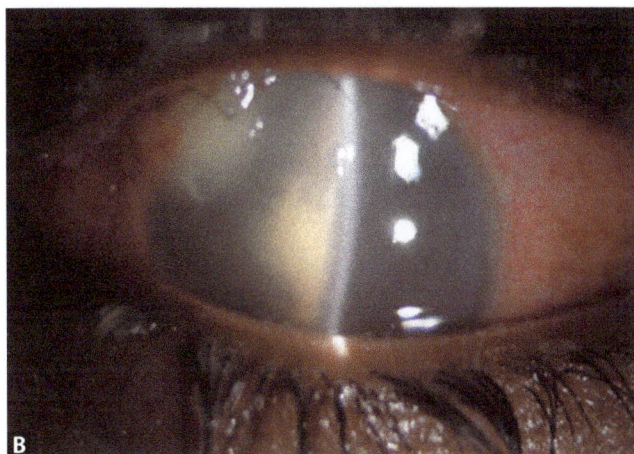

Figures 20.2A and B Bleb-associated endophthalmitis (Stage III). (A) Mucopurulent contents of the bleb with exposed sutures; (B) Severe inflammation in the anterior chamber, B-scan was suggestive of exudates in the vitreous cavity

to the bleb area and inflammatory cells may be visible in the anterior chamber on slit-lamp biomicroscopy **(Figs 20.1A and B)**. It is labelled as bleb-associated endophthalmitis (BAE) if there are exudates in the vitreous cavity along with features of blebitis **(Figs 20.2A and B)**.

Bleb-related infection can develop within days or years after glaucoma filtering surgery. It is categorized as *Early-onset BRI* when infection develops within 1 month after glaucoma filtration surgery and *Late-onset BRI* when infection develops 1 month after surgery.[11,12] Late-onset BRI is more commonly seen than early-onset BRI and is associated with a different spectrum of causative organisms.[11,13] In general, BAE is regarded as a more serious virulent infection than other post-operative endophthalmitis, thus mandating an early and aggressive treatment.

RISK FACTORS

Numerous risk factors have been implicated in bleb-associated endophthalmitis **(Table 20.2)**. Use of antimitotic agents (especially Mitomycin C or 5-fluorouracil) is the most important factor predisposing to the formation of thin cystic blebs and bleb-related infections. Other ocular risk factors include any locus of infection in the eye or adnexa such as conjunctivitis, blepharitis, dacryocystitis, etc. CBIITS revealed that bleb leakage and younger age were the main risk factors for bleb-related infections.

MICROBIAL SPECTRUM

The microbial spectrum may slightly vary between blebitis and bleb-associated endophthalmitis. In blebitis, the most commonly isolated organisms

Ocular Infections: Prophylaxis and Management

Table 20.2 Risk factors for bleb-related infections
Bleb-related factors
• Use of antimitotic agents like MMC, 5-FU[14]
• Thin walled, cystic bleb[5] **(Figs 20.3A and B)**
• Bleb leak/bleb sweating[5,7] **(Fig. 20.4)**
• Localized avascular bleb[5]
• Inferior bleb[4]
• Exposed sutures[15]
• Releasable sutures[15]
• Limbal based conjunctival flap[8]
Other ocular risk factors[16-18]
• Conjunctivitis[6]
• Blepharitis[6]
• Infections of lacrimal drainage system (dacryocystitis, canaliculitis)[16]
• Poor ocular surface
• Contact lens wear[17]
• Prolonged use of topical antibiotics[12]
• Lagophthalmos
General or systemic risk factors
• Young age[7]
• Black race[8]
• Diabetes[14]
• Immunosuppression
• Malnutrition
• Poor hygiene

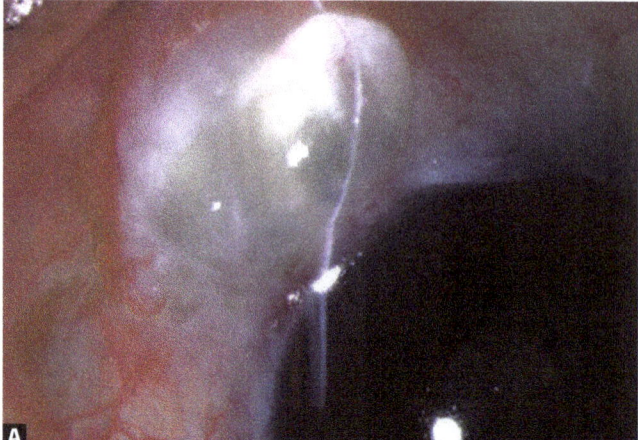
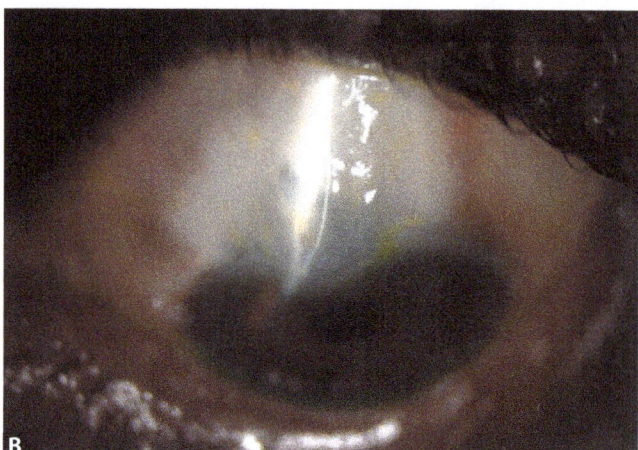

Figures 20.3A and B Thin-walled, elevated, cystic and avascular bleb

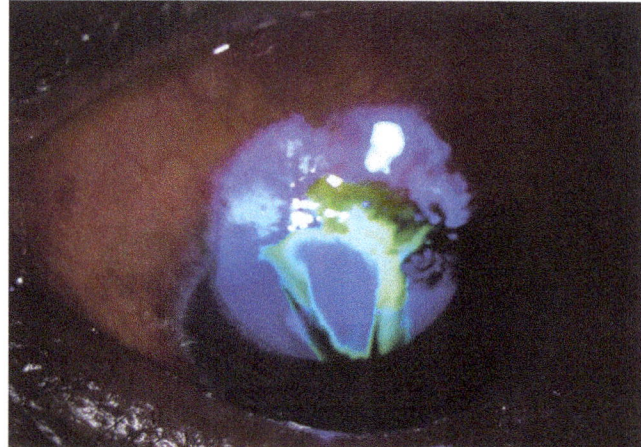

Figure 20.4 Bleb leakage visible after fluorescein staining (positive Siedel's test)

are *S. epidermidis, S. aureus, Streptococcus viridans* and *Streptococcus pneumoniae*.[19-21] Some of these commonly cultured organisms can be consistent with the normal flora. BAE on the other hand is most commonly associated with isolates of *Streptococcus sp.* followed by Gram-negative organisms (*Moraxella catarrhalis, Haemophilus influenzae, Serratia species*).[6,20,22]

The spectrum is also different for early (rare) and late onset infections. Studies have shown early onset endophthalmitis has causative organisms similar to post cataract surgery endophthalmitis which include coagulase-negative staphylococci (specifically *Staphylococcus epidermidis*) and *S. aureus*.[13,19] Late onset BAE is caused by more virulent organisms like *Streptococcus species* and gram-negative organisms.[23]

It is important to note here that bacteria isolated from conjunctival scraping may not be the same as obtained from vitreous tap. It is postulated that the bacteria causing BAE was present over the bleb surface for short time only, and thus the isolate from the bleb area may not be the causative organism.[19]

PROPHYLAXIS

Pre-operative

Similar to any other intraocular surgeries, it is important to rule out any nidus of infection involving the ocular surface or adnexa. In the presence of blepharitis, conjunctivitis, dacryocystitis, poor ocular surface or nasolacrimal duct obstruction, the glaucoma surgery should be deferred till the infection has been completely eradicated with appropriate medical and surgical therapy as required. Basic systemic work up of the patient must be done to exclude systemic diseases such as diabetes with appropriate physician consultation prior to surgery. Host immunosuppression is also an important risk factor for post-operative infection and must be ruled out. In case of unexplained fever or malaise, a thorough investigation should be done to look for an infective focus elsewhere in the body. Patient should be taken up for the surgery only after the blood sugar levels are controlled and written clearance has been obtained from the physician. Pre-operative topical broad spectrum antibiotics can be started 48–72 hrs prior to surgery. Any trichiatic lashes should be removed prior to surgery.

Intra-operative

Maintaining asepsis in the operating room is one of the most important requirements to prevent any post-operative infection. The details pertaining to the OT layout, ventilation, disinfection protocols, OT etiquettes and autoclaving have been covered elsewhere in this book.

In early onset bleb-related infections which are relatively rare, most common causative organisms come from the patients' own ocular flora. Thus, it becomes important to reduce the bacterial count in the ocular and periocular area. Use of 5% povidone iodine solution shows bactericidal action within one minute of application to the periocular area and the conjunctival surface. It kills 96.7% of the bacteria and the effect lasts for at least one hour.[24]

Late onset bleb-related infections are more common after glaucoma filtration surgery. Bleb leakage resulting from cystic, thin walled, avascular blebs is the single most important risk factor for developing blebitis or BAE.[7] Prevention of this serious complication requires controlled use of antifibrotic agents like MMC or 5-FU both in terms of concentration and duration. A wider area of MMC application also ensures a diffuse and good bleb morphology. A study comparing limbal versus fornix based flap in trabeculectomy found marked decrease in incidence of localized cystic blebs (90% vs 29%) and bleb-related infections (20% vs 0%) using fornix based conjunctival flaps.[8] Use of low dose mitomycin C (0.1 mg for 1 minute) or using biodegradable collagen implants as alternatives to MMC can help to reduce the risk of thin cystic blebs and risk of bleb-related infections.

Post-operative

A short course of antibiotic is imperative to prevent post-operative infection. However, the use of long-term antibiotics is discouraged to prevent the development of microbial resistance.[14] It is important to look for bleb leaks in the early post-operative phase and also in the later months, especially if the patient has developed a thin-walled avascular bleb. Early identification and management of bleb sweating or bleb leakage is the most important step in prophylaxis of bleb-related infections. The management options for bleb leak have been listed in **Table 20.3**. The success rates of non-surgical methods are mostly poor and the effect is short-term. Most cases require surgical intervention at some point. Studies have shown superiority of conjunctival advancement technique over other nonsurgical and surgical modalities such as amniotic membrane grafting.[25-27]

Table 20.3 Management of late onset bleb leaks

Non-surgical methods	Surgical methods
• Aqueous suppressants[28]	• Conjunctival advancement[34,35] (bleb excision or bleb sparing)
• Pressure bandage[29]	
• Oversize contact lens, Collagen shields, Glaucoma shells[29]	• Conjunctival pedicle graft[36]
	• Conjunctival free autograft[37]
• Tissue adhesives[30] (fibrin glue, cyanoacrylate glue)	• Hinged scleral flap reconstruction with conjunctival advancement[26]
• Injection of autologous blood into the bleb[31]	• Homologous scleral patch graft for scleral thinning post-trabeculectomy
• Lasers—Nd: YAG,[32] Argon[33]	

DIAGNOSIS AND MANAGEMENT

Early diagnosis and prompt aggressive treatment is the key in management of bleb-related infections. Patients with blebitis present with complaints of sudden onset pain, redness and slight diminution of vision. On examination conjunctival congestion, milky content of the bleb, loss of translucency and mild anterior chamber reaction is present. A characteristic "white on red" appearance is seen. In patients with bleb-associated endophthalmitis the clinical course is more accelerated and outcome is worse. In addition to the features of blebitis, patients with BAE show inflammatory cells and exudates in the vitreous cavity. Hypopyon may or may not be present; its absence should not preclude the diagnosis of BAE.

After the diagnosis of blebitis or bleb-related endophthalmitis has been made, samples should be sent for culture and polymerase chain reaction (PCR) **(Table 20.4)**. However, it is important that in the process of sending these investigations and awaiting their reports, there should be no delay in initiating treatment.

In both, blebitis and bleb-associated endophthalmitis, the patient should be immediately started on antimicrobial therapy. Fortified topical antibiotics such as 5% vancomycin/5% cefazolin and 1.3% tobramycin are started one hourly round the clock covering both gram-positive and gram-negative organisms. Another widely accepted regimen is one hourly use of topical fluoroquinolones like 0.5% moxifloxacin. Subconjunctival injection of antibiotics near the bleb site to dry the source of infection is also recommended. Oral fluoroquinolones which achieve high intraocular concentration like ciprofloxacin (250–500 mg twice a day) should also be considered.[33] Additional therapy includes cycloplegics and analgesics. Topical steroids to prevent scarring, should only be started after 48 hours of intense antibiotic therapy has been given with clear evidence of clinical improvement.[38]

In addition to the above treatment protocol, patients with bleb-associated endophthalmitis should also receive intravitreal antibiotics like ceftazidime (2.25 mg in 0.1 mL) and vancomycin (1 mg in 0.1 mL). Some surgeons have also suggested the role of intravenous antibiotics[39] including ceftazidime (100 mg/kg in two divided doses) and vancomycin (40 mg/kg in three divided doses). The results of endophthalmitis vitrectomy study (EVS) cannot be directly applied here, as the study groups (post-cataract surgery versus post-glaucoma filtration surgery) and microbiological profile (*Staphylococcus* vs *Streptococcus*) are different. In a study by Busbee et al.,[40] they found that in patients with culture positive BAE, visual outcomes were better with early pars plana vitrectomy (PPV) compared to the conventional therapy with antibiotics and intravitreal injections.

Management of Late Bleb Leak

Thin blebs without leaks should be carefully followed up and the patient counseled about the signs and symptoms of infection. Any episodes of conjunctivitis or blebitis or leaks mandate a bleb revision surgery for these patients.

In a bleb revision or repair surgery, the bleb area is covered by the surrounding healthy conjunctiva. Bleb sparing epithelial exchange[41] is done by staining of the dead conjunctiva by Trypan blue dye, peeling of the atrophic conjunctiva from bleb area, without disturbing the bleb and advancement of the conjunctiva over the bleb **(Figs 20.5A to D)**.

VISUAL OUTCOME AND PROGNOSIS

Bleb-related infection poses a significant threat to vision and can lead to adverse outcomes with loss of IOP control. The final visual outcome and prognosis depend upon the stage of infection. Patients presenting with blebitis have a better visual outcome as compared to the patients presenting with BRE.[42] Yamada et al estimated the rate of blindness to be 14% for the total cases with BRI (including blebitis) and 30% for the endophthalmitis subgroup. Highly virulent organisms such as *Streptococcus* spp. and gram-negative bacteria are associated with poor visual outcomes[42] and higher rates of evisceration and enucleation.[43] Stage III BRI and a positive vitreous culture have been associated with nil light perception vision.[41,42]

Table 20.4 Samples to be sent for microbiological profile	
Sample	
Conjunctival Swab	From area around the bleb, pus, discharge from the bleb surface
Aqueous tap	In cases of blebitis with marked anterior segment reaction. In all cases of bleb-associated endophthalmitis.
Vitreous tap	Only in cases of bleb-associated endophthalmitis

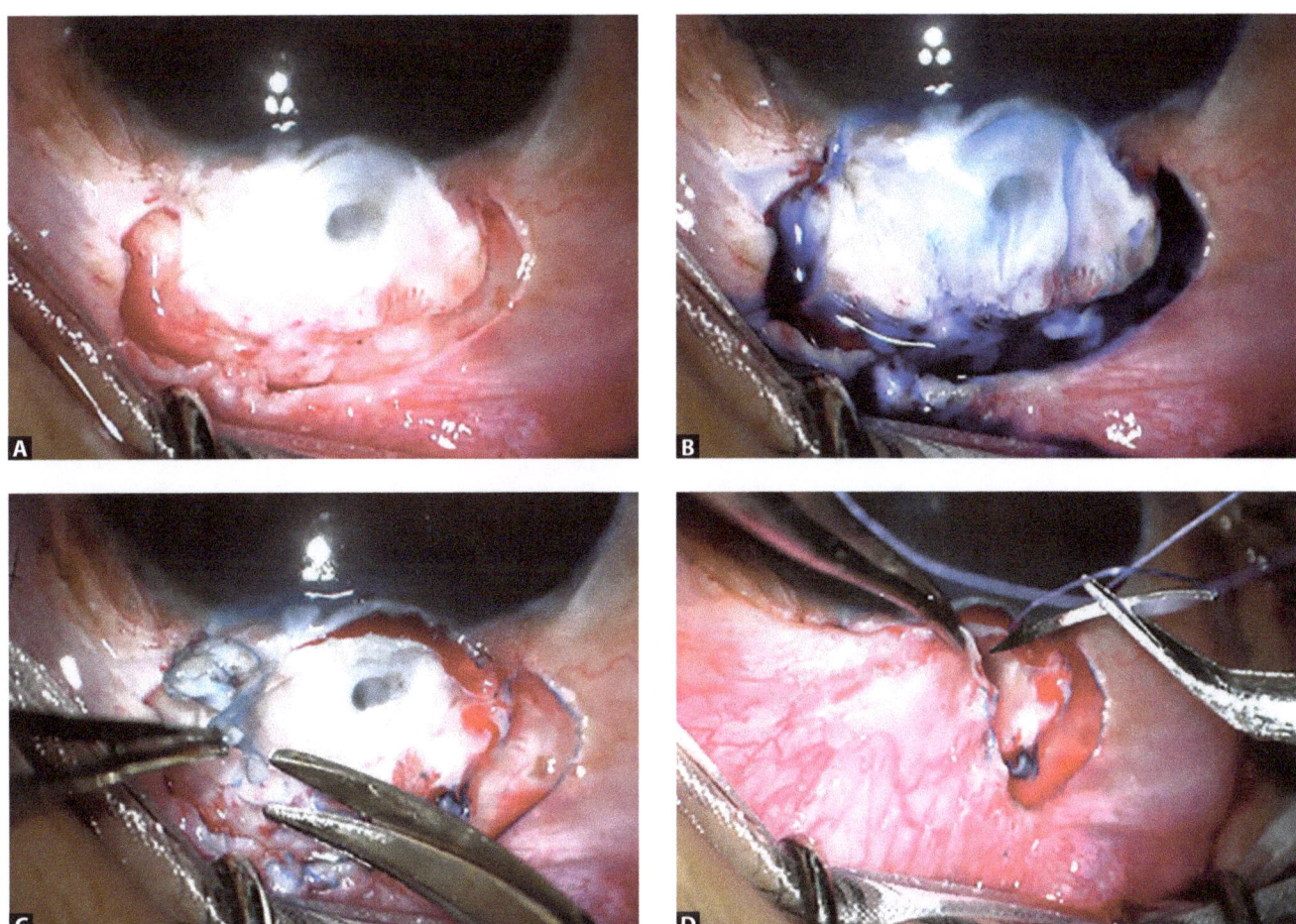

Figures 20.5A to D The conjunctiva around the bleb area is separated. The dead epithelium over bleb is stained using trypan blue dye and peeled off, leaving underlying bleb intact. The surrounding conjunctiva is advanced over the bleb

Good visual acuity post-BRI was correlated with shorter interval from onset of symptoms to treatment, better initial visual acuity, clear cornea at presentation, isolation of less virulent organisms and absence of diabetes mellitus.[44] Multiple studies have reported that a visual acuity better than 20/100 is obtained only in less than 50% of patients.

PATIENT EDUCATION AND COUNSELING

Patients should be explained regarding the danger signs related to bleb infections-"RSVP"-redness, sensitivity to light, visual loss and pain. In an event of delay in reaching an ophthalmologist, the patient should be educated to start topical antibiotics such as moxifloxacin 0.5%, till ophthalmic consultation is available. Patients who are using any eyedrops after trabeculectomy surgery should be explained proper instillation technique—avoid touching the tip of nozzle with eyelashes or conjunctiva and medications should be discarded after 30–45 days of opening the vial. It is important to emphasize on the need of regular, life-long follow-up for all glaucoma patients, who undergo a trabeculectomy.

REFERENCES

1. Kent DG. Endophthalmitis in Auckland 1983–1991. Aust NZJ Ophthalmol. 1993;21(4):227-36.
2. Mochizuki K, Jikihara S, Ando Y, et al. Incidence of delayed onset infection after trabeculectomy with adjunctive mitomycin C or 5-fluorouracil treatment. Br J Ophthalmol. 1997;81(10):877-83.
3. Collignon-Brach J. Surgery for glaucoma and endophthalmitis. Bull Soc Belge Ophtalmol. 1996;260: 73-7.

4. Higginbotham EJ, Stevens RK, Musch DC, et al. Bleb-related endophthalmitis after trabeculectomy with mitomycin C. Ophthalmology. 1996;103(4):650-6.
5. Wolner B, Liebmann JM, Sassani JW, et al. Late bleb-related endophthalmitis after trabeculectomy with adjunctive 5-fluorouracil. Ophthalmology. 1991;98(7):1053-60.
6. Greenfield DS, Suner IJ, Miller MP, et al. Endophthalmitis after filtering surgery with mitomycin. Arch Ophthalmol. 1996;114(8):943-9.
7. Sugimoto Y, Mochizuki H, Ohkubo S, Higashide T, Sugiyama K, Kiuchi Y. Intraocular Pressure Outcomes and Risk Factors for Failure in the Collaborative Bleb-Related Infection Incidence and Treatment Study. Ophthalmology. 2015;122(11):2223-33.
8. Wells AP, Cordeiro MF, Bunce C, Khaw PT. Cystic bleb formation and related complications in limbus- versus fornix-based conjunctival flaps in pediatric and young adult trabeculectomy with mitomycin C. Ophthalmology. 2003;110(11):2192-7.
9. Rai P, Kotecha A, Kaltsos K, Ruddle JB, Murdoch IE, Bunce C, Barton K. Changing trends in the incidence of bleb-related infection in trabeculectomy. Br J Ophthalmol 2012;96: 971-5.
10. Kuroda U, Inoue T, Awai-Kasaoka N, Shobayashi K, Kojima S, Tanihara H. Fornix-based versus limbal-based conjunctival flaps in trabeculectomy with mitomycin C in high-risk patients. Clin Ophthalmol. 2014;8:949-54.
11. Kangas TA, Greenfield DS, Flynn HW Jr, Parrish RK II, Palmberg P. Delayed-onset endophthalmitis associated with conjunctival filtering blebs. Ophthalmology. 1997;104:746-52.
12. Jampel HD, Quigley HA, Kerrigan-Baumrind LA, Melia BM, Friedman D, Barron Y. Risk factors for late-onset infection following glaucoma filtration surgery. Arch Ophthalmol. 2001;119:1001-8.
13. Brillat-Zaratzian E, Bron A, Aptel F, et al. FRIENDS Group: clinical and microbiological characteristics of post-filtering surgery endophthalmitis. Graefes Arch Clin Exp Ophthalmol. 2014;252:101-7.
14. Lehmann OJ, Bunce C, Matheson MM, Maurino V, Khaw PT, Wormald R, Barton K. Risk factors for development of post-trabeculectomy endophthalmitis. Br J Ophthalmol. 2000;84(12):1349-53.
15. Cohen JS, Osher RH. Endophthalmitis associated with releasable sutures. Arch Ophthalmol. 1997;115(2):292.
16. Tabbara KF. Late infections following filtering procedures. Ann Ophthalmol. 1976;8(10):1228-31.
17. Gupta N, Weinreb RN. Filtering bleb infection as a complication of orthokeratology. Arch Ophthalmol. 1997;115(8):1076.
18. Soltau JB, Rothman RF, Budenz DL, Greenfield DS, Feuer W, Liebmann JM, Ritch R. Risk factors for glaucoma filtering bleb infections. Arch Ophthalmol. 2000;118(3):338-42
19. Ciulla TA, Beck AD, Topping TM, Baker AS. Blebitis, early endophthalmitis, and late endophthalmitis after glaucoma-filtering surgery. Ophthalmology. 1997;104:986-95.
20. Mandelbaum S, Forster RK. Endophthalmitis associated with filtering blebs. IntOphthalmol Clin. 1987;27:107-11.
21. Brown RH, Yang LH, Walker SD, Lynch MG, Martinez LA, Wilson LA. Treatment of bleb infection after glaucoma surgery. Arch Ophthalmol. 1994;112:57-61.
22. Mandelbaum S, Forster RK, Gelender H, Culbertson W. Late onset endophthalmitis associated with filtering blebs. Ophthalmology. 1985;92:964-72.
23. Leng T, Miller D, Flynn HW Jr, Jacobs DJ, Gedde SJ. Delayed-onset bleb-associated endophthalmitis: causative organisms and visual acuity outcomes. Retina. 1996–2008;31:344-52.
24. Schmitz S, Dick HB, Krummenauer F, Pfeiffer N. Endophthalmitis in cataract surgery: results of a German study. Ophthalmology. 1999;106:1869-77.
25. Burnstein AL, WuDunn D, Knotts SL, Catoira Y, Cantor LB. Conjunctival advancement versus nonincisional treatment for late-onset glaucoma filtering bleb leaks. Ophthalmology. 2002;109(1):71-5.
26. Mandal AK. Management of the late leaking filtration blebs. A report of seven cases and a selective review of the literature. Indian J Ophthalmol. 2001;49(4):247-54.
27. Wadhwani RA, Bellows AR, Hutchinson BT. Surgical repair of leaking filtering blebs. Ophthalmology. 2000;107(9):1681-7.
28. Feldman RM, Altaher G. Management of late-onset bleb leaks. Curr Opin Ophthalmol. 2004;15(2):151-4.
29. Hill RA, Aminlari A, Sassani JW, Michalski M. Use of a symblepharon ring for treatment of over filtration and leaking blebs after glaucoma filtering surgery. Ophthalmic Surg. 1999;21:707-10
30. Asrani SG, Wilensky JT. Management of bleb leaks after glaucoma filtering surgery. Use of autologous fibrin tissue as an alternative. Ophthalmology. 1996;103:294-8.
31. Burnstein A, WuDunn D, Ishii Y, et al. Autologous blood injection for late-onset filtering bleb leak. Am J Ophthalmol. 2001;132:36-40.
32. Lynch MG, Roesch M, Brown RH. Remolding filtering blebs with the neodymium: YAG laser. Ophthalmology. 1996;103:1700-5.
33. Hennis HL, Stewart WC. Use of the argon laser to close filtering bleb leaks. Greases Arch Clint Exp Ophthalmol. 1992;230:537-41.
34. Budenz DL, Chen PP, Weaver YK. Conjunctival advancement for late-onset filtering bleb leaks: indications and outcomes. Arch Ophthalmol. 1999;117:1014-9.

35. Catoria Y, Wudunn D, Cantor LB. Revision of dysfunctional filtering blebs by conjunctival advancement with bleb preservation. Am J Ophthalmol. 2000;130:574-9.
36. Ye T, Li F, Li X. Revision of thin-walled cystic bleb by transposing conjunctival flap technique. Zhonghua Yan Ke Za Zhi. 2001;37:37-9.
37. Schnyder CC, Shaarawy T, Ravinet E, et al. Free conjunctival autologous graft for bleb repair and bleb reduction after trabeculectomy and nonpenetrating filtering surgery. J Glaucoma. 2001;11:10-6.
38. Chen PP, Gedde SJ, Budenz DL, et al. Outpatient treatment of bleb infection. Arch Ophthalmol. 1997;115:1124-8.
39. Ba'arah BT, Smiddy WE. Bleb-related Endophthalmitis: Clinical presentation, isolates, treatment and visual outcome of culture-proven cases. Middle East Afr J Ophthalmol. 2009;16(1): 20-4.
40. Busbee BG, Recchia FM, Kaiser R, Nagra P, Rosenblatt B, Pearlman RB. Bleb-associated endophthalmitis: clinical characteristics and visual outcomes. Ophthalmology. 2004;111(8):1495-503
41. Sihota R, et al. The Long-term Outcome of Primary "Bleb-sparing, Epithelial Exchange" in Dysfunctional Filtering Blebs. J Glaucoma. 2016;25(7):571-8
42. Al-Turki TA, Al-Shahwan S, Al-Mezaine HS, Kangave D, Abu El-Asrar AM. Microbiology and visual outcome of bleb-associated endophthalmitis. Ocul Immunol Inflamm. 2010;18:121-6.
43. Song A, Scott IU, Flynn HW Jr, Budenz DL. Delayed-onset bleb-associated endophthalmitis: clinical features and visual acuity outcomes. Ophthalmology. 2002;109:985-91.
44. Yamamoto T, Kuwayama Y, Nomura E, Tanihara H, Mori K. Changes in visual acuity and intraocular pressure following bleb-related infection: the Japan Glaucoma Society Survey of Bleb-related Infection Report 2. Acta Ophthalmol. 2013;91:420-6.

CHAPTER 21

Post-Strabismus Surgery Infections

Saranya Devi K, Rohit Saxena

INCIDENCE AND PREVALENCE

Infections following strabismus surgery are relatively rare.[1] The spectrum of infections can vary from milder forms such as preseptal cellulitis, subconjunctival abscess to the more severe vision threatening forms such as orbital cellulitis and endophthalmitis **(Flow chart 21.1)**. Periorbital infections affecting the conjunctiva and Tenon's capsule have also been reported.[2] Orbital cellulitis incidence was reported to be 1 per 1900 cases whereas that of endophthalmitis was 1 per 30,000 cases following strabismus surgery.[3] Various other studies reported the incidence of endophthalmitis following strabismus surgery to be varying from 1:3500 to 1:185,000.[4,5] The rarity of these infections may result in delayed diagnosis. Thus, the surgeon should carry high index of suspicion to identify and manage these complications following strabismus surgery.

MICROBIAL FLORA AND RISK FACTORS

The most common risk factor for infection following strabismus surgery is the patient's own normal conjuctival microbial flora. Other risk factors include contaminated sutures and needles, post-operative periocular abscess and transient endogenous bacteremia.[1] Immunocompromised patients such as those with diabetes, those on steroids or chemotherapy are also at higher risk of developing infections post-strabismus surgery owing to their inability to mount an adequate immune response.

It has been proven that surgeons speaking or shouting in the operating room can be a possible source of infections.[6] This study demonstrated the massive increase in the bacterial colony count on blood agar plates which was placed 30 cm from the surgeons' mouth and this increase was directly proportional to the volume at which the surgeon speaks.

Flow chart 21.1 Spectrum of ocular infections following strabismus surgery

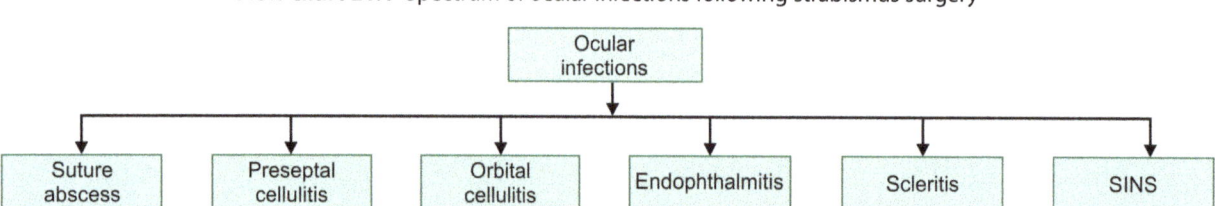

Abbreviation: SINS, surgically-induced necrotizing scleritis

Glove Perforation

Another important risk factor identified to be a major source of infection is glove perforation.[7] Glove perforation can be equally dangerous to both the patients and the surgeons. It has been reported that occult glove perforation is more common than the recognized perforation. The perforation may be that of surgeons, assistants or nurses' gloves.[8] Perforation was most common in retinal surgery and least common with strabismus surgery. It has been reported that the perforation was common in left gloves than the right gloves and thumb and index finger parts were commonly involved. The rate of glove perforation in ophthalmic surgery has been reported to be around 4%.[9]

Intra-operative Contamination

Infections can occur due to contamination of fluid used during the surgery. Instruments, sutures and supplies can act as a possible source of contamination. Needle contamination has been reported to be a major source of infection following strabismus surgery, the incidence of which was reported to be as high as 15.1%.[10] Carothers et al[11] have reported that needles and sutures can be contaminated despite proper precautions such as the use of pre-operative povidone iodine. This study reported the contamination rate of needles to be 19% and that of the sutures to be 25.2%. *Coagulase negative staphylococci* were the most recovered organism in this study. Eustis et al[12] conducted a randomized analysis to report the contamination rate of sutures in strabismus surgery. They assigned patients to three groups namely (1) a control without pretreatment sutures; (2) antibiotic/steroid-coated sutures; and (3) antiseptic-soaked and antibiotic/steroid-coated sutures. This study reported the contamination rate of the suture to be as high as 28% and this can be reduced by soaking the sutures in antiseptic solution before use. Another randomized clinical trial by Rossetto et al[13] assessed whether application of post-operative povidone iodine to the adjustable suture in strabismus surgery decreased the colonization rate. *Staphylococcus epidermidis* was the most common isolate in this study and the longer duration between the surgery and the adjustment was found to be associated with higher culture positivity. They concluded that the use of povidone-iodine at the end of adjustable strabismus surgery was not associated with reduction in colonization rate. Scleral perforation if occurs, should be promptly identified by the surgeon and the needle should be withdrawn immediately to avoid contamination at the perforation which would otherwise result in grave complications such as endophthalmitis.[11]

ENDOPHTHALMITIS

Various risk factors have been proposed to be responsible for post-strabismus surgery endophthalmitis. Scleral perforation is believed to be a major cause.[4] Some authors suggest that endophthalmitis can be endogenous[14] following strabismus surgery while others suggest partial obstruction of nasolacrimal duct and upper airway infection[15] to be the major risk factors. *Staphylococcus* and *Streptococcus* were the predominant organisms involved. Single cases of endophthalmitis have been reported following suture abcess[14] and reoperation[16] as well.

As most strabismus surgery is done in the pediatric age group, assessment of vision is difficult in such patients. The rarity of this condition and inability of the children to report the visual loss at the early stage makes the diagnosis all the more difficult. This makes the prognosis of endophthalmitis following strabismus surgery poor. Salamon et al[17] reported two cases of endophthalmitis following strabismus surgery, of which one had scleral perforation and was treated with cryopexy. Recchia et al[4] reported six cases in pediatric age group and reported that lethargy, asymmetric eye redness, eyelid swelling, or fever in the post-operative period should raise a suspicion of endophthalmitis.

ORBITAL AND PRESEPTAL CELLULITIS

Orbital and preseptal cellulitis are rare following strabismus surgery. Patients might present with proptosis, chemosis, eyelid swelling and pain. Very few single cases of orbital cellulitis have been reported following strabismus surgery.[18-23]

SCLERITIS

Scleritis is again a rare complication following strabismus surgery where patients can present with redness and ocular discomfort. Single cases of infectious scleritis have been following strabismus surgery. The pathogens isolated were *Proteus mirabilis*,[24] *Hemophilus influenzae*[25] and *Pseudomonas*.[26] These patients had evidence of nodular abscess, areas of scleral necrosis or evidence of sterile endophthalmitis.

SURGICALLY-INDUCED NECROTIZING SCLERITIS

Surgically induced necrotizing scleritis (SINS) is a destructive, inflammatory process resulting in scleral necrosis which occurs following ocular surgery. The mean interval reported for its occurrence varies from 9 months to 40 years after the surgery.[27] The common risk factors for the development of SINS include underlying autoimmune disease and multiple ocular procedures.[28,29] Single case reports of SINS following strabismus surgery in thyroid ophthalmopathy are also available in literature.[30-33]

PROPHYLAXIS AND MANAGEMENT

Prophylaxis

Surgeon Awareness

Despite the rarity of infections following strabismus surgery, surgeons should be aware of the risk factors, clinical presentation and treatment modalities to facilitate prompt diagnosis and management. A high index of suspicion and prompt, aggressive treatment of such infections would prevent the occurrence of sight-threatening complications such as endophthalmitis and orbital cellulitis.

Avoiding Glove Perforation

Glove perforation can result in exposure of surgeon's hands resulting in contamination during surgery. Majority of the glove perforation can occur during the loading of needle onto the needle holder. The surgeon should avoid suture handling with hands and should not pass it away from the field of surgery. Proper placement of needle onto the needle holder can be facilitated by holding the suture close to the needle. Similar practice should be followed by assistants and nurses to avoid glove perforation and contamination.

Avoiding Suture and Needle Contamination

Since contaminated needles and sutures have been proven to be a major source of infections in strabismus surgery, steps to reduce exposure to such contaminated needles and sutures become mandatory. These include separating the eyelids and lashes using an appropriate drape during the surgery. The surgeon should be careful enough to avoid sclera perforation while passing the sutures, especially during the reattachment of the sutures in the recession surgery. Care should be taken in patients with thin sclera such as those with myopia or systemic diseases such as Marfan's syndrome. Also if scleral perforation is suspected, the surgeon should immediately stop and withdraw the needle out, to avoid passage of contaminated needle through the perforation site. If the needle is already inside, the surgeon should cut the suture and remove it so that the contaminated suture does not pass through the perforation site. Also suturing should be done away from the perforation site to avoid contamination by the retained suture material.

Endophthalmitis Prophylaxis

Infection prophylaxis for strabismus surgery has not been established so far owing to the rarity of this complication. Literature review reveals lack of prospective or randomized contolled trials to report the infection prophylaxis following strabismus surgery. Available information is based mainly on the practice pattern surveys. One such survey[33] reported that there was no difference in outcome with or without pre-operative antibiotic administration or iodine preparation. Also, the use of post-operative topical antibiotics is not a routine for all strabismus surgeons.[34] Another prospective study reported that there was no difference in the incidence of post-operative infection or clinical appearance after strabismus surgery in children treated with or without post-operative topical antibiotics.[35]

Periocular Infection Prophylaxis

Good hygiene, hand washing and avoidance of eye rubbing should be advised following surgery to prevent the occurrence of periocular infections. Kivlin et al[21] suggested prescription of oral antibiotics to children having upper respiratory infection or infection elsewhere following strabismus surgery. This in turn reduced the risk of ocular or periocular infections.

Management

Suture Abscess

Immediate treatment of this condition is imminent to avoid complications such as slippage or loss of muscle[36] which can occur due to the fragility of tissues. Topical antibiotics should be prescribed to treat this condition immediately. If the condition persists one might consider draining the pus through an incision and the infected suture should be removed.

Preseptal Cellulitis

It is essential to differentiate between preseptal cellulitis and orbital cellulitis. These patients will show evidence of normal vision without proptosis/resistance to retropulsion, limitation of ocular motility, orbital pain, afferent pupillary defect, optic nerve edema, and posterior segment venous engorgement. Evaluation includes assessment of visual acuity, pupillary reactions, tonometry, slit lamp biomicroscopy and ophthalmoscopy. In case of suspected systemic toxicity, blood culture should be done and lumbar puncture is essential in patients with meningeal signs. Treatment includes empirical therapy with antibiotics initially, which can later be modified based on the culture results. Outpatient care would be sufficient in adults and children older than one year of age. If oral antibiotics fail to show clinical improvement, intravenous antibiotics may be administered for 7–10 days. Other coexisting infections such as sinusitis should also be promptly managed. Literature review advises antibiotic therapy to be directed against *Staphylococcus* and *Streptococcus* species.[37,38] Surgical management might rarely be required in patients with preseptal cellulitis. Eyelid abscess may be managed through incision and drainage followed by culture of the aspirated material which would guide towards the choice of antibiotics.

Orbital Cellulitis

These patients may present with severe eyelid edema, decreased vision, pain on ocular movements, proptosis, and ophthalmoplegia. Acute sinusitis or upper respiratory tract infection might precede the development of eyelid edema. Symptoms may progress rapidly, and as such, prompt diagnosis and aggressive therapy are essential. Apart from the routine evaluation, imaging might be essential to confirm the orbital extension, to diagnose associated sinus infections and also to look for orbital and subperiosteal abscesses.[39] This can be achieved by getting a computed tomography (CT) done. Magnetic resonance imaging (MRI) of the orbits can also be done to reduce the radiation exposure. MRI might be a useful tool in the evaluation of nonmetallic foreign body and also to rule out intracranial involvement.[40,41]

Treatment includes intravenous antibiotics to empirically cover the common causative organisms and later can be modified based on the culture sensitivity results. Since most of the *Staphylococcus* species are resistant to methicillin, vancomycin can be considered for empirical therapy. To achieve gram negative and anaerobic coverage, cefotaxime and metronidazole or clindamycin can be concurrently administered. Other commonly used antibiotics are piperacillin–tazobactam, ticarcillin–clavulanate, and ceftriaxone. For patients with penicillin resistance, vancomycin in combination with a fluoroquinolone can be considered.

Aggressive nasal hygiene should be advised for patients with associated sinusitis. Nasal decongestant and saline nasal irrigation might be of help in draining the sinuses and also have favorable results in subperiosteal abscess.[42] Treatment with intravenous corticosteroids is controversial. Studies prove that steroids decrease the mucosal edema and release of inflammatory cytokines[43] in patients with chronic sinusitis and also facilitates the drainage of subperiosteal abcess[44] if present.

Indications of surgical management in orbital cellulitis is shown in **Table 21.1**.

Endophthalmitis

Most surgeons follow the treatment guidelines provided by the endophthalmitis vitrectomy study (EVS). This study suggested that immediate vitrectomy is of benefit in patients with vision of light perception only.[50] However, the results of this study cannot be translated to non cataract surgery endophthalmitis. Most of the strabismus surgery is being done in children and the

Table 21.1 Indications of surgical management in orbital cellulitis
Failure of response to medical therapy
Worsening visual function despite the medical therapy
Development of orbital abscess[45]
Subperiosteal abscess[46]
Retained orbital foreign body[47]
Associated adnexal infections such as dacryocystitis
Associated endophthalmitis
Elderly with opacified sinuses
Severe mucormycosis[48] or aspergillosis[49]

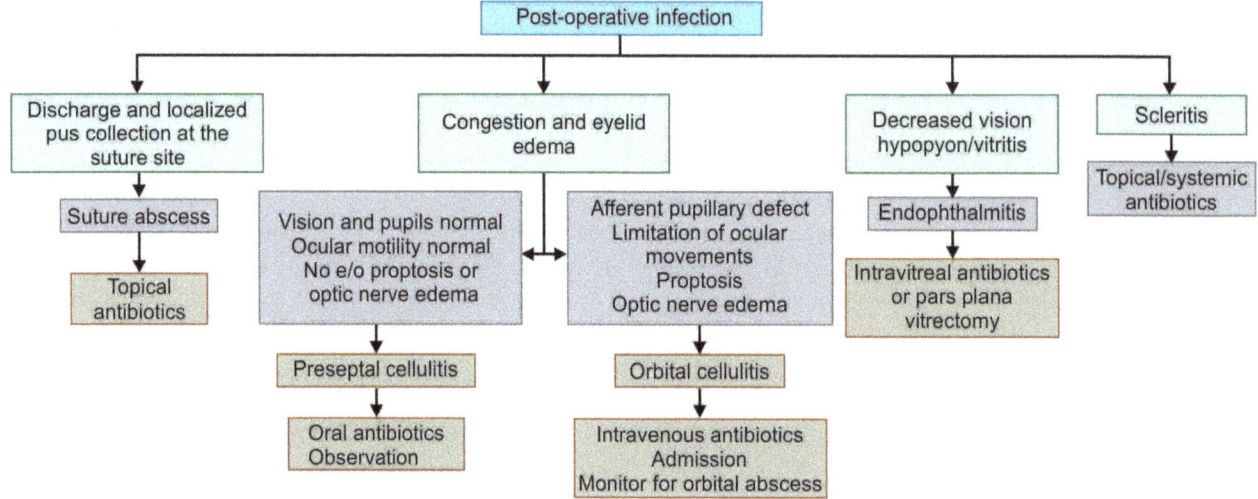

Flow chart 21.2 Summary of management of infections following strabismus surgery

inability of children to report decreased vision along with the extreme rarity of this condition makes the diagnosis difficult. High index of suspicion, prompt diagnosis and management is essential in such cases. Management includes administration of intravitreal antibiotics or vitrectomy depending upon the severity of the condition.

Scleritis and Surgically-induced Necrotizing Scleritis

Infectious scleritis can be treated effectively with empirical antibiotics which may be topical, oral or intravenous depending upon the severity of infection and its response to therapy. The antibiotic therapy can later be modified based on the culture and sensitivity results. Failure of response to antibiotics should prompt the diagnosis of SINS which is caused by autoimmune reaction. SINS can be effectively treated with topical or oral corticosteroids. The summary of management of infections following strabismus surgery is shown in **Flow chart 21.2**.

CONCLUSION

Infections following strabismus surgery are extremely rare. The clinical presentation may be subtle, especially in pediatric age group. High index of suspicion is essential to facilitate prompt diagnosis and management to prevent sight-threatening complications.

REFERENCES

1. Olitsky SE, Coats DK. Complications of strabismus surgery. Middle East Afr J Ophthalmol. 2015;22(3):271-8.
2. Yau GL, Warder D, Farmer JP, Urton T, Strube YN. A child with rapidly progressive necrotizing group a streptococcal Tenon's capsule infection one day afterstrabismus surgery. J AAPOS. 2015;19(5):470-3.
3. Ing MR. Infection following strabismus surgery. Ophthalmic Surgery, Lasers and Imaging Retina. 1991; 22(1):41-3.
4. Recchia FM, Baumal CR, Sivalingam A, Kleiner R, Duker JS, Vrabec TR. Endophthalmitis after pediatric strabismus surgery. Arch Ophthalmol. 2000;118(7):939-44.
5. Weinstein CS, Mondino BJ, Weinberg RJ, Biglan AW. Endophthalmitis in the pediatric population. Ann Ophthalmol. 1979;11(6):935-43.
6. Schiff FS. The shouting surgeon as a possible source of endophthalmitis. Ophthalmic Surg. 1990;21(6):438-40.
7. Apt L, Miller KM. Occult glove perforation during ophthalmic surgery. Trans Am Ophthalmol Soc. 1992; 90:71-95.
8. Wright JG, McGeer AJ, Chyatte D, Ransohoff DF. Mechanisms of glove tears and sharp injuries among surgical personnel. JAMA. 1991;266(12):1668-71.
9. Nakazawa M, Sato K, Mizuno K. Incidence of perforations in rubber gloves during ophthalmic surgery. Ophthalmic Surg. 1984;15(3):236-40.
10. Olitsky SE, Vilardo M, Awner S, Reynolds JD. Needle sterility during strabismus surgery. J AAPOS.1998;2:151-2.

11. Carothers TS, Coats DK, McCreery KM, Rossman SN, Wilson P, Wu TG, Paysse EA. Quantification of incidental needle and suture contamination during strabismus surgery. Binocul Vis Strabismus Q. 2003;18(2):75-9.
12. Eustis HS, Rhodes A. Suture contamination in strabismus surgery. J Pediatr Ophthalmol Strabismus. 2012;49(4):206-9.
13. Rossetto JD, Suwannaraj S, Cavuoto KM, Spierer O, Miller D, McKeown CA, Capo H. Evaluation of postoperative povidone iodine in adjustable suture strabismus surgery to reduce suture colonization: A randomized clinical trial. JAMA Ophthalmol; 2016.
14. Rosenbaum AL. Endophthalmitis after strabismus surgery. Arch Ophthalmol. 2000;118:982-3.
15. Good WV, Hing S, Irvine AR, Hoyt CS, Taylor DS. Postoperative endophthalmitis in children following cataract surgery. J Pediatr Ophthalmol Strabismus. 1990;27:283-5.
16. Kushner BJ, Meyers FL. Good visual outcome after endophthalmitis in an eye previously treated successfully for amblyopia. J Pediatr Ophthalmol Strabismus. 1989;26(2):69-71.
17. Salamon SM, Friberg TR, Luxenberg MN. Endophthalmitis after strabismus surgery. Am J Ophthalmol. 1982;93(1):39-41.
18. Von Noorden GK. Orbital cellulitis following extraocular muscle surgery. Am J Ophthalmol. 1972;74:627-9.
19. Wilson ME, Paul TO. Orbital cellulitis following strabismus surgery. Ophthalmic Surg. 1987;18:92-4.
20. Weakley DR. Orbital cellulitis complicating strabismus surgery: a case report and review of the literature. Ann Ophthalmol. 1991;23:454-7.
21. Kivlin JD, Wilson ME Jr. Periocular infection after strabismus surgery. The Periocular Infection Study Group. J Pediatr Ophthalmol Strabismus. 1995;32:42-9.
22. Palamar M, Uretmen O, Kose S. Orbital cellulitis after strabismus surgery. J AAPOS. 2005;9:602-3.
23. Hoyama E, Limawararut V, Leibovitch I, Pater J, Davis G, Selva D. Blinding orbital cellulitis: a complication of strabismus surgery. Ophthal Plast Reconstr Surg. 2006;22:472-3.
24. Hemady R, Sainz de la Maza M, Raizman MB, Foster CS. Six cases of scleritis associated with systemic infection. Am J Ophthalmol. 1992;114(1):55-62.
25. Sykes S, Riemann C, Santos C, Meisler D, Lowder C, Whitcher J, Cunningham E. *Haemophilus influenzae* associated scleritis. Br J Ophthalmol. 1999;83(4):410-3.
26. Chao DL, Albini TA, McKeown CA, Cavuoto KM. Infectious Pseudomonas scleritis after strabismus surgery. J AAPOS. 2013;17(4):423-5.
27. O'Donoghue E, Lightman S, Tuft S, Watson P. Surgically induced necrotising sclerokeratitis (SINS) – precipitating factors and response to treatment. Br J Ophth. 1992;76:17-21.
28. de la Maza MS, Foster CS. Necrotizing scleritis after ocular surgery: a clinicopathologic study. Ophthalmology. 1991;98:1720-6.
29. Bloomfield SE, et al. Bilateral anterior necrotising scleritis with marginal corneal ulceration after cataract surgery in a patient with vasculitis. Br J Ophth. 1980;64:170-4.
30. Kaufman LM, Folk ER, Miller MT, Tessler HH. Necrotizing scleritis following strabismus surgery for thyroid ophthalmopathy. J Pediatr Ophthalmol Strabismus. 1989;26(5):236-8.
31. Kearney FM, Blaikie AJ, Gole GA. Anterior necrotizing scleritis after strabismus surgery in a child. J AAPOS. 2007;11(2):197-8.
32. Gross SA, von Noorden GK, Jones DB. Necrotizing scleritis and transient myopia following strabismus surgery. Ophthalmic Surg. 1993;24(12):839-41.
33. Baumal CR, Levin AV, Read SE. Cytomegalovirus retinitis in immunosuppressed children. Am J Ophthalmol. 1999;127:550-8.
34. Folk ER. Antibiotics and timing of follow-up visits in routine postoperative care: a survey of 25 strabismus surgeons. Binocular Vis Q. 1990;57.
35. Wortham E, Anandakrishnan I, Kraft SP, Smith D, Morin JD. Are antibiotic-steroid drops necessary following strabismus surgery? A prospective, randomized, masked trial. J Pediatr Ophthalmol Strabismus. 1990;27:205-7.
36. McNeer K. Three complications of strabismus surgery. Ann Ophthalmol. 1975;7(3):441-6.
37. Howe L, Jones NS. Guidelines for the management of periorbital cellulitis/abscess. Clin Otolaryngol. 2004;29:725-8.
38. Israele V, Nelson JD. Periorbital and orbital cellulitis. Pediatr Infect Dis J. 1987;6:404-10.
39. Shah NB, Platt SL. ALARA: is there a cause for alarm? Reducing radiation risks from computed tomography scanning in children. Curr Opin Pediatr. 2008;20(3):243-7.
40. Mills RP, Kartush JM. Orbital wall thickness and the spread of infection from the paranasal sinuses. Clin Otolaryngol. 1985;10(4):209-16.
41. Mills DM, Tsai S. Pediatric ophthalmic computed tomographic scanning and associated cancer risk. Am J Ophthalmol. 2006;142(6):1046-53.
42. Brown CL, Graham SM. Nasal irrigations: good or bad? Curr Opin Otolaryngol. Head Neck Surg. 2004;12:9-13.
43. Fu SY, Su GW. Cytokine expression in pediatric subperiosteal orbital abscesses. Can J Ophthalmol. 2007;42(6):865-9.
44. Yen MT, Yen KG. Effect of corticosteroids in the acute management of pediatric orbital cellulitis with

subperiosteal abscess. Ophthal Plast Reconstr Surg. 2005;21(5):363-6.
45. Chaudhry IA, Shamsi FA. Outcome of treated orbital cellulitis in a tertiary eye care center in the middle East. Ophthalmology. 2007;114(2):345-54.
46. Ryan JT, Preciado DA. Management of pediatric orbital cellulitis in patients with radiographic findings of subperiosteal abscess. Otolaryngol. Head Neck Surg. 2009;140(6):907-11.
47. Green BF, Kraft SP. Intraorbital wood. Detection by magnetic resonance imaging. Ophthalmology. 1990;97:608-11.
48. McCarty ML, Wilson MW. Manifestations of fungal cellulitis of the orbit in children with neutropenia and fever. Ophthal Plast Reconstr Surg. 2004;20:217-23.
49. Dhiwakar M, Thakar A, Bahadur S. Invasive sino-orbital aspergillosis: surgical decisions and dilemmas. J Laryngol Otol. 2003;117:280-5.
50. Results of the Endophthalmitis Vitrectomy Study. A randomized trial of immediate vitrectomy and of intravenous antibiotics for the treatment of post-operative bacterial endophthalmitis. Endophthalmitis Vitrectomy Study Group Arch Ophthalmol. 1995;113: 479-96.

CHAPTER 22

Post-Pterygium Surgery Infections

Neelima Aron, Divya Agarwal, Prafulla K Maharana, Namrata Sharma

INTRODUCTION

Pterygium surgery is one of the most commonly performed procedures aiming at better cosmetic and visual outcomes. Though recurrence is the most common complication of pterygium surgery, postoperative infections with corneo-scleral melts are of major concern. Pterygium surgery is a common predisposing factor for infectious scleral ulcers in areas where prevalence of pterygium is high like India, Taiwan, and China.[1] Poor prognosis of these cases was much emphasized earlier but early diagnosis and aggressive medical and surgical therapy can salvage the eye.[1]

INCIDENCE AND MICROBIAL SPECTRUM

The overall incidence of scleral necrosis after pterygium surgery has been reported to be 0.2–4.5%.[2] This includes both infectious and non-infectious cases. The etiology of scleral melts after pterygium surgery includes:
- Scleromalacia or a quiet scleral melt which is detected on routine examination. The patient may be totally asymptomatic.
- Non-infectious necrotizing scleritis with a localized area of scleral melt which may or may not be associated with pain. It is diagnosed by an absence of infiltrates and anterior chamber reaction.
- Infectious corneoscleral melts associated with pain, redness, discharge associated with infiltrates with or without anterior camber reaction and hypopyon. Of all the cases of scleral necrosis that have been reported, 58.6% cases have been attributed to infection.[3]

The most common microorganism isolated in post-pterygium surgery infections is *Pseudomonas aeruginosa* accounting for almost 60% of cases. Other isolates include *Staphylococcus* species, *Nocardia*, *Escherichia coli* and fungal keratitis of which the most common is *Aspergillus* species or mixed infection.[3,4]

RISK FACTORS

One of the most important and commonest cause of post pterygium corneoscleral melts is the injudicious use of intra-operative mitomycin-C especially when conjunctival closure is not done and higher doses are applied on to bare sclera.[5-8] Further, conjunctival closure with sutures may increase the chances of infection due to retention of sutures within the eye for a prolonged period of time **(Figs 22.1A and B)**. Sutureless conjunctival closure with the use of fibrin glue may reduce this risk. Other adjuncts which are used intra-operatively and increase the chances of post-operative melts include thiotepa[9] and beta-irradiation.[10,11-15] Further, faulty surgical techniques such as excessive cauterization,[10,14] excessive tissue destruction and prolonged exposure of bare sclera may lead to post-operative scleral melts.

PATHOGENESIS

Various mechanisms have been proposed for the occurrence of scleral melts post pterygium surgery though the exact pathogenesis has not been elucidated.

Vascular deprivation[16,17] has been proposed as a probable cause for melting of sclera. It is believed that β irradiation causes obliterative endarteritis whereas

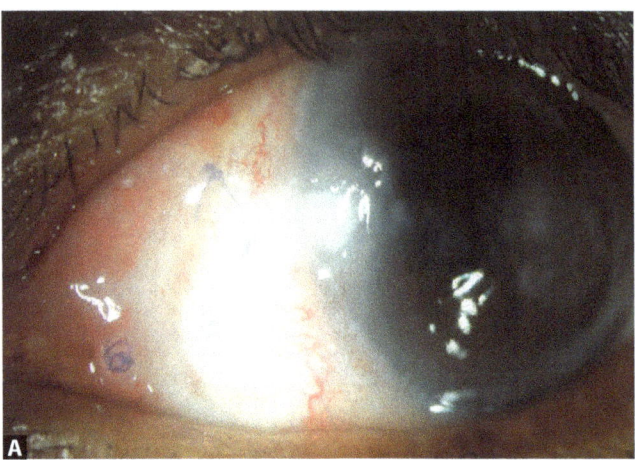
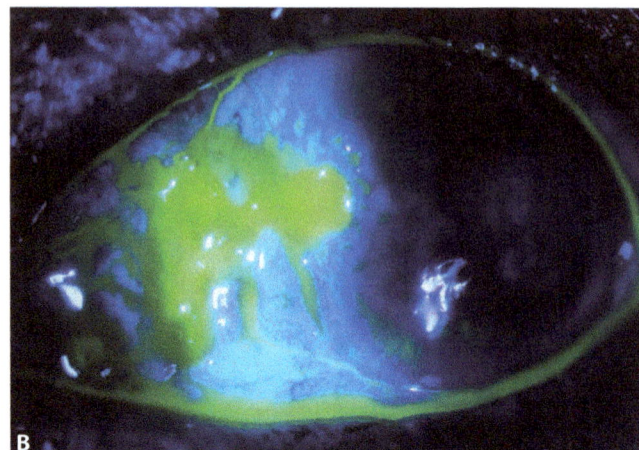

Figures 22.1A and B Clinical photograph (A) and fluorescein staining (B) of post-operative bacterial keratitis 4 days after pterygium surgery. Note the presence of 8-0 vicryl sutures used for conjunctival closure which may be a potential source of infection in this patient

thiotepa and mitomycin cause inhibition of mitosis of capillary endothelial cells, both leading to ischemic damage. Another hypothesis for vascular damage is ischemia at the site due to lack of episcleral vessels especially seen in cases operated by the bare sclera technique. Excessive cauterization of the scleral bed also leads to an avascular scleral bed. However, sclera is an avascular tissue without any significant nutritional requirements, thus ischemia alone may not be responsible as a sole factor for causing scleral necrosis. This was proved by David et al. by demonstrating that when silicone was placed between the episcleral plexuses and choroid and sclera resulting in a portion of sclera being 'sandwiched' to deprive both sides of the blood supply to sclera, it did not induce any scleral change in the form of sequestroid or smudgy necrosis.[16]

Another hypothesis proposed is the enzymatic degradation of the sclera by collagenases at the site of pterygium excision. Faulty surgical techniques like extensive tissue destruction and prolonged operative time resulting in prolonged exposure of bare sclera can stimulate host collagenases and other proteolytic enzymes resulting in loss of epithelial integrity. This enzymatic degradation results in immediate massive wound ulceration following surgery.[18,19] These weakened barriers are predisposed to invasion by microorganisms leading to exaggerated lysis by microbe released proteases and hydrolytic enzymes released by host neutrophils. Microbes can either cause direct invasion by releasing lytic enzymes or induce microangiopathy of the vessels.[1,3]

In addition, a defective epithelial cover and use of cytotoxic therapies like Mitomycin-C and irradiation that inactivate the host immune defenses by killing the leukocytes and other inflammatory cells lead to increased risk of wound infection.[3]

It has been seen that infectious scleritis may occur as long as 20 years (average delay of 90 months) after the surgery at the site of pterygium excision.[1] It is uncommon for infection to occur in an operative site after a long and uneventful post-operative period. A trigger mechanism is required for ulceration to develop at the site after a long period of latency. Necrotizing scleritis has been known to get activated any time after the surgical procedure.[3] It has been hypothesized by Lin et al. that probably after the initiation of surgically induced necrotising scleritis, the microorganisms can invade and cause the late onset postsurgical infectious scleritis.[1]

CLINICAL PRESENTATION

Presence of mucopurulent discharge with corneal/scleral ulcers or abscess points towards an infectious etiology especially in cases with hypopyon in the setting of post-operative scleral necrosis.[3]

Typical scleral ulcers are 2–3 mm in width with 1–2 mm corneal edge from limbus with surrounding white avascular sclera and avascular conjunctiva.[10] Episcleral vessels partly cover the ulcer base. Superficial scleral ulcers involve less than one third of the sclera. Moderate ulceration involves till two thirds of sclera.

Severe ulcer involves depth more than two third of scleral thickness with dark base. The frequency and severity of symptoms do not differ greatly among the three groups. There is no correlation between area and depth of the ulcer.[10]

Multiple scleral abscesses may also be seen appearing as yellowish nodules covered by normal conjunctival epithelium scattered superiorly or inferiorly along an area of 3-4 mm around limbus. A black arc shaped band may be seen to spread from initial ulcer site to scattered abscesses suggesting scleral thinning. These findings suggest a direct intrascleral dissemination and not an immunological phenomenon. The abscesses can extend resulting in corneal abscesses, anterior uveitis or to the extraocular muscle mimicking orbital cellulitis or pseudotumor. Few reports of retinal detachment and choroidal detachment have been documented with intrascleral dissemination.[20]

Cases of corneal ulceration do occur after complicated pterygium surgeries. These ulcers may be sterile, indolent and have necrotic margins characterized by absence of inflammation or vascularization.[10] These sterile epithelial defects can persist upto one year and can develop secondary infection with symptoms of infective keratitis.

Endophthalmitis can develop as a rare complication after pterygium excision. *Pseudomonas aeruginosa* is the most frequent organism cultured in post pterygium endophthalmitis.[11] Most of the cases have associated deep scleral ulceration. They have large avascular sclera surrounding the ulcer site. Management is based on the lines of management of post-operative endophthalmitis.

Aspergillus panophthalmitis has been reported in literature following pterygium surgery.[12] The patient had received post-operative beta radiation and developed a scleral ulcer in the area of treatment. The difficulty in diagnosing superficial mycotic infections and treatment of radiation scleritis which worsens fungal infections makes the management of these infections highly difficult.

INVESTIGATIONS

All cases of post-pterygium infections should be subjected to scraping followed by microscopic examination using Gram's stain and KOH stain. A part of the scraping material should be sent for culture-sensitivity examination. Confocal microscopy may be performed to rule out fungal etiology.

MANAGEMENT

Infectious scleritis is difficult to treat because of poor penetration of antimicrobial agents into the tightly bound collagen fibers of the scleral layer which result in prolonged sequestration of organisms within the intrascleral lamellae. The avascularity of sclera further makes it difficult for the antibiotics to reach the microbes stationed deep within the sclera. Infectious scleral necrosis thus tends to have poorer outcomes than noninfectious counterparts. This warrants prolonged and aggressive institution of topical fortified antibiotics especially in patients where intrascleral dissemination of infection is suspected. Early surgical debridement of the infected foci should be carried out to allow externalization of the wound enhancing the penetration of antibiotics. All devitalized, necrotic, and infective soft tissues and sclera should be excised with preservation of healthy adjacent conjunctiva. The dissection should be carried out until a clean scleral/choroidal bed is obtained free of infection.

Early restoration of epithelial integrity by conjunctival or amniotic membrane grafts (AMG) may be done to prevent further worsening of the condition. Early grafting also reduces the risk of superadded infections.[13,21] AMG should be avoided where infection has already occurred in the area of scleral melt. AMG promotes conjunctival re-epithelialization and reduces scleral melting and inflammation. It should be considered as an alternative biomaterial to improve wound healing in scleral and corneoscleral ulcerations with persistent stromal melting despite recurrent debridement and adequate antibiotic therapy.[22] However, AMG may not be able to provide adequate tectonic support in cases of deep scleral ulceration since it is just a thin membrane lacking rigidity. Such cases require scleral or corneal grafting for providing anatomical support.

In cases of non-resolution of infection, impending perforation and frank perforations, surgical management of the infection becomes necessary. Further in cases of severe scleral melting, restoration of integrity of the globe is required to prevent endophthalmitis. The basic principle in restoring tectonic integrity is to place a scleral patch, either lamellar or full thickness, depending upon the presence or absence of perforation **(Figs 22.2A to C)**. If infection is already present, surgical debridement of the area is required before scleral grafting to prevent graft infection.

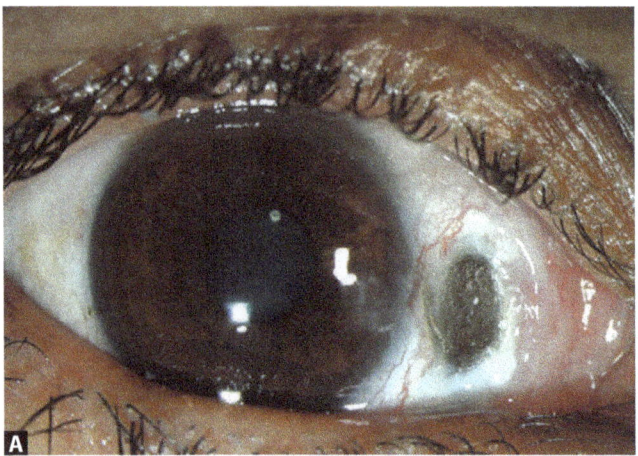
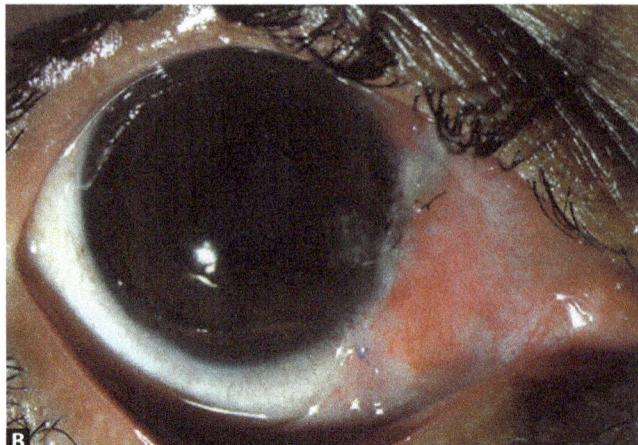
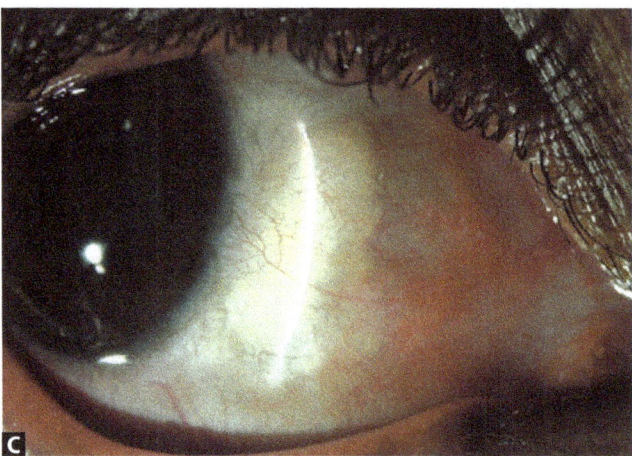

Figures 22.2A to C (A) Sterile severe scleral melt 3 months after pterygium excision with conjunctival autograft; (B) Post-operative Day 1 of operated full thickness scleral patch graft with conjunctival advancement to cover the scleral defect; (C) At 1 month postoperatively, the scleral patch graft is well apposed with a healthy overlying conjunctiva

A failure of adequate surgical debridement along with antibiotic therapy may lead to graft sloughing and necrosis.[13] Involvement of the adjacent cornea warrants a corneoscleral patch graft. Patch grafts have also been recommended early in the course of treatment if there are no signs of improvement within the first few days of initiating antibiotic therapy.

Apart from sclera, other materials such as pericardium[23] and dura[24] have been used to cover the scleral defect. However, the major drawback of these tissues is the high cost and limited surgical experience. Also, large scleral rim may not be readily available for scleral grafting in view of more number of in-situ cadaveric corneoscleral rim excisions being carried out instead of whole globe excision. Hence, the use of corneal tissue has been advocated to cover the scleral defects to provide tectonic support.[2] Some of the advantages of using cornea over sclera are that corneal tissue is thicker with a higher rigidity than scleral tissue thus providing better tectonic support thereby reducing the risk of graft melting or future ectasia. Further, in cases of infection, the more tightly packed lamellae of corneal tissue offer a higher resistance to infection in comparison to sclera.

Surgical procedures are much easier to perform with better post-operative outcomes in cases of sterile melts as compared to infectious melts. In the absence of infection, the surgery is considerably less complex without extensive areas of purulent scleral necrosis, inflammation or hemorrhage, which are invariably present with infective scleritis. Further, infected cases require an intensive perioperative antibiotic therapy with oral or intravenous antibiotics, copious antibiotic irrigation of the scleral bed and adjacent soft tissues before placement of the graft and subconjunctival injections of broad-spectrum antibiotics or antifungal agents at the end of surgery.

Poor visual acuity outcomes (≤20/200) are seen in more than one third cases of postsurgical scleral necrosis. Out of all the cases, 10% are usually not salvageable and the eye is lost to evisceration.[3] Due to prolonged and severe inflammation, there is high risk of development of cataract, glaucoma, retinal detachment, choroidal detachment and endophthalmitis.[3,4]

PROPHYLAXIS [4,5,20,23]

All preventive measures should be taken to avoid post-operative scleral melt and infections. Intra-operatively, all sterile precautions should be maintained by the surgeon with respect to scrubbing, gowning, gloving, cleaning and draping the patient to avoid contamination of the surgical field. As far as the surgical technique is concerned, conjunctival closure with autograft should be the procedure of choice after pterygium excision. Bare sclera should be avoided. Antimetabolites such as mitomycin-C and β-irradiation should be used judiciously to avoid scleral melts. Excessive cauterization of scleral vessels should not be performed during the surgery.

Post-operatively, the patients should be followed up regularly to monitor the healing of donor site from where the graft has been harvested and the recipient site where the pterygium excision has been performed. The area was the graft is placed and re-epithelialization of the surrounding areas should be examined on slit lamp microscopy. Detailed anterior segment and posterior segment evaluation along with monitoring of visual acuity and intraocular pressure should be done. Corticosteroids should be used cautiously and should be tapered on a weekly basis. Prophylactic patch graft for scleral thinning, bare sclera or sterile scleral necrosis can be done to prevent secondary infections.[20]

REFERENCES

1. Lin C, Shih M, Tsai M. Clinical experiences of infectious scleral ulceration: a complication of pterygium operation. Br J Ophthalmol. 1997;81(11):980-3.
2. Ti SE, Tan DT. Tectonic corneal lamellar grafting for severe scleral melting after pterygium surgery. Ophthalmology. 2003;110(6):1126-36.
3. Doshi RR, Harocopos GJ, Schwab IR, Cunningham ET Jr. The spectrum of postoperative scleral necrosis. Surv Ophthalmol. 2013;58(6):620-33.
4. Jain V, Garg P, Sharma S. Microbial scleritis-experience from a developing country. Eye (Lond). 2009;23(2):255-61.
5. Roy SR, Roswell RP, Raymond MS, Stephen F, Neil FM, Samnel S, et al. Serious complications of topical mitomycin-C after pterygium surgery. Ophthalmology. 1992;99:1647-54.
6. Fukamachi Y, Hikita N. Ocular complication following pterygium operation and instillation of mitomycin C. Folia Ophthalmol Jpn. 1981;32:197-201.
7. Yamanouchi U, Takaku I, Tsuda N, Kajiwara Y, Mine M, Ueno Y, et al. Scleromalacia presumably due to mitomycin C instillation after pterygium excision. Jpn J Clin Ophthalmol. 1979;33:139-44.
8. Singh G. Postoperative instillation of low-dose mitomycin C in the treatment of primary pterygium. Am J Ophthalmol. 1989;107:570-1.
9. Farrell PLR, Smith RE. Bacterial corneoscleritis complicating pterygium excision. Am J Ophthalmol. 1989;107:515-7.
10. Tarr KH, Constable IJ. Late complications of pterygium treatment. Br J Ophthalmol. 1980;64:496-505.
11. Tarr KH, Constable IJ. Pseudomonas endophthalmitis associated with scleral necrosis. Br J Ophthalmol. 1980;64(9):676-9.
12. Margo CE, Polack FM, Hood CI. Aspergillus panophthalmitis complicating treatment of pterygium. Cornea. 1988;7(4):285-9.
13. Reynolds MG, Alfonso E. Treatment of infectious scleritis and keratoscleritis. Am J Ophthalmol. 1991;112(5):543-7.
14. Mackenzie FD, Hirst LW, Kynaston B, Bain C. Recurrence rate and complications after beta irradiation for pterygia. Ophthalmology. 1991;98:1776-81.
15. Altman AJ, Cohen EJ, Berger ST, Mondino BJ. Scleritis and Streptococcus pneumoniae. Cornea. 1991;10:341-5.
16. David S. Necrogranulomatous scleritis—effects on the sclera of vascular deprivation. Br J Ophthalmol. 1968;52:453-60.
17. David LO, James EP, John GM, Mark LM. Scleral flap necrosis and infectious endophthalmitis after cataract surgery with a scleral tunnel incision. Ophthalmology. 1993;100:159-63.
18. Gordon JM, Bauer EA, Eisen AZ. Collagenase in human cornea. Immunologic localization. Arch Ophthalmol. 1980;98:341-5.
19. Kreger AS, Gray LD. Purification of Pseudomonas aeruginosa protease and microscopic characterization of pseudomonal protease-induced rabbit corneal damage. Infect Immun. 1978;19:630-48.

20. Hsiao, Chen J, Huang S, Ma H, Chen P, Tsai R. Intrascleral dissemination of infectious scleritis following pterygium excision. Br J Ophthalmol. 1998;82(1):29-34.
21. Huang FC, Huang SP, Tseng SH. Management of infectious scleritis after pterygium excision. Cornea. 2000;19(1):34-9.
22. Ma DH, Wang SF, Su WY, Tsai RJ. Amniotic membrane graft for the management of scleral melting and corneal perforation in recalcitrant infectious scleral and corneoscleral ulcers. Cornea. 2002;21(3):275-83.
23. Schein OD. The use of processed pericardial tissue in anterior ocular segment reconstruction. Am J Ophthalmol. 1998;125:549-52.
24. Brandt JD. Patch grafts of dehydrated cadaveric dura mater for tube-shunt glaucoma surgery. Arch Ophthalmol. 1993;111:1436-9.

CHAPTER 23

Infections after Ocular Surface Reconstruction Surgery

Amreen Aslam, Renu Venugopal, Neelima Aron, Prafulla K Maharana, Namrata Sharma

INTRODUCTION

Amniotic membrane transplantation (AMT) has been successfully used as an epithelial surrogate for ocular surface reconstruction, after excision of large ocular surface neoplasms, in severe or refractory neurotrophic ulcers and acute chemical burns as a better alternative to previously used conjunctival flaps and tarsorrhaphy. AMT functions by various ways starting from the epithelium which produces various growth factors, the basement membrane which facilitates migration of epithelial cells, reinforces adhesion of basal epithelial cells, and may promote epithelial differentiation and stroma, which downregulates major inflammatory complexes that are found in many ocular surface conditions leading to scarring. It further prevents scar tissue formation by trapping polymorphonuclear cells thereby preventing them from infiltrating the corneal stroma suppressing the transforming growth factor β (TGF β) signaling system and myofibroblast differentiation of normal fibroblasts.[1]

Stem cells in the palisades of Vogt participate in regeneration and preservation of corneal transparency and avascularity. Limbal stem cell deficiency is associated with conjunctivalization of the cornea and can be complicated with persistent epithelial defects, vascularization, scarring, ulceration, melting, and perforation of the cornea. Patients with these abnormalities are poor candidates for conventional corneal transplantation. Lamellar or penetrating keratoplasty provides only a temporary replacement of the host's corneal epithelium and does not permanently restore limbal function. In cases with diffuse corneal stem cell deficiency, limbal transplantation, autologous in case of unilateral, and allogeneic in case of bilateral cases, is now considered essential for corneal surface reconstruction.[2] Cultivated limbal epithelial transplantation (CLET) has been successfully used in patients with diffuse limbal stem cell deficiency and severe ocular surface disease, including Stevens–Johnson syndrome, advanced ocular cicatricial pemphigoid, chemical and thermal burns. It involves culture of a small portion of limbal stem cells on an amniotic membrane ex-vivo in the first stage followed by the transplantation of the sheet with proliferated stem cells onto the diseased eye in the second stage. Simple limbal epithelial transplantation (SLET) combines these two stages by transferring the amniotic membrane with multiple cut limbal stem cell tissue onto the fellow eye in a single stage.[2] Another emerging option for this subset of patients is the use of noncorneal cells such as cultivated mucosal grafts (oral/buccal/vaginal/nasal).

Cornea being more vulnerable to infections from otherwise nonpathogenic organisms must first be rendered free of bacterial colonization before transplanting any graft. This requires an effective decontamination process.

INCIDENCE

The incidence of post-AMT microbial infections is as low as 1.6%.[3] The incidence, however, rises with the use of non-preserved AMT.[4] Gram-positive organisms are the most frequent isolates.

The most consistently reported adverse events following tissue cultured limbal stem cell allograft transplantation is bacterial infection. The incidence of this complication ranged from 7% (1/13) eyes,[5] through 10% (1/10) eyes,[6] to 15% (2/13) eyes.[7]

RISK FACTORS

Factors influencing postocular-surface-reconstruction infection include host factors and donor factors.

Host Factors

Local Factors

- *Ocular surface problems:* The risk of microbial infection is higher in patients with poor ocular surface.[8] Poor ocular surface disturbs the tear film thereby decreasing the antimicrobial action of tear fluid. The tear film provides antimicrobial action by specific substances namely lysozyme, lactoferrin, immunoglobulins and betalysin. Meibomian gland dysfunction affects the lipid layer of the tear film leading to instability and rapid evaporation of tears. Absence of goblet cells in cases of severe chemical burns or Stevens–Johnson syndrome leads to decreased corneal wettability and tear film instability.
- *Lid abnormalities:* Foreign bodies and micro-organisms get flushed from the ocular surface by the blink action of the eyelids. Presence of lid pathologies like lagophthalmos and ectropion cause corneal exposure and predispose to infection. Entropion and trichiasis cause breach in the epithelium leading to persistent epithelial defects.

Socioeconomic Status

Lower socioeconomic status, poor living conditions and inadequate hygiene are also reported to predispose to infection.

Systemic Factors

Systemic factors include the immune status of the person, presence of coexisting diabetes, any condition that requires prolonged immunosuppression like malignancies and autoimmune conditions.

Donor-related Factors

Donor factors include contaminated tissue, contaminated storage medium, use of nonpreserved tissue[4] and prolonged duration of storage. Amniotic membrane graft (AMG) procured without proper screening of the donor for conditions like syphilis, septicemia, HIV and hepatitis, can lead to transmission of infection to the host.

Intra-operative Factors

Intra-operative factors, including poor sterilization of instruments, faulty OT sterilization techniques and improper handling of tissues can lead to infection.

Post-operative Factors

- *Suture-related problems:* Post-operatively, suture-related problems like loose suture can attract mucin and act as a nidus for microbial adhesion and proliferation.
- *Persistent epithelial defect:* Persistent epithelial defect increases the chance of microbial invasion. It is caused due to conditions that delay wound healing like diabetes mellitus, lid abnormalities like trichiasis, entropion or usage of toxic preservative containing topical medications.
- *Symblepharon ring- and contact lens-related problem:* Symblepharon ring acts as a nidus for invasion of micro-organisms predisposing the eye to infection. Bandage contact lens used to promote wound healing can cause local tissue hypoxia, decreased local immunity and promote microbial adhesion.
- *Medications:* Indiscriminate use of topical steroids and topical antibiotics has been associated with increased incidence of post-operative infections, especially fungal. They also reactivate any latent viral infection in the host.

CLINICAL FEATURES

Symptoms

The patient presents with pain, photophobia, discharge and excessive stickiness of eyelids.

Clinical Signs

Conjunctival signs include congestion, chemosis, dilated vasculature, discharge and ulceration. Presence of epithelial defect with infiltrates and anterior chamber reaction is suggestive of keratitis. Rapid corneal melts occur in the presence of already compromised surface **(Figs 23.1 and 23.2)**. Sterile hypopyon secondary to inflammation may be present. Adnexal tissue may show signs of inflammation like lid edema, lymphadenopathy, dacryoadenitis and scleritis.

Infections after Ocular Surface Reconstruction Surgery

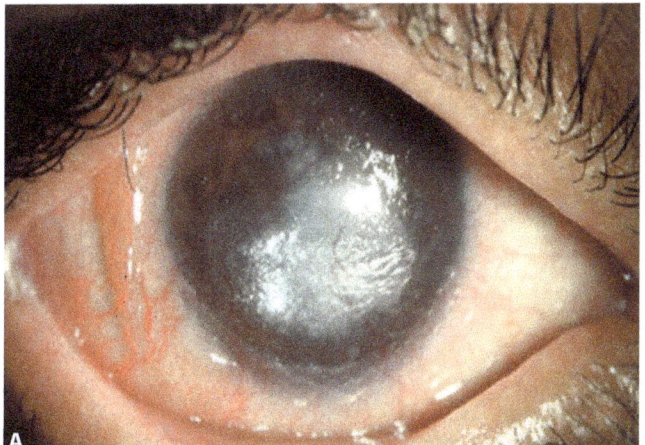
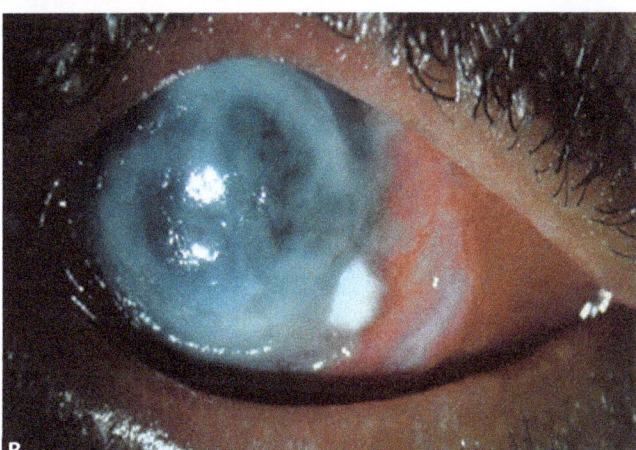
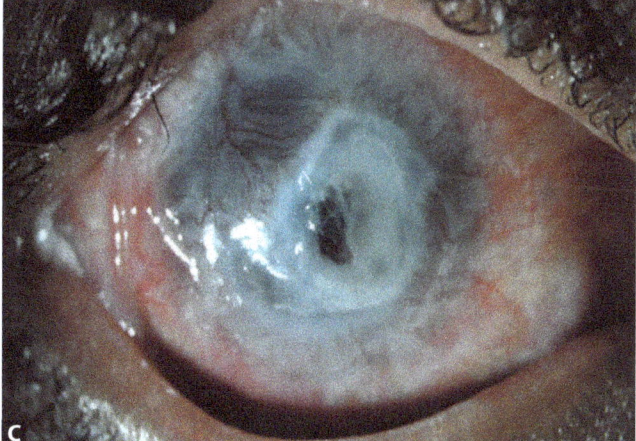

Figures 23.1A to C Post-cultivated oral mucosal transplantation (COMET) infection: (A) Pre-operative clinical photograph of the left eye with 360° limbal stem cell deficiency; (B) Post-COMET at one week, corneal ulcer with infiltrates developed at the inferotemporal limbus; (C) A rapid corneal melt developed despite starting topical antibiotic therapy

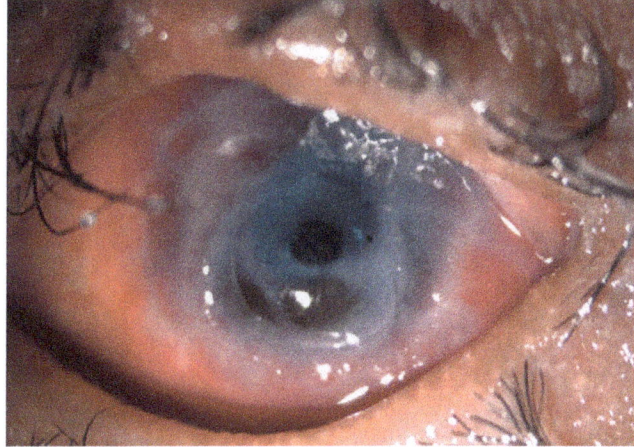

Figure 23.2 Post-simple limbal epithelial transplantation (SLET) infection: A rapid corneal melt with lens extrusion occurred at 1 month post-surgery

INVESTIGATIONS

Conjunctival Swab

Conjunctival swab must be obtained and sent for both bacterial and fungal culture.

Corneal Scraping

In case of corneal ulcer, corneal scraping using a number 15 blade or Kimura's spatula is done and smear is prepared. The material obtained is examined under the microscope by using Gram's stain, Giemsa stain and potassium hydroxide and inoculated on various culture medium that will facilitate growth of fungi, bacteria and protozoa. In case of negative cultures and progressive suppuration, punch/suture biopsy is done to increase the yield of the organism.

Confocal Microscopy

Tandem scanning confocal microscope is a new modality for quickly and accurately identifying the organism thereby facilitating prompt and appropriate treatment.

Ultrasonography B Scan

For the assessment of posterior segment in the presence of corneal ulcer, ultrasonography B scan should be done. Details like retinal detachment, choroidal detachment and presence of vitreous exudation help in prognosticating the condition and optimizing the management option.

Systemic Investigations

Systemic investigations to assess the immune status of the individual such as complete blood count and fasting blood sugar are done. Liver and renal function tests before instituting systemic antibiotics are mandatory.

PROPHYLAXIS

There is, therefore, a need for microbiological quality control of tissue procurement and preservation as well as prevention of transmission of infection from the donor.

Procurement and Storage of AMG

For long-term tissue preservation, the method used must reliably disinfect the stored biological tissue. Antibiotic disinfection is currently the method of choice to preserve the tissue matrix. Amniotic membrane should be prepared according to Good Tissue Banking Practice set forth by the FDA.[3] A detailed medical history and clinical condition of the potential donor should exclude the risk of tissue-transmissible infections and unsuitability of the donors. The clinician responsible for collecting the tissue must ensure that the donor has been asked about any activities or other risk factors, which may suggest that the donor is unsuitable. Donors are screened for human immunodeficiency virus (HIV) type 1 and 2, Hepatitis B virus (HBV), hepatitis C virus (HCV) and *Treponema pallidum* infections. Competent laboratories should perform these tests, and the records should be maintained for 11 years post-transplantation.[9] Upon confirmation of the HIV-negative status of the donor by repeat serology done 3–4 months after the collection of AM,[10] the membranes are released. The AM is best procured from elective cesarean delivery to avoid labor, rupture of membranes and internal monitoring. The AM should be obtained under sterile conditions. Tissue must be handled, processed, and transported at all times in a way that minimizes contamination from exogenous sources as far as practically possible. The obstetrician must place the placenta in a sterile stainless steel 12-inch diameter basin, preferably covered with a sterile lid. During placement, the clamp from the cord should not be removed to avoid the AM getting covered with blood. In the clean atmosphere of the operating room or the clean laminar flow workbench, the AM is dissected from the placenta in two large bits. As much of the chorion as possible should be peeled out before the bits are dropped into a sterile, wide mouthed 125 mL screw-capped reagent bottle containing 50 mL transport medium. The transport medium generally used is the commercially available Eagles' minimum essential medium (EMEM) supplemented with 3.3% L-glutamine and antibiotics (50 µg/mL gentamicin, 100 units/mL penicillin, 200 µg/mL ciprofloxacin and 1 mg/mL amphotericin B). The media and the antibiotic preparations should be of recognized quality manufactured as per the ISO 9002 standards and certified by a competent certifying authority. The membrane must be transported immediately to the laboratory. In the laboratory, under the laminar flow hood, the AM is washed free of blood clots with EMEM containing antibiotics. Any leftover chorion attached to the AM and blood clots are gently peeled off the epithelial cell layer using round-ended forceps. With the epithelial/basement layer surface up, the AM is spread uniformly without folds or tears on individually sterilized 0.22 µm nitrocellulose membranes of the required size (47 mm or 25 mm).[11] A random bottle from the batch is left at the work bench at room temperature for about an hour and about 5 mL of the same is inoculated into 100 mL of brain heart infusion medium and 100 mL of thioglycollate broth medium to check the bacterial and fungal sterility. These media are incubated for 21 days and if no growth of bacteria or fungus is observed, the batch should be considered as preserved free of cultivable microbial agents. The prepared membrane should be handled properly avoiding microbial contamination during transportation to the operating room in ice. The color of the storage medium after thawing should be light pink. A change towards yellow should be taken as suggestive of microbial contamination; any such membrane is discarded. The AM can be preserved in glycerol, by irradiation, cryopreservation or lyophilization techniques. Cryopreservation at –80°C is done with either glycerol or dimethyl sulfoxide (DMSO).[12]

After AMT, the patient is started on preservative free prednisolone acetate 1% eye drops four times a day and preservative-free chloramphenicol 0.5%, both tapered off in 1 month. A close follow-up is needed till the epithelium heals.

Improvement of the Ocular Surface

All attempts should be made to improve the ocular environment with tear substitutes, punctal occlusion or lid surgery if required. Adequate eyelid closure should be ensured. Preexisting Meibomian gland disease should be treated before any procedure.

Role of the Operating Team

Optimal precautions must be taken by the operating team to prevent intra-operative transfer of infection. Good handwashing practices should be followed. One should use sterile instruments and maintain sterility throughout the procedure. Daily cleaning and standard fumigation technique must be carried out after the operating session gets over.

Pre-operative preparation of the patient is a must. Pre-operative usage of povidone iodine plays the most important role.

TREATMENT

Medical Management

Topical Medications

In all cases of suppurative infections, topical steroid therapy is stopped immediately and intensive broad spectrum combination therapy with fortified cefazolin sodium 50 mg/mL and fortified tobramycin 14 mg/mL is instituted every 1 hour round the clock for the first 48 hours and then gradually tapered off depending upon the response. Antifungal medication, topical natamycin 5% one hourly is added only if there is microbiological evidence of fungus. In worsening fungal keratitis, topical amphotericin B 0.15% or topical voriconazole 1% is added.

Supportive Therapy

Supportive therapy with topical cycloplegics to relieve pain by decreasing the ciliary spasm and antiglaucoma medications to combat the rise in intraocular pressure secondary to inflammation should be initiated.

Systemic Therapy

Systemic antibiotics are started in case of impending/frank perforation, scleral involvement, large-sized ulcer (>5 mm) involving >50% depth of stroma and endophthalmitis. Systemic antifungals is given in cases with large ulcers, deep keratitis, scleral involvement and endophthalmitis. Most common drug used is ketoconazole 200–400 mg per day given for 4–6 weeks. Liver function test is to be monitored constantly. Other drugs used are itraconazole (200 mg/day), fluconazole (200 mg/day) and voriconazole (200 mg BD).

Monitoring

The patient should be examined daily to monitor the clinical details and medication is altered depending upon the clinical response and culture reports if needed. The ulcer size, extent of infiltrates, anterior chamber reaction, epithelialization and vascularization is looked for. In case of negative culture reports and progressive infection, topical medications are stopped for 48 hours and a repeat scraping is done. Alternate techniques to improve the yield of organisms like enhanced medium culture, suture biopsy or punch biopsy are considered.

Surgical Management

Surgical Debridement

Debridement works by debulking the tissue thereby decreasing the organism load and enhancing the response to topical medications. By removing the dead necrotic tissue, it enhances the penetration of topical medications. This is effective, especially in case of fungal keratitis. It is performed under topical anesthesia on slit lamp with blade or spatula. It can be repeated every 48 hours.

Tissue Adhesives and Corneal Transplantation

In cases of small perforations or descemetocele <3 mm size, tissue adhesives like cyanoacrylate glue with bandage contact lens is applied. Apart from securing the perforation, cyanoacrylate glue has antibacterial properties. It is bacteriostatic against most of the Gram-positive organisms. Patch graft is done for perforation up to 5 mm in size. For perforations larger in size, a therapeutic keratoplasty is performed. Non-resolving keratitis is also managed by keratoplasty after all the options of medical therapy have been exhausted.

COEXISTING ENDOPHTHALMITIS

In case of coexisting endophthalmitis, a diagnostic vitreous tap is done and intravitreal injection containing 1 mg of 0.1 mL vancomycin and 2.25 mg in 0.1 mL of ceftazidime is given for bacterial endophthalmitis. The response is monitored in 24–48 hours. In case of no response, a repeat injection may be given. If fungal organisms are suspected, then 10 μg/0.1 mL amphotericin B or 50 μg/0.1 mL voriconazole is given. Topical therapy with fortified antibiotics and cycloplegics is continued. Due to the poor visualization of posterior segment structures, vitrectomy is the last option which can be done with the help of a temporary keratoprosthesis.

Thus, infections post-ocular surface surgeries, though uncommon, are usually severe with poor anatomical and visual outcomes due to the presence of an already compromised ocular surface. This prevents wound healing and a prolonged course of infection. Prophylaxis, thus, plays the most important role in preventing the occurrence of these infections in the first place.

REFERENCES

1. Faulk WP, Matthews RN, Stevens PJ, et al. Human amnion as an adjunct in wound healing. Lancet. 1980;i:1156.
2. Shimazaki J, Yang H-Y, Tsubota K. Amniotic membrane transplantation for ocular surface reconstruction in patients with chemical and thermal burns. Ophthalmology. 1997;104:2068-76.
3. Marangon FB, Alfonso EC, Miller D, Remonda NM, Marcus S, Tseng SC. Incidence of microbial infection after amniotic membrane transplantation. Cornea. 2004;23:264-9.
4. Khokhar S, Sharma N, Kumar H, Soni A. Infection after use of nonpreserved human amniotic membrane for the reconstruction of the ocular surface. Cornea. 2001;20:773-4.
5. Koizumi N, Inatomi T, Suzuki T, et al. Cultivated corneal epithelial stem cell transplantation in ocular surface disorders. Ophthalmology. 2001;108:1569-74.
6. Daya SM, Watson A, Sharpe JR, et al. Outcomes and DNA analysis of ex vivo expanded stem cell allograft for ocular surface reconstruction. Ophthalmology. 2005;112:470-7.
7. Shimazaki J, Aiba M, Goto E, et al. Transplantation of human limbal epithelium cultivated on amniotic membrane for the treatment of severe ocular surface disorders. Ophthalmology. 2002;109:1285-90.
8. Sujata Das, Balasubramanya Ramamurthy, Virender S Sangwan. Fungal keratitis following amniotic membrane transplantion. International ophthalmology. 2009;29:49-51.
9. Dua HS, Blanco AA. Amniotic membrane transplantation. Br J Ophthalmol. 1999;83:748-52.
10. Committee Microbiological Safety of Blood and Tissues for Transplantation. Guidance on the microbiological safety of human tissues and organs used in transplantation. London: Department of Health.
11. Tseng SCG, Prabhasawat P, Lee SH. Amniotic membrane transplantation for conjunctival surface reconstruction. Am J Ophthalmol. 1997;124:765-74.
12. Tsubota K, Toda I, Saito H, et al. Reconstruction of the corneal epithelium by limbal allograft transplantation for severe ocular surface disorders. Ophthalmology. 1995;102:1486-96.

CHAPTER 24

Infections after Oculoplasty Surgery

Amar Pujari, Rachna Meel, Neelam Pushker

INTRODUCTION

Oculoplasty surgeries unlike intraocular surgeries often involve entering/encroaching on areas of the body which may harbor pathogenic microorganisms, such as lacrimal sac, the paranasal sinuses or nose. This may increase the risk of post-operative wound infections after oculoplasty surgeries as compared to other intraocular or ocular surface surgeries. Post-operative wound infection not only causes patient morbidity but also hampers the effective outcome of the surgical procedure.

However, the risk of infections following eyelid and lacrimal drainage system surgeries may be avoided by performing a meticulous pre-operative assessment, following proper intra-operative aseptic measures and maintaining post-operative hygiene. The need for universal antibiotic coverage of oculoplastic surgery in the post-operative period is controversial.

PRE-OPERATIVE ASSESSMENT

A meticulous local and systemic pre-operative assessment is crucial in avoiding or minimizing post-surgery infection. The operating surgeon must look carefully for any potential sources of infection in/around the area of surgery. For example, the sinuses and the nose should be evaluated using X-ray of paranasal sinuses and an evaluation by otorhinologist must be done to rule out any infection in the sinuses or the nose when a lacrimal surgery such as dacryocystorhinostomy (DCR) surgery is being planned. The regurgitant from the lacrimal sac in cases of nasolacrimal duct blockade should be sent for microbiology examination. Similarly, in cases of elective eyelid surgeries, operating surgeon must rule out sources of infection like an external or internal hordeolum or an infective blepharitis, etc. Elective procedures should be withheld till acute infection is taken care of, for example, if there is acute dacryocystitis, it should be treated first with oral antibiotics followed by DCR (elective surgery) once the infection is cured.[1,2]

Also systemic examination and evaluation to rule out any disease condition that may compromise the immune system, such as metabolic diseases (diabetes), valvular diseases, patients on immunosuppressants, etc. should be documented and these should be marked as high risk cases for post-operative wound infection. Oculoplastic surgeries for post-traumatic repairs are also at high risk for post-operative wound infection. A swab for bacterial culture should be sent, especially if the wound is dirty with signs of infection. Copious saline irrigation should be done before proceeding for surgery.

INTRA-OPERATIVE PRECAUTIONS

Universal intra-operative aseptic precautions have to be observed for all oculoplasty surgeries. A sterile field is established and maintained for all surgical procedures to avoid wound contamination and minimize risk of post-operative infection. Appropriate measures should be taken to avoid accumulation of blood or fluid in dead spaces created by surgical removal of large masses, such as after orbitotomy as they may be potential site for growth of pathogens.

POST-OPERATIVE CARE AND ANTIBIOTIC PROPHYLAXIS

Oculoplasty surgeries routinely have skin sutures that need to be cleaned with antiseptics like betadine. In case of placement of drain, monitoring to look for any signs of infection and removal of drain at the earliest is critical to avoid infections. Skin sutures must be removed on time (within 5–7 days) not only to reduce scarring, but also to minimize risk of post-operative suture-related wound infection. There are no universal guidelines regarding the use of prophylactic antibiotics. Different surgeons follow different protocols.

MICROBIOLOGY PROFILE

Several studies in literature have tried to evaluate the pathogens commonly isolated from the field of surgery in an effort to guide the antibiotic prophylaxis for post-operative wound infection. According to a study, authors found culture positivity in 8.3% cases of nasolacrimal duct obstruction. The gram-positive organisms cultured from intrasaccular samples during DCR surgery were *Staphylococcus aureus, Streptococcus pneumoniae* and *Staphylococcus saprophyticus* and gram-negative organisms were *Haemophilus influenzae, Serratia marcescens* and *Pseudomonas aeruginosa*. The rate of positive culture was higher in patients with mucocele, mucopyocele and recurrent dacryocystitis. The post-operative infection of surgical wound was found in 8.7% cases.[1] In another study on use of prophylactic antibiotics in plastic and reconstructive surgery, the rates of post-operative infection ranged between 1.3% and 7.3%. The common organisms isolated were *Staphylococcus aureus, Pseudomonas aeruginosa, Staphylococcus epidermidis, Streptococcus pneumoniae,* and α-hemolytic *Streptococcus*.[3] **Table 24.1** summarizes the most common pathogens isolated in various studies in patients with nasolacrimal duct obstruction.

ANTIBIOTICS FOR PROPHYLAXIS

Prophylactic antibiotics have been in use for more than 50 years to prevent surgical site infections, but still no general agreement exists regarding the use of pre- or post-operative antibiotic prophylaxis. Considerable debate exists for the use of prophylactic oral antibiotics before surgery, but topical antibiotics are routinely used pre-operatively in almost all cases. In a study on antibiotic prophylaxis in external DCR, authors reported no difference in the rates of infection between those patients receiving and not receiving antibiotics. However, they found higher rates of infection in patients with preexisting acute dacryocystitis, mucocele, and mucopyocele.[1] In another study on antibiotic use in plastic and reconstructive surgery, the nature of surgery was grouped under 4 categories, viz., trauma cases, cosmetic lid surgery, flap/ graft procedures and use of alloplastic implants. No significant association of infection rates was found with the nature of the surgery which ranged between 1.3% and 7.3%.[3] A multinational survey study conducted by Fay et al. concluded the following points regarding the use of prophylactic antibiotics for eyelid surgery.[7]

- Among the topical, oral or intravenous routes, topical route was the most commonly preferred way to prevent infections in all regions with rates of 85.2% immediately after surgery and 87.9% as post-operative care.
- There is a wide variation in post-operative oral antibiotic prescription rates by region ranging from 86.7% in India to 2.9% in the United Kingdom. Some government agencies in the US and Europe are strongly against prescribing systemic antibiotics in the absence of definite indication.
- For uncomplicated eyelid surgical procedures, post-operative oral antibiotics were prescribed more commonly followed by intravenously.
- About 34.6% of respondents reported an estimated wound infection in routine, elective eyelid surgeries

Table 24.1 Commonly isolated gram-positive and negative organisms from different studies in patients with dacryocystitis[1,4-6]				
Authors/ year	Number of cases	Sample site	Gram positive	Gram negative
Pinar-Sueiro et al, 2010[1]	697	Intrasaccular samples during DCR	S. aureus	H. influenzae
Delia et al, 2008[4]	421	Intrasaccular samples during DCR	S. epidermidis	P. aeruginosa
Bharathi et al, 2008[5]	1891	Regurgitant	S. aureus	P. aeruginosa
Mills et al, 2007[6]	89	Regurgitant/Intrasaccular samples	S. aureus	P. aeruginosa

Table 24.2 Common antibiotics which are sensitive and resistant to gram-positive as well as gram-negative organisms in dacryocystitis[1]

	Gram-positive organism	Gram-negative organism
Sensitive	100% sensitivity was found with fusidic acid, cefazolin, cefuroxime axetil, chloramphenicol, levofloxacin, tobramycin and vancomycin	100% sensitivity was found with ciprofloxacin, ceftriaxone, cloxacillin, gentamycin, norfloxacin, piperacillin-tazobactam
Resistant	Cefazolin, ciprofloxacin, penicillin, ampicillin,	Cefazolin, clindamycin, nitrofurantoin, cefazolin

without the use of oral/intravenous antibiotics as 1%, which is quite low.

The authors concluded that there are no universal guidelines for antibiotic use. The choice is based on individual surgeon's training and apprehension of risk of post-operative infection versus antibiotic-related complications which are usually under estimated by most surgeons. Most large-scale studies discourage use of any antibiotic prophylaxis beyond 24 hours post-operatively.[8]

DIAGNOSIS AND MANAGEMENT

Post-operative signs of infection include erythema around the sutures, purulent discharge from the incision/wound or fistula formation. Treatment involves treatment with antibiotics based on culture sensitivity of the discharge or pus from the infected area with or without surgical drainage. In a study on external DCR, authors also studied the sensitivity of antibiotics which is mentioned in **Table 24.2**. They also concluded that the most commonly used antibiotics (cefazolin and amoxicillin-clavulanate) showed poor overall sensitivity for the bacteria.[1] In another study, the antibiotics selected for prophylaxis were cephalexin or erythromycin which provided excellent cover against Gram-positive organisms but less potent against gram-negative organisms but authors justified the use as they found that the samples from the sac mostly grew gram-positive organisms (65%).[2]

To conclude, use of topical antibiotics as antibiotic prophylaxis is widely accepted but judicious use of oral/intravenous antibiotics in clean cases is important to prevent antibiotic resistance, Stevens Johnson syndrome and other dreaded complications, in addition to cost burden.

In scenarios such as systemic immune compromised patients, patients with valvular diseases, kidney or metabolic diseases, trauma cases, operations on surgical sites that are likely to be contaminated such as DCR and previous history of infection at the surgical site, perioperative antibiotic prophylaxis may be used. Use of prophylactic antibiotics also depends on the surgeon's preference and experience and the likely compliance of post-operative wound care and maintenance of hygiene by the patient.

REFERENCES

1. Pinar-Sueiro S, Fernandez-Hermida RV, Gibelalde A, Martinez-Indart L. Study on the Effectiveness of Antibiotic Prophylaxis in External Dacryocystorhinostomy: A Review of 697 Cases. Ophthal Plast Reconstr Surg. 2010;26(6):467-72.
2. Walland MJ, Rose GE. Factors affecting the success rate of open lacrimal surgery. Br J Ophthalmol. 1994;78:888-91.
3. Baran CN, Sensöz O, Ulusoy MG. Prophylactic antibiotics in plastic and reconstructive surgery. Plast Reconstr Surg. 1999;103:1561-6.
4. Delia AC, Uuri GC, Battacharjee K, et al. Bacteriology of chronic dacryocystitis in adult population of Northeast India. Orbit. 2008;27:243-7.
5. Bharathi MJ, Ramakrishnan R, Maneksha V, et al. Comparative bacteriology of acute and chronic dacryocystitis. Eye (Lond). 2008;22:953-60.
6. Mills D, Bodman MG, Meyer DR, Morton AD III: ASOPRS Dacryocystitis Study Group. The microbiological spectrum of dacryocystitis: a national study of acute versus chronic infection. Ophthal Plast Reconstr Surg. 2007;23:302-6.
7. Fay A, Nallasamy N, Bernardini F, Wladis EJ, Durand ML, Devoto MH, Meyer D, Hartstein M, Honavar S, Osaki MH, Osaki TH, Santiago YM, Sanz M, Vadala G, Verity D. Multinational comparison of prophylactic antibiotic use for eyelid surgery. JAMA Ophthalmol. 2015;133(7):778-84.
8. Zhang Y, Dong J, Qiao Y, He J, Wang T, Ma S. Efficacy and safety profile of antibiotic prophylaxis usage in clean and clean-contaminated plastic and reconstructive surgery: a meta-analysis of randomized controlled trials. Ann Plast Surg. 2014;72:121-30.

Index

Page numbers followed by *f* refer to figure and *t* refer to table.

A

Acanthamoeba 106, 107, 115, 116, 118, 124
    infection 125
    keratitis 107
    trophozoites 106
Acquired immunodeficiency syndrome 41
Active air sampling, disadvantages of 81*t*
Acute post-cataract surgery endophthalmitis 91
Acute post-operative endophthalmitis 92, 92*f*
Adequate sterilization 75*f*
Adjunctive therapy 112
Aggressive medical therapy 125
Air
    conditioning 22
        ducts 53
    filtration 24
    flow system 22
        maintenance of 24
    handling unit 23*f*, 24, 24*f*
    sampling 80
        advantages of active 81*t*
    velocity 23
Airborne dispersion 47
American Operating Room Nursing 26
American Society for Testing and Materials 27
Amies' transport medium 79
Amniotic membrane
    grafts 145, 150
    transplantation 149
Amoxicillin-clavulanate 157
Ampoules
    single dose 97
    single use 97*f*
Anesthesia, mode of 29
Anterior chamber 129*f*

Anterior lamellar
    graft removal 125
    keratoplasty 123, 124
Antibiotic 156
    prophylaxis 156
Anti-microbial agents 92*t*
Antiretroviral therapy 36
Aspergillus 87, 124, 145
    flavus 124
Autoclaves 61
    types of 60
Automated endothelial keratoplasty 123*f*
Automated instrument rinsing systems 57

B

Bacillus atrophaeus 74
    spores 77
Bacteria 124
    washing-off of 34
Bandage contact lens 115, 123
Barraquer thickness law 110
Bevacizumab 98, 99
Biological indicator test, positive 78
Biomedical waste 68
    management register 32
Bleb leakage visible after fluorescein staining 130*f*
Bleb-associated endophthalmitis 128, 129, 129*f*, 132
Bleb-related infection 128, 129*f*, 131
    risk factors for 130*t*
Blepharitis 96
Blood agar 112
Bowie dick test 74, 76, 77*f*

C

Candida 87
Candida infections 124

Candida keratitis 111
Candida parapsilosis 111
Carbolic acid 53
Cataract
    surgery 96
    type of 88
Cefazolin 103, 157
Ceftriaxone 139
Cefuroxime 50
Centers for Disease Control and Prevention 42
Central corneal ulcer 117*f*
Channel infection 111
Chemical disinfectant 53, 53*f*, 54*f*
Chemical indicators 75
    types of 75
Chemical waste 69
Chemosis 150
Chlorine 7, 9
    compounds 7, 9
Chlorofluorocarbon 62
Chocolate agar 112
Ciprofloxacin 103
Cleaning, mechanical method of 58*f*
Clostridium perfringens 111
Clostridium tetani 79
Coagulase negative staphylococci 87, 137
Coexisting endophthalmitis 153
Collection of swabs, method of 79
Colony-forming units 80
Common antibiotics 157*t*
Compounding pharmacy 97
Confocal microscopy 106, 151
Conjunctival flaps 131
Conjunctival sac 34
Conjunctival swab 132, 151
Contact lenses, use of 120
Corneal collagen cross-linking 114
Corneal incision, clear 88
Corneal perforation, infection with 106*f*

Corneal scraping 151
Corneal transplantation 153
Corneal ulcer 107f, 122f, 151f
   large 117f
   small 122f
Corynebacterium diphtheriae 87, 115
Cuff method
   closed 44
   open 45
Cuff technique
   closed 44
   open 44
Cultivated limbal epithelial transplantation 149
Cytotoxic waste 69, 70

D

Dacryocystitis 157t
Dacryocystorhinostomy 155
Diabetes mellitus 102
Diathermy 66
Dimethyl sulfoxide 152
Disinfection 4, 5t
   low-level 4
   methods of 6
Donor corneal tissue 119
Donor tissue 120, 125
Drug, dispensing of 97f
Dry heat 60, 65, 74

E

Eagles' minimum essential medium 152
Early onset infectious keratitis 105
Endophthalmitis 94, 95, 99, 101, 102, 136, 137, 139
   prophylaxis 138
   vitrectomy study 90, 95, 132, 139
Epithelial defect 113, 114, 121, 122f
Erythema 129f
Escherichia coli 26, 115, 143
Ethylene oxide 2, 62, 65, 75
   method 62
   sterilization 62f
European Society of Cataract and Refractive Surgeons 88
Extracapsular cataract extraction 88
Eye protection goggles 40, 41f
Eyelashes 99f

F

Flash sterilization 61, 65, 74, 83
Fluoroquinolones 33
Fogging method 54
Formaldehyde 9
Formaldehyde fumigation 53
Formaldehyde steam 64
Fungal keratitis 106
Fungi 124
Fusarium 87

G

Gas plasma
   method 63t
   sterilization 63f
Geobacillus stearothermophilus 74, 83
   spores 77
Giemsa stain 112
Glove perforation 137
Gloving 43, 44
   technique 45f
Glue, deterioration of 8
Glutaraldehyde 10
Good manufacturing practice 97
Gowning 43
   technique 44f
Graft dehiscence 121
Graft infection 119, 121, 124
Graft rejection, history of 121
Graft-host junction 122f
Graft-related problems 121
Gram's stain 106, 112
Gram-negative organisms 130, 156, 156t, 157, 157t
Gram-positive cocci 124
Gram-positive organism 156t, 157
   resistant to 157t

H

Haemophilus influenzae 130, 137, 156
Hand scrubbing technique 43f
Heat 60
   method 60t
Heavy metals 12
Hepatitis
   B 41, 56
      virus 37, 152
   C 41, 56
      virus 41, 152
Herpes simplex 106, 124
Herpes zoster 106
Herpetic eye disease 119
Herpetic keratitis 121
High level disinfection 4
Hospital infection control 68
Hospital sterilization and disinfection policy 82
Hospital waste management 68t
Host-related problems 120
Hot air oven 60, 65, 74
   types of 61
Human immunodeficiency virus 36, 41, 56
Humidity control register 32
Hydrochlorofluorocarbons 62
Hydrogen peroxide 10, 11
   gas plasma 65, 74
   method 62
Hypochlorous acid 9
Hypo-osmolar CXL procedure 117f

I

In vivo confocal microscopy 112
Incision
   location of 88
   type of 88
Infections, management of 140
Infectious corneoscleral 143
Infectious keratitis 111, 126
Infectious waste 69, 70
Infective keratitis 106f, 122f
Inflammation, severe 129f
Intensive care unit 16
Intermediate level disinfection 4
Intracameral cefuroxime, role of 90t
Intracameral use of vancomycin 89
Intracapsular cataract extraction 88
Intraocular lens 66, 88
   nature of 88
Intra-operative contamination 137
Intra-operative mitomycin-C 143
Intra-operative precautions 98, 155
Intrastromal corneal ring segments 110
   infections after 110
Intrastromal ring implantation 111f
Intravitreal administration, dosage for 92t
Intravitreal biopsy, technique of 96f
Intravitreal injection 99f
Iodophors 10
Ionising radiation 63
Iritis post-CXL treatment 115

K

Keratitis post-keratoplasty 124
Keratoplasty 112
Klebsiella pneumoniae 23, 124
Klebsiella species 111

Index

L
Lacrimal sac 34
Lamellar keratoplasty, 124
Laminar air flow 23
Laser *in situ* keratomileusis 105, 108
Late bleb leak, management of 131*t*, 132
Left eye 151*f*
Lid abnormalities 150
Listeria monocytogenes 115

M
Macular degeneration, age-related 94
Medical and surgical therapy, treatment of 108
Medical therapy 112
Medical waste 69
Medications 150
Meibomitis 96
Metabolic diseases 155
Methicillin-resistant *Staphylococcus aureus* 36, 87
Methicillin-resistant *Staphylococcus epidermidis* 87
Meticulous planning 21
Microincision vitrectomy surgery 102
Microbial air 82
Microbial flora 136
Microbial keratitis 110
Microbial spectrum 105, 129
    of post-operative endophthalmitis 87
Microbiological spectrum 124
Microbiology profile 156
Minor operation theatre 20
Mitomycin c 129, 144
Moist heat 60
Moraxella catarrhalis 130
Mucopurulent discharge 144
Multi-parameter indicators 76
Multiple scleral abscesses 145
Mycobacterium species 105, 115, 117

N
National Accreditation Board for Hospitals and Healthcare Providers 16, 22, 68
Nebulization of disinfectant 54
Neisseria gonorrhoeae 115
Nocardia 105, 108, 143
    species 110
Non-infectious necrotizing scleritis 143
Nonsteroidal anti-inflammatory drugs 116

O
Ocular surface
    disorders 120
    improvement of 152
    problems 150
    reconstruction surgery, infections after 149
Oculoplasty surgery, infections after 155
Operating room
    milieu 98
    sterilization of 98
Operating surgeon 31, 38
Operating team, role of 153
Operation theatre 26, 29, 31, 33, 35, 38, 47, 50, 52, 72*t*, 78
    assistant 49
    attire 34, 38
    cleaning 52
    design 15
    disinfection 53
    layout 15, 16*t*
    occupancy 38
    setting up 15
    setup of 56
    sterilization 52, 53
    techniques 93
Ophthalmic instrument sterilization 57
Ophthalmic operation theatre 22, 26
Ophthalmic viscoelastic devices 51
Optical penetrating keratoplasty 120
Orbital cellulitis 137, 139
    management in 139*t*
Ortho-phthalaldehyde 11
Osmosis 27
Ozone 2, 63

P
Pars plana vitrectomy 101, 132
Passive air sampling 81, 82*t*
Patient-related factors 88
Peel pouch packaging 59*f*
Peracetic acid 11, 65, 74
    method 63
Performic acid 64
Peribulbar anesthesia 20*f*
Peri-injection precautions 98
Periocular cleaning of left eye 36*f*
Periocular infection prophylaxis 138
Persistent epithelial defect 121, 150
Phacoemulsification instruments 51
Pharmaceutical waste 69
Pharmacological wastes 70
Phenol 53
Photophobia 150
Photorefractive keratectomy 106
Piperacillin 103, 139
Plasma sterilization 76*f*
Plasmodium 57
Polyethylene 69
Polymerase chain reaction 106, 107, 132
Polyvinylpyrrolidone 10
Poor visual acuity outcomes 147
Post optical penetrating keratoplasty 122*f*
Post pars plana vitrectomy endophthalmitis 101*f*
Post penetrating keratoplasty 122*f*
Post-AMT microbial infections 149
Post-cataract surgery endophthalmitis 87, 92
    incidence of 88
Post-collagen cross-linking infection 114, 115
Post-cultivated oral mucosal transplantation infection 151*f*
Post-CXL keratitis 115, 117*f*
Post-intravitreal injection
    endophthalmitis 94
    fulminant endophthalmitis 95*f*
    infections 94, 95*t*
Post-keratoplasty infections 119, 125
Post-lamellar keratoplasty infections, treatment of 125
Post-LASIK
    infections 105
    infectious keratitis 106
    keratitis 107*f*
        risk factors for 106*t*
    period 105
Post-operative care 156
Post-operative endophthalmitis 94
    preventing 90*t*
Post-operative period 90, 116
Post-operative precautions 98
Post-operative steroids 116
Post-pterygium surgery infections 143
Post-simple limbal epithelial transplantation infection 151*f*
Post-strabismus surgery infections 136
Potassium hydroxide 112
Pouring sterile solution 49

Povidone iodine 35, 36f
    in patient preparation, role of 89
Precorneal tear film 111
Pre-operative antisepsis 89
Pre-operative assessment 155
Pre-operative factors 114
Pre-operative medications 115
Pre-operative period 88, 115
Preseptal cellulitis 137, 139
Prevent transmission of infection 42
Prompt aggressive treatment 132
Prophylactic antibiotics 107
Prophylactic topical antibiotics 98
Prophylaxis 96, 102, 107, 112, 115, 131, 138, 147, 152, 154
    and management 138
    of post-cataract surgery endophthalmitis 88, 91
Propionibacterium 101
    acnes 87
Proteus mirabilis 137
Pseudomonas 137
    aeruginosa 23, 87, 105, 106f, 115, 124, 143, 145, 147, 156
    infection 116
    species 101, 110
Pterygium surgery 143
    after 144f

Q

Quaternary ammonium compounds 12

R

Rapid corneal melt 151f
Recovery room 19
Recurrence of previous infection 120
Regurgitation on pressure over lacrimal sac 33
Resolving graft infection 122f
Reverse osmosis 26, 27
Rhegmatogenous retinal detachment 29
Rhodotorula 124
Riboflavin solution 115

S

Sabouraud's dextrose agar 112
Sclera 146
Scleritis 137, 140
Scleromalacia 143
Scrub 39
    room 19, 42
Septic operation theatre 55
    setup of 55
    sterilization of 55
Serratia marcescens 156
Serratia species 130
Siedel's test, positive 130f
Simple limbal epithelial transplantation 149
Single-parameter indicators 76
Socioeconomic status 120, 150
Spaulding's classification 4t
    system 2
Staphylococcus aureus 88, 105, 106, 107f, 110, 111, 115, 117, 117f, 118, 124, 156
Staphylococcus epidermidis 87, 111, 130, 137
Staphylococcus saprophyticus 156
Staphylococcus species 95, 105, 115, 124, 132, 137, 139, 143
Steam under pressure 60, 65, 74
Stem cell deficiency 151f
Sterile items, storage of 83
Sterile plastic drape, use of 99f
Sterile severe scleral 146f
Sterile speculum, use of 99f
Sterilization 2t, 4, 5, 5t, 57, 59, 73
    and quality control 98
    cycle of 57f
    method of 61, 65, 66t, 82
    practices 6
    procedures 74t
    process 75f
    register 31
    technologies 65t
    time of 60-62
Sterilizers, monitoring of 83
Steroids, use of 115
Stevens-Johnson syndrome 149
Strabismus surgery 136, 140
Streptococci 103
Streptococcus 132
Streptococcus oralis 115
Streptococcus pneumoniae 87, 105, 111, 124, 130, 156
Streptococcus salivarius 115
Streptococcus species 115, 117, 130, 132, 139
Streptococcus viridans 95, 105, 110, 130
Subconjunctival antibiotic injection, role of 90
Superior bleb 128
Superoxidized water 9
Supportive therapy 153
Surgeon
    awareness 138
    factors 98
    learning curve 102
    preparation of 89, 116
Surgery, types of 30
Surgical complications 88
Surgical debridement 153
Surgical field, preparation of 116
Surgical gloves 41
Surgical gowns 40
Surgical mask 39
Surgical plan 29
Surgical preparation 35
Surgical scrubbing 42
Surgical site infection 22
Surgical therapy 112
Surgically induced necrotizing scleritis 136, 138, 140
Suture abscess 138
Suture-related problems 121, 150
Swab
    collection of 79
    processing of 79
Symblepharon ring 150
Systemic antibiotics 153
Systemic diseases 120
Systemic therapy 153

T

Tazobactam 103, 139
Temperature 32
Therapeutic penetrating keratoplasty 119
Ticarcillin 139
Tissue adhesives 153
Topical antibiotics 90
    role of 89
Topical broad spectrum antibiotics 33
Topical medications 153
Topical steroids 120
Total organic carbons 27
Toxic anterior segment syndrome 64, 95
Transconjunctival sutureless vitrectomy 101
Transforming growth factor β 149

Treating pre-existing
    diseases 115
    ocular conditions 88
Treponema pallidum infections 152
Tunnel infection 111*f*

U

Ultrasonic cleaner 58*f*
Ultrasonography B scan 151
Ultraviolet radiation 12
Ultraviolet rays 55
Ultraviolet-A light 114

V

Validation of system 25
Vancomycin 50
Vancomycin-resistant *Staphylococcus aureus* 88
Vancomycin-resistant *Staphylococcus epidermidis* 88
Vaporized hydrogen peroxide 64
Vascular deprivation 143
Vascular endothelial growth factor 94
Ventilation 22
Venting incisions 121
Vernal keratoconjunctivitis 115
Viruses 124
Visual outcome and prognosis 132
Vitreous cavity 129*f*
Vitreous exudates 101*f*
Vitreous tap 132
Vitreous wick syndrome 102

W

Waste
    categorization of 68, 69
    disposal 68
    handlers 72
    treatment of 71
    types of 70*t*
Water
    analysis and culture register 32
    recommended quality of 28
Wound
    dressings 49
    gape 113
    leak 121

Z

Ziehl-Neelsen stain 106

www.ingramcontent.com/pod-product-compliance
Lightning Source LLC
Chambersburg PA
CBHW040540220526
45473CB00016B/2987